Advanced
ECG

Advanced
ECG:
Boards and Beyond
SECOND EDITION

BRENDAN P. PHIBBS, MD

Professor of Clinical Medicine
Section of Cardiology
University of Arizona Medical Center

Chief of Medicine
Director of Cardiology
University-Kino Hospital
Tucson, Arizona

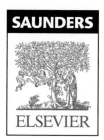

SAUNDERS

ELSEVIER

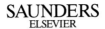

SAUNDERS
ELSEVIER

1600 John F. Kennedy Blvd.
Ste 1800
Philadelphia, PA 19103-2899

ADVANCED ECG: BOARDS AND BEYOND

ISBN-13: 9781416024026
ISBN-10: 1-4160-2402-6

Second edition

Library of Congress Cataloging-in-Publication Data

Phibbs, Brendan.
  Advanced ECG : boards and beyond / Brendan P. Phibbs.— 2nd ed.
      p. cm.
  Rev. ed. of: Advanced ECG. Boston : Little, Brown, c1997.
  Includes index.
  ISBN 1-4160-2402-6
  1. Electrocardiography. I. Title: Advanced electrocardiography. II. Title.
  RC683.5.E5P48 2006
  616.1'207547—dc22
                                          2005051175

ISBN-13: 9781416024026
ISBN-10: 1-4160-2402-6

Acquisitions Editor: Susan Pioli
Developmental Editor: Vera Ginsburgs
Publishing Services Manager: Frank Polizzano
Project Manager: Natalie Ware
Design Direction: Steven Stave

Printed in the United States of America

Last digit is the print number: 9 8 7 6 5 4 3 2 1

To the memory of T. K. of Loughrea, County Galway

Preface to the Second Edition

My dear and esteemed colleagues, I guarantee you can understand everything in this book. I've spent a great deal of my professional life reducing the facts about electrocardiography to simple basic English. For example . . .

Gobbledygook: "antegrade propagation of the depolarizing impulse"

English: "The wave goes down."

Gobbledygook: "The fast track exhibits preferential retrograde conduction."

English: "The fast track likes to conduct backward."

And so on.

All the essentials about electrocardiographic interpretation can be reduced to simple, clear English if one makes the effort. This book is a sustained effort to do just that. (As Richard Sheridan said in the 18th century, "Easy writing is curs'd hard reading." This book is an exercise on the other face of that coin.)

Everything I said in the Preface to the First Edition is still true in the United States today. Whole generations of cardiologists and internists are going forth into practice without adequate ECG training. In programs across the country, young physicians are expected to learn about ECG interpretation by osmosis or maybe by intuition. Most major centers don't have adequate organized ECG training. (A couple of intensive conferences a month would be a minimum recommendation. Did you have them where you trained?)

There's a tendency to rush to the EP laboratory whenever a significant disorder of impulse formation or conduction pops up. Ninety percent of the time this is wasted motion because a simple ECG can provide all the information. For instance:

- There's a benign type of wide-beat tachycardia that never threatens life; you can recognize it with complete accuracy on the ECG. You know prognosis and treatment at once.
- Does a patient need a pacemaker? The ECG is all you need. You can diagnose all the varieties of heart block and make accurate decisions about the need for a pacemaker entirely from the ECG. Forget the EP laboratory.
- Narrow-beat tachycardias, mechanism and treatment?
- Atrial fibrillation with very rapid response? Pre-excitation?
- Myocardial infarction in the presence of left bundle-branch block? (Yes, sometimes you can make a diagnosis!)
- Complete A-V dissociation—benign or life threatening?

All these and more are distinctions and diagnoses you can make correctly and only from the ECG.

Some of my students have thought that they would start out with simple ECG abnormalities in practice, and they have been horrified to be confronted with a snarling complex arrhythmia that demanded a life-or-death decision on their first night in the emergency department. Be prepared!

Special note! Ignore the computer! Computer ECG programs are a medical and medicolegal quagmire: I've analyzed a number of programs and I find that anything beyond the simplest disorder sends the computer circuits into terminal collapse.

Electrocardiography is an elegant, basically simple, totally logical means of diagnosis that gives more pragmatically significant information than any other diagnostic mode in cardiology.

Learn it!

Slain leath! (That's Irish for long life and health and it also implies good hunting!)

Brendan P. Phibbs, MD

Preface to the First Edition

If you're a physician who trained in the United States, you were cheated. You've been neglected. You're entitled to a sense of outrage.

Electrocardiography is a basic life-and-death skill that's going to confront you with harrowing decisions throughout your professional life, but chances are that all through your residency and fellowship training you never had any organized formal training in it. Your instructors thought you were going to learn electrocardiography by osmosis or by ionic exchange or by breathing the air of the university hospital.

How do I know this? I know it because I served several terms on the ECG Interpretation Committee of the ACC and because, on my own, I surveyed teaching hospitals across the country from Boston to San Francisco. *Eighty percent of teaching hospitals have no organized ECG-arrhythmia training in residency or fellowship programs.*

Whenever I lecture to residents and fellows I hear the same complaint: "Why don't we get more of this stuff? We really need to know it!"

Okay chaps,* you're right. You certainly do need to know this stuff. That's what *Advanced ECG: Boards and Beyond* is for. It's based on the tutorial sessions I lead with the fellows in our program at the Veterans Hospital in Tucson.

This book isn't going to waste your time with baby steps: it's assumed you know how the leads are hooked up and what a P wave is. This is a book for you to use when you're ready to start functioning in the real world as a clinician. In fact, the first arrhythmia illustrated in the book is one I guarantee you'll run into as a question on the Internal Medicine Boards.

In your clinical life you're not going to start with simple cases and go on to complex ones: your very first night in the emergency room or in the coronary care unit may bring you face to face with some incredibly complex *gemisch* of wide and narrow beats, anomalies of AV conduction, and variations of aberrancy, and you'd better be able to dissect the ECGs and react intelligently. I think I can honestly say this text will help you do just that. I say so on the basis of responses from students, residents, and fellows I've trained over the years using exactly these methods and many of the figures in this book.

The language of *Advanced ECG: Boards and Beyond* is deliberately simple. Don't be surprised when you read that "the fast AV nodal channel likes to conduct backward" instead of "the fast AV nodal channel exhibits preferential retrograde conduction." The two statements are in fact identical, and the simple language is chosen with considerable care. This book is written to be as different as possible from the gibberish that came with your computer!

Electrocardiography is an elegant, basically simple, totally logical means of diagnosis that gives more pragmatic information than any other diagnostic mode in cardiology.

Learn it!

Good hunting!

B. P. P.

---

*"Chaps" is a unisex term.

Contents

One

Sinus Rhythms: Two Benign Variations

Wandering Pacemaker

This is a completely harmless, totally insignificant variation of a sinus rhythm. The shape of the P wave changes from beat to beat, but the timing of the beats doesn't. The rhythm is regular and uninterrupted even though the P waves look different. Sometimes the contour of the P wave will change from upright to inverted and then back to upright (Fig. 1–1A and B). You distinguish this from ectopic firing by a simple observation. There are no premature beats. The rhythm doesn't change. All that changes is the shape of the P waves.

This phenomenon is important only because it is sometimes confused with significant arrhythmias (one text even refers to it as a form of sick sinus syndrome!).

The peculiar change in P wave shape is a result of "wandering" of the sinus impulse in the region around the sinoatrial node. The deeply inverted P waves suggest that the pacing site has "wandered" toward the upper reaches of the AV node—a region often described as the "coronary" node.

I have seen cardiologists confuse this harmless phenomenon with multifocal atrial tachycardia, a really significant arrhythmia. This is inexcusable! In multifocal atrial tachycardia, there are showers and runs of premature beats from many different sites in the atria (more about this later). With a wandering pacemaker—to say it one more time—the rhythm is *regular*; all that changes is the shape of the P waves.

Change in Sinus P Wave Morphology with Rate

When the rate increases, the sinus P waves sometimes "peak," assuming a taller, steeper shape. When it slows, they resume their more rounded shape (Fig. 1–2). This is another sinus variant of absolutely no significance; don't confuse it with ectopic atrial rhythms.

Figure 1–1.
A and **B**, Two examples of wandering pacemaker. In each strip, the P wave changes its shape from upright to inverted and back again *with no change in rhythm*. This consistent rhythm is important because it distinguishes the innocuous wandering pacemaker from true ectopic firing.

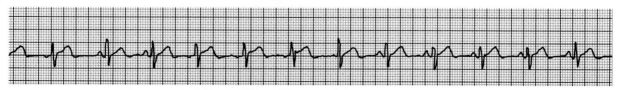

A

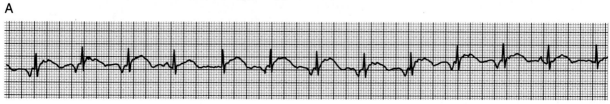

B

1

Figure 1–2.
Strip from an event
recorder with sinus rate
varying from 59 on the left
to 110 on the right. Note
the striking increase in
amplitude of P waves. (The
loss in R wave amplitude
was not rate related but
was simply due to a
change in body position
when the patient turned on
the recorder.)

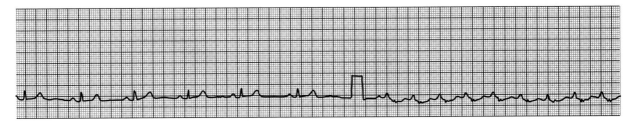

Sinus Arrhythmia

Take your pulse; now take a deep breath in and then exhale. Your pulse rate probably slowed when you exhaled. This is the normal type of variation in sinus node discharge associated with the breathing cycle (Fig. 1–3). It may be quite exaggerated, especially in young people, but it's harmless.

The clinically significant disturbances of sinus node function are described in Chapter 15, The Sick Sinus Syndrome.

Figure 1–3.
Sinus arrhythmia.
Sometimes respiratory
variations in rhythm can be
quite striking, as in this
strip, but they are
harmless. Some rare
forms of sinus arrhythmia
are independent of the
breathing cycle.

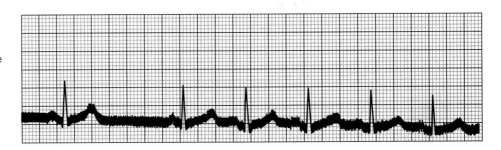

Two

Ectopic Beats and Sustained Ectopic Rhythms: Mechanisms of Idiorhythms and Paroxysmal Tachycardia

If you are an internist or a cardiologist, sooner or later you will find yourself taking an electrocardiogram (ECG) competency test. It may come as part of the Internal Medicine Boards or the Cardiovascular Boards, the American College of Cardiology (ACC) Competency Test, or a hospital ECG privileges examination. In every case, you can be certain you'll confront a problem like the one shown in Figure 2–1. Is the right answer obvious? Read on!

When you study ectopic beats and sustained ectopic rhythms, you have to acquire two sets of skills. First, you have to be able to decide where the ectopic focus lies anatomically. Is it atrial, junctional, or ventricular? Most of the time, this is a simple diagnosis, but it can get tricky.

Second, you have to decide what kind of ectopic firing is going on. Ectopic beats and ectopic rhythms will always be the result of one of two mechanisms: reentrant or automatic. It's critical to decide which mechanism is at work because treatment and prognosis are completely different; fortunately, it's usually easy to make the distinction.

Determining the Source of Ectopic Beats

You probably already know how to localize ectopic beats, but here are some fine points.

Atrial Ectopic Beats

You need to remember three facts. First, if a beat arises in an atrial ectopic focus, it will generate a P wave with a different shape from the sinus P wave. This difference in shape may be slight or extreme, but it will always be detectable (Fig. 2–2).

Second, the P-R interval of the atrial ectopic beat will always be 0.12 second or more, never less. It will usually be longer than the P-R interval of the sinus beats. In other words,

Figure 2–1.
A patient has suffered an inferior wall myocardial infarction. Eighteen hours later, the rhythm illustrated here appears. The blood pressure is 130/80 mm Hg, the patient is pain free, and all vital signs are normal. Choose one of the following treatments: (1) lidocaine, (2) isoproterenol, (3) atropine, (4) pacemaker, or (5) no treatment.

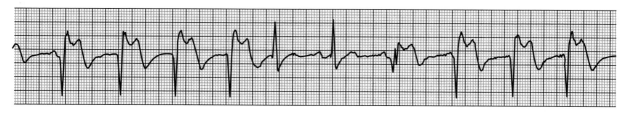

Figure 2–2.
Premature atrial beats from a number of foci. Note the difference in P wave morphology—sometimes striking, sometimes minimal, but always different from the sinus P waves.

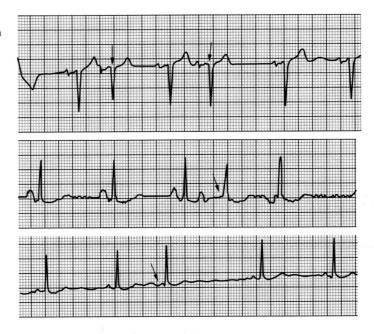

the track from sinus node to atrioventricular (AV) node is the most efficient track from atria to ventricles. If a beat arises somewhere else in the atria, it will usually take longer than the sinus beat to reach and traverse the AV node.

Third, a beat arising at any given site in the atria will produce a characteristic P wave specific for that site. This is important in the diagnosis of multifocal atrial tachycardias (Fig. 2–3).

These are small points, but they may be important in analyzing complex arrhythmias.

Junctional Beats

Most beats arising in the junction will be conducted *forward* (antegrade) into the ventricles and *backward* (retrograde) across the atria. As a result, there will be some combination of a normal narrow QRS with a retrograde P. The retrograde P may come just before, during, or after the QRS (Fig. 2–4). The relation of the atrial and ventricular complexes depends on the speed of conduction *back* across the atria compared with the speed of conduction *forward* across the ventricles.

If the retrograde impulse excites the atria before the antegrade impulse excites the ventricles, the P wave will come just ahead of the QRS. The P-R interval will always be less than 0.12 second. When you see a fixed short P-R interval (less than 0.12 second), you're looking at junctional beats (see Fig. 2–4A).

At this point, you interrupt: "Wait a minute! What about preexcitation? That will certainly produce a fixed short P-R." Good question. The difference is that the P wave of the junctional beat will have a "retrograde" morphology—completely different from the shape of the sinus P waves. It will usually be inverted in the inferior leads. With preexcitation, you see normal sinus P waves with a short P-R.

If the retrograde impulse excites the atria at the same instant that the antegrade impulse excites the ventricles, you won't see the P wave because it will be hidden in the QRS. Thus,

Figure 2–3.
Multifocal atrial rhythm. This is when P wave morphology becomes critical. You can identify at least four different atrial foci from the shape of the ectopic P waves.

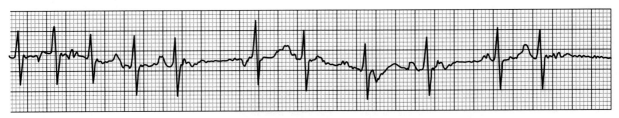

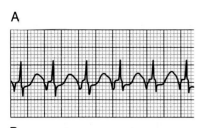

A

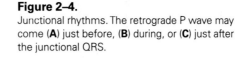

Figure 2–4.
Junctional rhythms. The retrograde P wave may come (**A**) just before, (**B**) during, or (**C**) just after the junctional QRS.

B

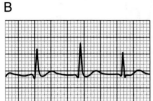

C

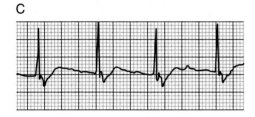

a narrow QRS not preceded by a P wave must be junctional (see Fig. 2–4B). If the retrograde impulse reaches the atria *after* the antegrade impulse reaches the ventricles, the retrograde P wave will follow the QRS (see Fig. 2–4C).

Odd and unexplained fact: In theory, the QRS of a junctional beat should look exactly like the QRS of the sinus beat; after all, both impulses come down the same ventricular track. However, sometimes the QRS of a junctional beat will be quite different from the QRS of the sinus beat. Nobody is sure why this happens, although it may be that the junctional beat breaks out into the bundle branch system from an eccentric point of entry. The practical point is that even though the shape of the QRS is different, the beats are still junctional (Fig. 2–5).

Ventricular Ectopic Beats

The bizarre QRST and the absence of a preceding P wave are obvious and need no further discussion. However, there is one critical difference between junctional and ventricular ectopic beats; learn this difference now, and it will help you on many dark nights in the emergency room when you're looking at a wide-beat tachycardia. During a junctional tachycardia, the junctional beats are practically always conducted retrogradely across the atria. This retrograde impulse discharges the sinus node before it can fire. The ventricles and the atria are activated from the same source: the junction. In contrast, about half of all ventricular ectopic beats, whether single or occurring during a tachycardia, are not conducted back up through the AV node. The sinus node is *not* affected and goes on firing independently. The atria and ventricles are dissociated for one beat, the atria responding to the sinus node and the ventricles to the ectopic beat. In Figure 2–6, you can see the sinus P wave inscribed near the end of the T of the ventricular premature contraction (VPC).

Figure 2–5.
There are a number of junctional beats on this strip. Most of them have a different contour from this sinus QRS. All the beats after the first beat are junctional with a QRS that is taller and different in composition from the sinus beats. (There's no S wave in the junctional beats.) Sometimes the difference is more striking than this.

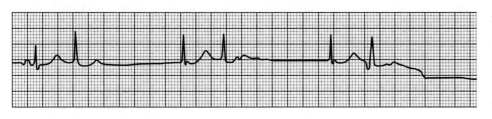

Figure 2–6.
Ventricular ectopic contraction with a dissociated sinus P wave. As a result, the interval from the P wave ahead of the VPC to the one after it is an exact double interval, or full compensatory pause.

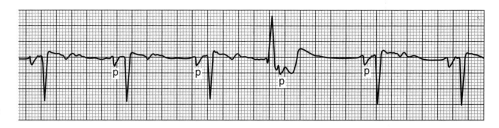

Figure 2–7.
Ventricular ectopic beats with retrograde P waves.

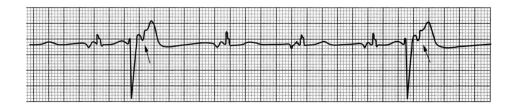

Because the sinus impulse marches undisturbed right through the VPC, and the next sinus beat comes in right on time, you will see a "full compensatory pause"—that is, a pause that is exactly double the sinus interval. Remember, about half of all VPCs are dissociated from the sinus rhythm, so when you see dissociated P waves during a wide-beat tachycardia, the diagnosis is *ventricular* tachycardia. Keep this simple observation in mind; you'll use it later in this chapter.

The other half of all VPCs are conducted retrogradely across the atria, just like the junctional beats, except that the atrial impulse always follows the QRS (Fig. 2–7).

If an ectopic beat arises out in the subendocardium of the ventricle, it will always be at least 0.12 second wide in the adult heart—sometimes more, but never less. This is a surprisingly consistent finding. (Formerly, there was a lot of speculation about "narrow" VPCs; it turns out that these are really "fascicular" beats, arising in the fascicles of the bundle branch system, hence the more rapid propagation. Fascicular VPCs and fascicular tachycardias are covered later in this chapter.)

Determining the Mechanism of Ectopic Beats

Reentry

Pick up any strip in your cardiac care unit (CCU) with a lot of VPCs on it and look at it carefully (Fig. 2–8). Note that the VPCs come at a precisely fixed interval after the sinus beat. The ectopic beats are "linked" to the preceding sinus beat with an exact, unchanging coupling interval. You'll find this kind of linkage about 98% of the time, whether the ectopic beats are atrial, junctional, or ventricular.

Any mathematician will tell you that when you see that kind of precise association more than five or six times, it can't possibly be a coincidence. There has to be a *causal connection*

Figure 2–8.
Reentrant ventricular ectopic beats. Note the precisely fixed interval to the preceding sinus beats.

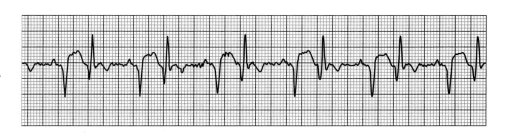

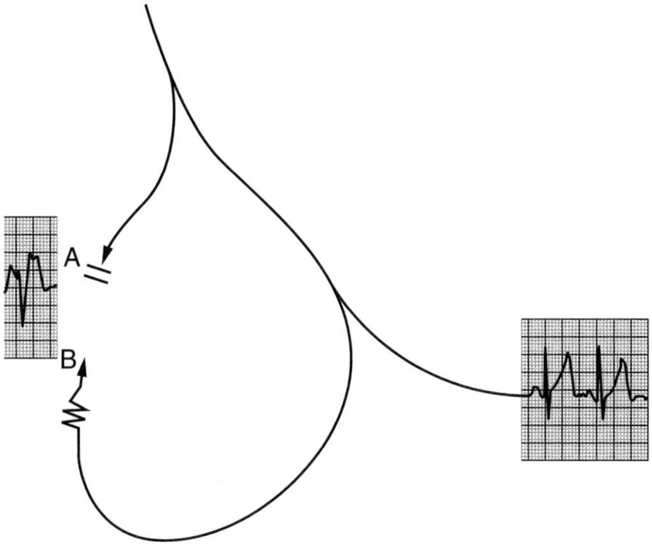

Figure 2–9.
Diagram of reentry.

between the sinus beat and the ectopic beat. Somehow the passage of the sinus impulse "triggers" the ectopic beat.

We now know how that happens; it's called *reentry* (Fig. 2–9). To set up reentry, there must be an area of one-way block somewhere in the Purkinje fibers (see Fig. 2–9A). (One-way block is fairly common; you'll see an obvious example of it later in this chapter.) There must also be an area of very slow conduction (see Fig. 2–9B). Because of the one-way block, the outgoing activating impulse isn't conducted forward normally in one small area. As a result, this area of conducting tissue remains unactivated, still ready for stimulation. In most parts of the chamber, the normal activating impulse moves swiftly, at 4 m/second. However, there's that slowly conducting area mentioned earlier; it's moving so slowly that it "reenters" and activates the blocked part of the system *after* the rest of the chamber has recovered and is ready to conduct again. This reentrant impulse breaks out into the chamber and produces the ectopic beat. Thus, the ectopic beat is in fact caused by the passage of the sinus impulse— that's why the two beats are linked. It's as if the sinus impulse flipped a little pinwheel that went through one rotation and fired at a fixed interval after the sinus beat. You'll see this constant linkage whether the reentrant ectopic beats are atrial, junctional, or ventricular.

Reentry may produce single ectopic beats; on the other hand, the reentry circuit may produce paroxysmal tachycardia when it goes on firing rapidly and regularly. Reentrant ectopic beating is always abnormal and sometimes dangerous (Fig. 2–10).

Automatic Ectopic Beats

Far back in the evolution of life, God or somebody saw to it that the heart had a "fail-safe" system. If the sinus node fails (and it can), there has to be some other means of generating a heartbeat, or the species will die off very quickly.

Fortunately, there are hundreds of "reserve" pacemakers scattered through the heart, chiefly in the AV node and junction and in the ventricles. These are small areas of tissue in the subendocardium that can fire as pacemakers (Fig. 2–11). They can build up a potential and discharge just the way the cells in the sinus node do. They may discharge one beat, or

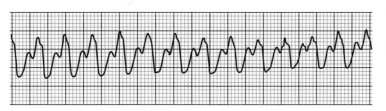

Figure 2–10.
Paroxysmal ventricular tachycardia, a reentrant rhythm.

Figure 2–11.
An automatic ectopic focus. At **A**, the passage of the normal sinus impulse has suppressed the ectopic focus. At **B**, something has halted the normal activating impulse; after a certain fixed period, the automatic focus is "released" to begin discharging, setting the rhythm of the heart.

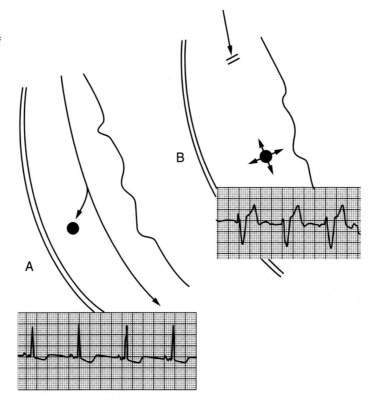

they may go on firing, producing a sustained ectopic rhythm. These sustained ectopic rhythms are the "idio" rhythms: idiojunctional or idioventricular. They practically always fire in the low to high-normal range.

There are several kinds of automatic rhythms. It's important to distinguish between them because they have very different clinical implications.

Automatic-Demand. This is the way an automatic focus is supposed to function. It fires only when the heart rate falls below a certain critical number, exactly like an implanted demand pacemaker. The ectopic focus "waits" for a certain preset interval before it fires. If a normal impulse doesn't come along during that period, the ectopic rhythm takes over.

Automatic ectopic foci are suppressed by the passage of the normal activating impulse. To use an intern's phrase, the passage of the normal activating impulse keeps the automatic ectopic pacemakers "pounded down." When the normal impulse fails, the ectopic focus is said to escape from the dominance of the sinus impulse. The length of time that must pass before the ectopic focus can fire is called the *escape interval* of the ectopic pacemaker.

To reiterate, these automatic foci fire only when the normal impulse fails. They're often life-saving.

Automatic rhythms may be idiojunctional or idioventricular (Fig. 2–12 A to C). (One of many errors you'll find in some texts is the statement that idioventricular rhythms are inherently slower than idiojunctional rhythms. In fact, the two types of rhythm overlap in rate, and there's no definitive difference.)

When a slow idiorhythm appears, of course, you have to ask what's wrong with the normal mechanism. Heart block? Sick sinus? Look for the cause whenever you see an idiorhythm.

Accelerated Automatic-Demand: Accelerated Idiorhythms. For reasons that are not clear, these automatic-demand pacemakers may become overactive; that is, they may fire when they're not really needed. Imagine an overenthusiastic lifeguard who comes dashing out to rescue you when you're only knee-deep and don't need rescuing. Or imagine a thermostat that's set too high so that the furnace keeps turning on when the house is already warm enough. To be more exact, imagine a demand pacemaker that's set to fire whenever the heart rate drops below 80. The problem with these accelerated-demand pacemakers is

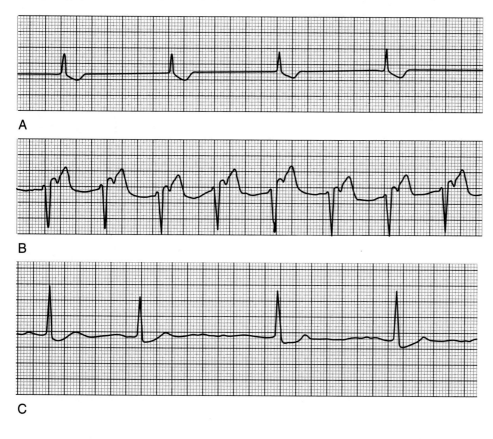

A

B

C

Figure 2–12.
A, Idiojunctional rhythm, rate 50. There is no sign of atrial activity, so it's clear that failure of the sinus node is the reason for the appearance of the idiorhythm. Perhaps it's a sick sinus? **B**, Idioventricular rhythm. Note the retrograde P waves. The ectopic focus is discharging the atria by retrograde conduction, thus suppressing sinus node activity. Part **B** presents a particular problem that can arise with idioventricular rhythms. Notice the retrograde P waves. The atria are contracting *after* ventricular systole, thus, atrial systole is hitting closed atrioventricular valves. There will be venous regurgitation into the pulmonic and systemic veins with symptoms of vertigo, syncope, or even failure. This is the *pacemaker syndrome* that appeared with the old single-electrode ventricular pacemakers when there was intact retrograde conduction. Those pacemakers are rare now, but idioventricular rhythms are common, and this problem will turn up. Treatment: If circulation is seriously compromised: speed the sinus rhythm with atropine, and if that doesn't succeed, pace the atria with a temporary pacing wire. (The results will be dramatic.) **C**, A sinus pause followed by an idiojunctional rhythm, rate about 30. The sinus pause was caused by retching, a powerful vagal stimulant. Here the idiojunctional rhythm is essential to maintain hemodynamics.

that they don't wait long enough before they start firing—their escape interval is too short. The normal pause after a premature beat or a slight slowing of the sinus rhythm is often all it takes to release one of these automatic foci. The accelerated idiorhythm begins firing and often takes over the rhythm of the heart for some time (Fig. 2–13A and B).

Accelerated idiorhythms may perform a useful function. If there's failure of normal conduction, such as AV block, the escape rhythm that takes over may fire in the "accelerated" mode—that is, in the range 55 to 110. When you see an accelerated idiorhythm, always look for the cause. Was there some serious failure of the normal rhythm that let the idiorhythm escape? Or is the idiorhythm simply an example of an "overexcited" ectopic focus getting in the way of a perfectly adequate normal rhythm? Either way, in most cases, these accelerated idiorhythms are harmless—if not actually helpful—and require no treatment.

Now go back to Figure 2–1 and mark the right answer—it's "no treatment," of course. You'd be surprised to learn how many candidates get that specific question wrong every year!

Very rarely, a sustained accelerated idiorhythm can cause problems in a hemodynamically compromised patient because of loss of atrial "kick." In those cases, the answer is to get rid of the slight pauses that are the cause, by eradicating the premature beats or speeding the sinus rate by drugs or pacing. This is rarely necessary.

Automatic Tachycardias. Rarely, an automatic focus may fire in the paroxysmal tachycardia range, 130 or higher. Automatic tachycardias may arise in the atria, the junction, or the ventricles. These are relatively rare arrhythmias with special characteristics; they will be described in a later chapter.

Automatic-Parasystolic. The other type of automatic firing is parasystolic. A parasystolic focus is a tiny area of tissue somewhere in the subendocardium that behaves like a totally independent pacemaker. It fires at its own rate and breaks out to produce a beat whenever it happens to hit the right instant between beats—when the tissues are out of their refractory period and receptive to stimulation.

The curious thing about parasystolic foci is that there's an area of "protection block," or one-way block, around them so that they aren't affected by the passage of the normal

Figure 2–13.
A, Accelerated idiojunctional rhythm. There are occasional sinus beats competing with an idiojunctional focus firing at a rate of 75. Note that as soon as there is a slight pause in the sinus rhythm, the junctional focus "escapes" and takes over. It's not serving any useful purpose, but it's probably not hurting anything.
B, The first five beats are sinus beats. Then there's a sinus pause, and the junctional focus escapes and begins discharging at a rate of 65, just fast enough to "get in the way" of the sinus impulses. The sinus node recaptures the rhythm in the last two beats. Harmless, no treatment needed.

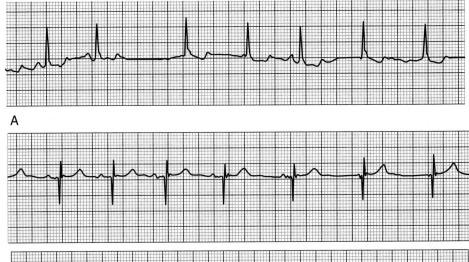

A

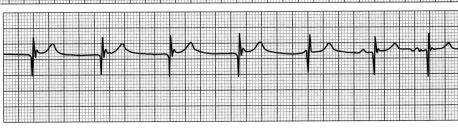

B

activating impulse (Fig. 2–14). The parasystolic focus is a little anarchist that bangs away at its own independent rate and captures the rhythm of the heart whenever it gets a chance.

Parasystolic beats differ from reentrant beats and automatic-demand beats in that they have no connection whatsoever with the preceding sinus beat. The interval from the sinus beat to the ectopic beat varies wildly (Fig. 2–15). This is one of the markers of parasystolic firing.

There's another way you can recognize parasystole: Because the parasystolic focus goes on firing at its own rhythm, the beats will always appear at an interval that's a multiple of the basic rate of the focus. In other words, you can reduce the interval between parasystolic beats to a least common denominator that represents the basic rate of the focus.

Parasystolic rhythms are rare. They have no particular function, although they may serve a useful purpose if they happen to be firing when the normal mechanism fails—but it's accidental when they do.

Figure 2–14.
Parasystole. A parasystolic focus is illustrated at **A**. It fires away at its own rate with no relation to the normal heart cycle. At **B**, the protection block around the parasystolic pacemaker is illustrated. The normal activating wave can't get in to discharge the ectopic focus, but the focus can and does get out whenever the surrounding tissues are out of their refractory period.

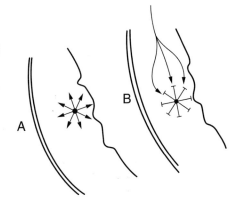

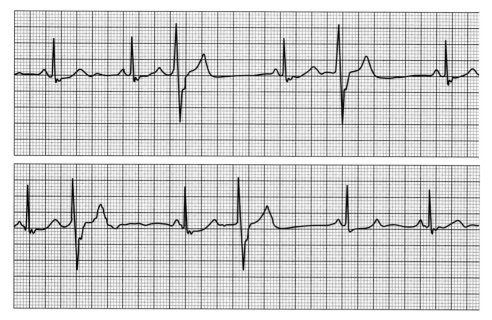

Figure 2–15.
Ventricular parasystole. The ventricular ectopic beats have no fixed relation to the preceding sinus beats, and they appear at their own regular rhythm.

To summarize, ectopic beating may be the result of one of the following mechanisms:

1. *Reentrant:* Always abnormal and sometimes dangerous. Paroxysmal tachycardia is usually caused by sustained reentry.

2. *Automatic-demand:* A physiologic and often life-saving response, idiojunctional or idioventricular, exactly like a demand pacemaker. Rate slow to low-normal, 40 to 60.

3. *Accelerated automatic-demand (accelerated idiorhythms):* An automatic focus that fires in the normal to high-normal range. Usually they're not needed; they're like demand pacemakers that are set too high, so that they interrupt a perfectly normal heart mechanism. Rate low to high-normal, 60 to 110.

4. *Automatic tachycardia:* A rare phenomenon with special clinical features, this occurs when an automatic focus in the atria, junction, or ventricles fires in the tachycardia range, 130 or higher.

5. *Automatic-parasystolic:* An independent automatic rhythm, unaffected by the normal activation of the heart. No consistent linkage to conducted beats; parasystolic beats appear at intervals that are multiples of the basic rate of the parasystolic focus. Locus may be atrial, junctional, or ventricular. Parasystolic rhythms may serve a useful purpose if one happens to be discharging when the normal mechanism fails, but it's an accident when they do. Rate low to high-normal, 40 to 110.

Three

Differential Diagnosis of Wide-Beat Tachycardia

It's 2 AM in the emergency room, and you confront an electrocardiogram (ECG) like the one shown in Figure 3–1. You see a rapid succession of wide QRS complexes without obvious P waves, rate 180. Your mental computer flashes two possible diagnoses:

> 1. **Ventricular tachycardia**
> 2. **Junctional tachycardia with bundle-branch block**

Prognosis and treatment are at opposite poles; the distinction may well be of life-and-death importance.

You need some basic tools, some specific ECG skills, to tackle this problem. You must be able to recognize the following:

> 1. **Bundle-branch block**
> 2. **Rate-dependent bundle-branch block**
> 3. **Dissociation**
> 4. **Fusion beats**
> 5. **Capture**

Bundle-Branch Block

This is a topic that is often made needlessly complex. In theory and practice, it's simple: V1 is the defining lead in bundle-branch block. The logic consists of three elements:

> 1. **If a supraventricular beat produces a QRS that is 0.12 second or more in width, one bundle branch must be blocked.**
> 2. **If V1 consists of a wide S wave, left bundle-branch block is present (Fig. 3–2).**
> 3. **If V1 consists mainly of a wide terminal R wave, right bundle-branch block is present (Fig. 3–3A, B, and C).**

As you can see, right bundle-branch block V1 may consist of a small r followed by a wide, tall R (rR′), a plain R wave, or a qR. The essential point is that the last two thirds of the

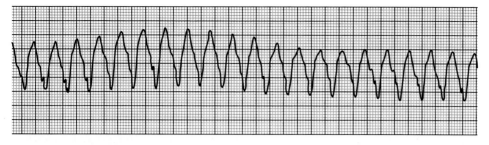

Figure 3–1.
Wide-beat tachycardia. Is it ventricular or junctional with bundle-branch block? You couldn't possibly make a diagnosis from this strip alone.

V1–V2–V3

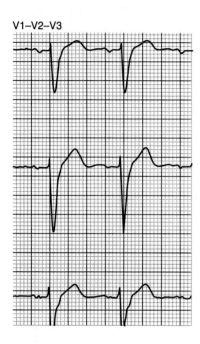

Figure 3–2.
Left bundle-branch block is defined by a wide S wave in V1; duration of total complex, 0.12 second or greater.

complex consist of a wide R wave. In simple terms, the wide R wave is over the blocked ventricle. There will of course be a corresponding wide S wave over the normally activated bundle-branch area.

(Some descriptions of this topic are fantastically complicated with vectors and mean electromotive force [EMF] and interfaces, but you can safely ignore all this. Look at V1, apply the simple differentiation above, and you're on solid ground.)

Rate-Dependent Bundle-Branch Block

This is the simplest form of transient aberrancy. (Remember, the word *aberrant* means "deviating from normal form or pathway." Bundle-branch block is the extreme form of ventricular aberrancy.) Rate-dependent bundle-branch block means that one bundle branch has a prolonged refractory period; that is, it takes longer than normal for it to recover from each transmission. If the next impulse comes along before the "tired" bundle branch has time to recover, it can't transmit, and the ECG will record bundle-branch block.

Figure 3–4A and B illustrates rate-dependent bundle-branch block. In Figure 3–4A, the difference in rate is substantial, but in Figure 3–4B, the first three beats are normally conducted at a rate of 73 (whereas bundle-branch block appears at a rate of 75). As you can see, the difference in rate between normal conduction and rate-dependent bundle-branch block may be very slight. In Figure 3–4, there is normal conduction at a rate of 75 and bundle-branch block at a rate of 78.

Curious phenomenon: Figure 3–5 was recorded during treadmill testing. In the top strip of Figure 3–5, you see normal conduction at a rate of 90. The patient went into rate-dependent

Figure 3–3.
Variations of right bundle-branch block patterns in V1. At **A**, there's the classic rR'; at **B**, there's a simple R wave; and at **C**, there's a qR because the patient has had an anterior myocardial infarct. The wide terminal R is the defining phenomenon for right bundle-branch block.

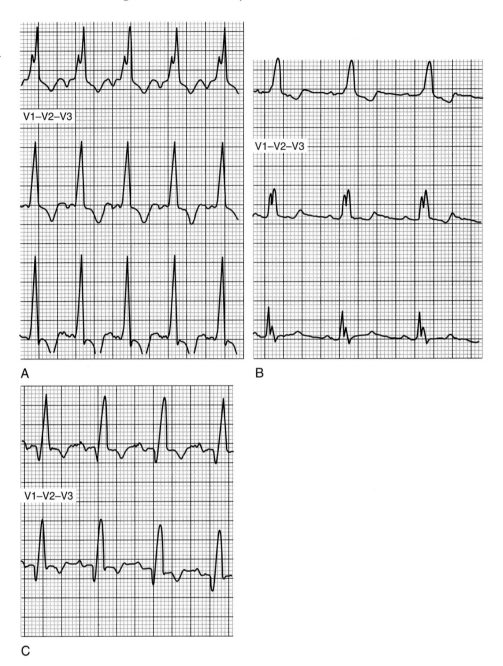

Figure 3–4.
A, Abrupt slowing of rate from 62 to 43: the bundle-branch block disappears. It resumes when the rate goes to 68 for one beat and then disappears when the rate falls to 54.
B, Rate-dependent bundle-branch block.

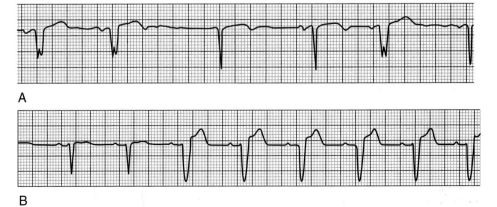

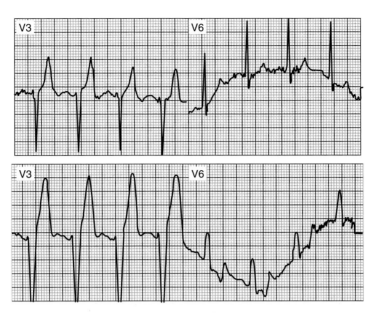

Figure 3–5.
Paradoxical persistence of rate-dependent bundle-branch block.

left bundle-branch block at a rate of 100, and the test was stopped. In the bottom strip of Figure 3–5, you see the pattern of left bundle-branch block *still present at a rate of 90.* For some reason, it often requires a slower rate to come out of bundle-branch block and back to normal conduction than it did to go into bundle-branch block in the first place.

In Figure 3–6, there's a typical example of rate-dependent bundle-branch block coming and going with slight variations in sinus rate; aberrancy also disappears with the pause after a ventricular ectopic beat. There is normal conduction in the beats marked N, at a rate of 65. The first aberrant beat (A) in the top strip comes at an R-R interval equivalent to a rate of 75. In the bottom strip, aberrant conduction persists at a rate of 71. When you're puzzling over wide beats and narrow beats, you must be ready to recognize "critical" rate-dependent aberrancy, which comes and goes with very small differences in rates.

From all this comes a first step in logic when you're looking at an intermittent wide-beat tachycardia. When you see wide QRS complexes at a rapid rate and normal ones at a slower rate, you can consider rate-dependent aberrancy. On the other hand, when you see wide QRS complexes at a slower rate than the narrow ones, forget about rate-dependent aberrancy. The wide beats must be ventricular (Fig. 3–7).

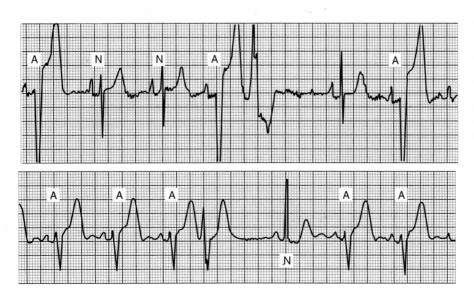

Figure 3–6.
Rate-dependent bundle-branch block. The beats labeled A are aberrant; the beats labeled N are normally conducted. Note the very small difference in rate that sets up the aberrancy.

Figure 3–7.
Strips recorded a few minutes apart on the same patient. The wide beats in the top strip appear at a rate of 140. The narrow beats in the bottom strip appear at a rate of 150. You can't attribute the wide beats in the top strip to rate-dependent aberrancy; they must be ventricular.

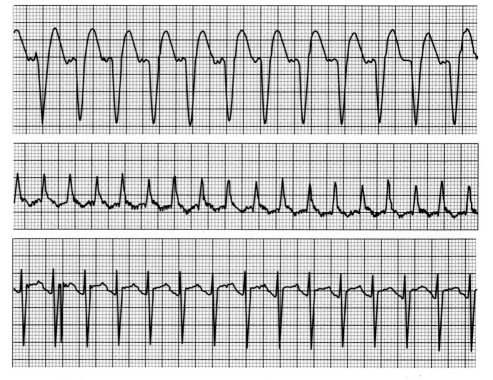

Dissociation

In Chapter 2, we discussed the phenomenon of atrioventricular (AV) dissociation. Dissociation means that the atria are being driven by one pacemaker (usually the sinus node) while the ventricles are being driven by an ectopic rhythm in the junction or the ventricles. The two rhythms are independent. This is a critical observation in the diagnosis of wide-beat tachycardia because about 50% of the time ventricular tachycardia is dissociated from an independent sinus rhythm. There are discernible independent P waves "marching through" the ventricular complexes.

With rare exceptions, junctional tachycardia is not dissociated. The ectopic focus lies at the edge of the atria, so the impulse is conducted back across the atria discharging the sinus node.

Here's a one-way correlation: If you see a dissociated sinus rhythm during a wide-beat tachycardia, the tachycardia is ventricular (accuracy about 98%). On the other hand, if you don't see dissociation, the tachycardia could still be ventricular. About 50% of all ventricular tachycardias are not dissociated.

Sometimes the dissociated P waves are obvious, sometimes not. In Figure 3–8, the P waves are sharp and well defined with a double "spike." You can put your calipers on them and march them through the wide-beat tachycardia; the unmistakable sharp deflection is obvious at the points marked *P*.

It's not always that easy. Sometimes you have to turn to the *Old Testament*: "Doth the leopard change its spots?" Obviously not; the author of Jeremiah was trying to make a point. Look at Figure 3–9. There's a wide-beat tachycardia. The T waves keep changing their shape.

Figure 3–8.
Dissociated sinus P waves "marching through" a short run of ventricular tachycardia.

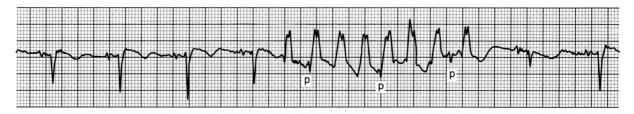

Leopards don't change their spots, and T waves don't change their shape. Further, the Q-T interval will be fixed at any given rate.

In Figure 3–9, the T waves are changing their shape from beat to beat, and the Q-T interval seems to be varying wildly. There's only one possible answer: AV dissociation is present, and the changing shape of the T waves means that there are dissociated P waves marching through them. Learn to look for changes in T wave morphology and Q-T interval in a wide-beat tachycardia. That's how you can spot dissociation and make a precise diagnosis.

Fusion Beats

When I talk to audiences of internists about arrhythmias, I often ask if anyone would like me to review fusion. Invariably, a great many hands go up.

Fusion beats are the 100% infallible marker for a ventricular source of wide beats. They are also called "Dressler beats" for the man who first described them. Figure 3–10A and B shows what happens.

To have a fusion beat, you must have AV dissociation—the atria must be beating independently. In Figure 3–10A, you see a normal sinus impulse at A. This impulse has traversed the atria and is part way through the AV node when an ectopic ventricular focus fires at B. Now the ventricle is invaded by two impulses that meet, or "fuse," somewhere in the ventricular network. The result will be a beat like the one shown in Figure 3–10B, labeled C.

The QRS will be a hybrid, with a morphology that lies somewhere between the shape of the sinus QRS and the shape of the ventricular ectopic beat. Note that beat C has a general outline like the ectopic beat, except that it's narrow. The ventricular ectopic beat has been "normalized" to some extent by the invading sinus impulse. For fusion to take place, the

Figure 3–9.
Wide-beat tachycardia. Note the striking change in T wave morphology. Sometimes you can see well-defined peaks; these are obviously dissociated P waves. The tachycardia is probably ventricular.

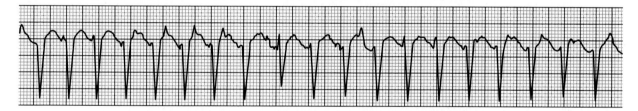

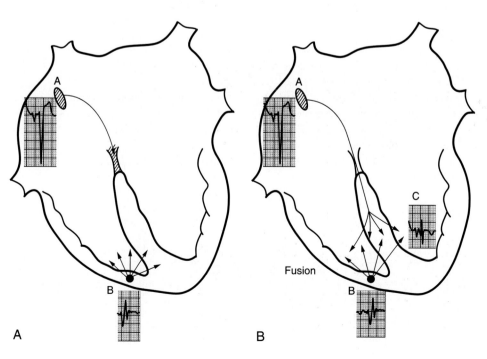

Figure 3–10.
A, Beginning of a fusion beat. **B**, Fusion beat. The sinus impulse (A) and the ventricular ectopic beat (B) have "collided" or fused in the ventricles, producing a hybrid beat at C.

Fusion

A

B

Figure 3–11.
The beats marked N are normal sinus beats. The beats marked with a question mark might be ventricular, or they might be junctional beats with aberrant conduction. The beat marked F is the answer. It has a shorter P-R and a QRS that's intermediate in shape between the sinus beats and the wide beats. Obviously, it's a fusion beat, and the wide beats must be ventricular.

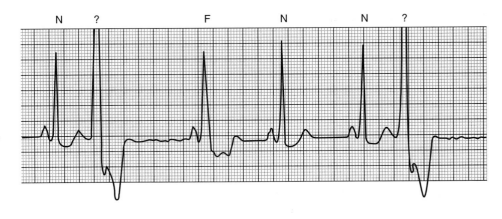

Figure 3–12.
You saw this strip in the last chapter. It's reproduced here again because it's such a good example of a fusion beat (f). Obviously, the beats marked with a question mark must be ventricular.

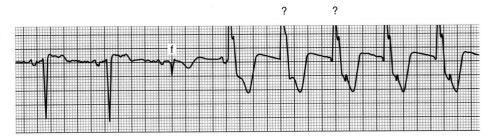

ventricular focus has to discharge while the sinus impulse is still in the AV node. Therefore, the P-R interval will always be shorter than the P-R of normal sinus beats.

One more time: Fusion beats will be characterized by a short P-R compared with the sinus beats. The QRS will be intermediate in shape between the QRS of the sinus beats and the QRS of the ventricular ectopic focus.

The fusion beat may look like a slightly widened and distorted sinus beat, or it may look like a slightly narrowed and normalized ventricular premature contraction (VPC). It all depends on which impulse penetrates farther into the ventricle. Figures 3–11, 3–12, 3–13, and 3–14 are all examples of fusion beats. Study them carefully. This is a basic skill you'll exercise in many tense moments in the coronary care unit.

Figure 3–13.
Normal sinus rhythm with occasional wide beats (V). At F, there's an obvious fusion beat. The 9th and 14th beats are also fusion beats.

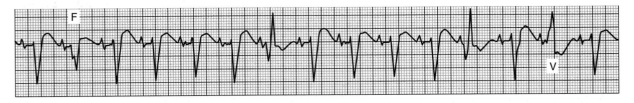

Figure 3–14.
Sinus rhythm. At F, one obvious fusion beat.

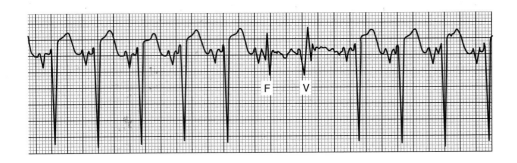

Capture

Fusion beats represent a partial capture of the rhythm by the sinus node. Sometimes the sinus impulse "sneaks through" between the beats of a ventricular tachycardia and penetrates the entire ventricular network, actually producing a normal sinus beat right in the midst of the ventricular arrhythmia. To have capture beats, of course, you must have a dissociated sinus rhythm.

When you see a capture beat, you use the logic you used to detect rate-dependent aberrancy. If you see a normal narrow QRS appearing at the same R–R interval as the wide beats, you have ruled out rate-dependent aberrancy as a cause of the wide-beat tachycardia. Logic!

The tracing in Figure 3–15 illustrates all the criteria for the precise diagnosis of ventricular tachycardia. There are short runs of wide beats. If you look closely, you can see dissociated sinus P waves marching through the wide-beat rhythms. The beat marked C is a capture beat. The QRS of the capture beat is normal even though it appears at the same R–R interval as the wide beats. The beats marked f are obvious fusion beats with a short P–R and an intermediate QRS morphology.

With all this information, you can make a 100% infallible diagnosis of ventricular tachycardia. Try making the same observations in Figure 3–16.

So far, this has been a one-way street. The criteria listed up till now are diagnostic of ventricular tachycardia. However, you won't find them in more than 50% of cases of ventricular tachycardia (some investigators put the percentage as low as 35% to 45%). If none of these criteria are present, it doesn't mean that you're not dealing with ventricular tachycardia. In at least half of all cases of ventricular tachycardia, the ectopic impulses are conducted back up through the AV node and across the atria. There's no dissociation, so there's no chance for capture or fusion. How do we establish a diagnosis in these cases?

At this point, I can predict the reader's question: "How about morphology? Can't you tell the difference between ventricular beating and aberrancy by the way the QRS looks? You

Figure 3–15.
Four-beat runs of ventricular tachycardia interrupting a sinus rhythm. You can see dissociated sinus P waves marching through the tachycardia with fusion beats (f) and a capture beat (C) with a normal QRS. This strip illustrates all the criteria for the precise diagnosis of ventricular tachycardia.

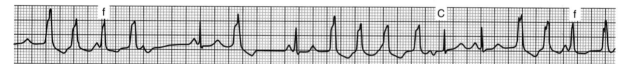

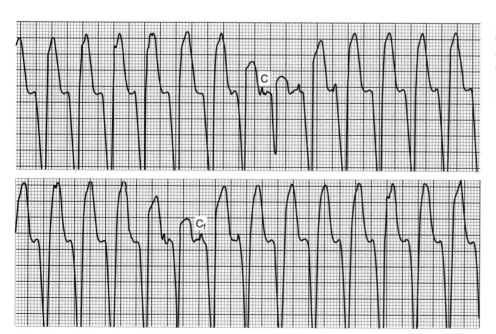

Figure 3–16.
Ventricular tachycardia with dissociated sinus P waves, capture with fusion (C_f) and capture with normal QRS (C).

certainly hear enough about it." Back in the 1960s, Marriott launched an attempt to differentiate ventricular ectopic beats from aberrantly conducted supraventricular beats by the *shape* of the complexes. Over the intervening years, many other investigators, including Wellens, Lie, Akhtar, Brugada, and Josephson, have pursued this possibility.

There are indeed some characteristics of QRS morphology that enable you to say, with about 98% accuracy, that a given wide-beat tachycardia is in fact ventricular:

1. **Wide QRS complexes: more than 0.15 second**

2. **Uniform, totally positive or negative complexes across the precordium. No R/S complexes in the precordium**

3. **Extreme axis (see Appendix II on axis measurement)**

4. **Deep S V6**

5. **R/S complexes with a prolonged interval from R to bottom of S (more than 100 m/second)**

6. **Notching near the nadir of the S wave in V1 when V1 consists of a wide S**

Figures 3–17, 3–18, and 3–19 illustrate many of these features.

How about QRS morphology in aberrancy? There's an enormous and frustrating overlap between ventricular tachycardia and junctional tachycardia with aberrancy when it comes to QRS morphology. *If* none of the above characteristics is present, and *if* there is a three-component R wave in V1 (rsR′), then there's a chance—no better than 80%—that the wide beats are caused by aberrancy. There are no specific characteristics of QRS morphology that

Figure 3–17.
QRS morphology of ventricular tachycardia. The ventricular beats are about 0.16 second wide. (Note the frequent fusion beats.)

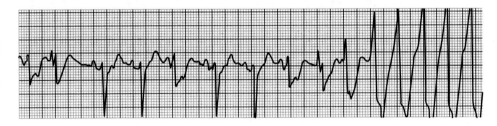

Figure 3–18.
Ventricular tachycardia. The distance from the beginning of the R to the bottom of the S is 0.16 second (Brugada's sign of ventricular ectopic complexes).

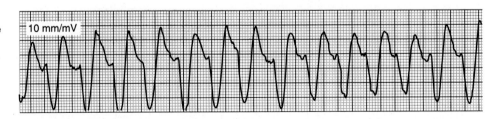

Figure 3–19.
Ventricular tachycardia, lead V1. Note the slurring just before the nadir of the S waves. This is evidence of ventricular tachycardia (Josephson's sign). Note that these beats look narrower than usual for ventricular tachycardia, but part of the QRS is "buried" in the baseline—they're really 0.12 second wide.

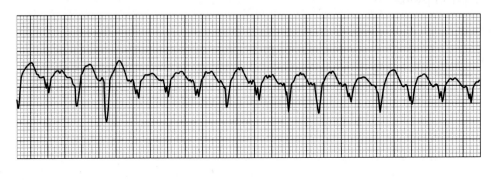

permit you to say, with acceptable accuracy, that a given wide-beat tachycardia is in fact due to aberrancy—80% simply isn't good enough for what may be a life-and-death decision. You can often very accurately rule ventricular tachycardia *in*, but you can't rule it *out*. This chapter is therefore going to conclude with an editorial.

The Aberrancy Aberrancy

Ventricular tachycardia is a dangerous arrhythmia; it practically always connotes significant organic heart disease. Conversely, junctional tachycardia with or without aberrancy is relatively benign. It frequently occurs in otherwise normal individuals. Because of the various studies trying to differentiate the two on the basis of QRS morphology, there's a dangerous and deplorable tendency for physicians in emergency departments and intensive care units to look at a wide-beat tachycardia, mutter that it "looks aberrant," and order potentially lethal treatment. Ventricular fibrillation, death, and malpractice suits are likely to follow in horrid swift succession.

Always apply these steps in logic:

1. **Treatment for supraventricular tachycardias includes verapamil, digitalis, and phenylephrine. Any one of these is likely to be lethal if the tachycardia is really ventricular.**

2. **On the other hand, drugs used to treat ventricular tachycardia (lidocaine, procaine amide, and amiodarone) will not do any harm if the rhythm is in fact junctional. Procainamide or amiodarone may well stop a junctional tachycardia.**

3. **There are many criteria, as listed previously, that enable you to say that a given wide-beat tachycardia is in fact ventricular. These criteria are specific, but they're not sensitive. Many cases of ventricular tachycardia—possibly half—won't fit any of these criteria, so you're stuck with a diagnosis of "wide-beat tachycardia, possibly ventricular."**

4. **On the other side of the coin, there are no criteria that permit you to say with acceptable accuracy that a given wide-beat tachycardia is not ventricular and is in fact caused by aberrancy. In other words, it's a one-way correlation—a fact that often escapes many clinicians and investigators. (Many of my colleagues are brilliant observers but not very good logicians.)**

There's only one sure way to diagnose aberrancy in this setting. *If you find a previous tracing with sinus rhythm and bundle-branch block and if the contours of the wide-beat tachycardia are the same as the bundle-branch configuration when the patient was in sinus rhythm, then and only then can you diagnose aberrancy with confidence.*

Here's a reasonable protocol for a wide-beat tachycardia:

First, always try vagal stimulation by carotid sinus massage, the diving reflex, or the Valsalva maneuver. If the tachycardia stops, you can be absolutely sure it was supraventricular.

Second, if vagal stimulation doesn't work, try adenosine. If this stops the tachycardia, you can be sure it was supraventricular.

Third, if none of these maneuvers works, if there's no previous ECG for comparison, and if you value your patient's life, *treat for ventricular tachycardia!*

Four

The Supraventricular Tachycardias

There are six different, well-defined types of supraventricular tachycardia:

1. **Atrioventricular (AV) nodal reentrant tachycardia—the most common cause of paroxysmal supraventricular tachycardia**

2. **AV nodal reciprocating tachycardia—the term *reciprocating* means that there's a bypass tract that forms a reentrant circuit with the AV node**

3. **Automatic or "nonparoxysmal" junctional tachycardia**

4. **Ectopic atrial tachycardia of childhood (relatively rare)**

5. **Sinus node reentrant tachycardia—the rarest of the six**

6. **Multifocal atrial tachycardia**

AV Nodal Reentrant Tachycardia or Two-Track AV Nodal Reentry

It's only in the past decade that we've learned what really happens in this very common arrhythmia. Figure 4–1 is a good illustration of the underlying pathophysiology. (This isn't the best-preserved electrocardiogram in my collection—we had to rescue it from the wastebasket at our Veterans' Hospital, but it's such a rare and striking example of dual AV

Figure 4–1.
Dual AV nodal pathways. In the top strip, the P-R interval is 0.20 second. In the middle strip, the P-R has abruptly lengthened to 0.48 second. These two intervals varied back and forth erratically even though the heart rate remained the same. There are obviously two separate pathways through the AV node, one fast and one slow. (Tracing courtesy of Dr. Samuel Goldfein.)

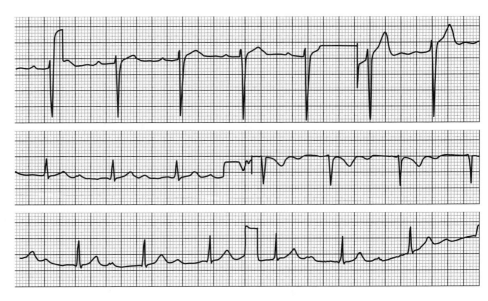

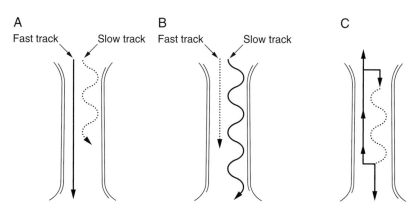

A Fast track Slow track

B Fast track Slow track

C

Figure 4–2.
Mechanism of AV nodal reentrant tachycardia. In 30% of patients, there is a slow track and a fast track. Normally, the activating impulse comes down the fast track (**A**). Sometimes the impulse comes down the slow track (**B**). Part of this impulse then enters the fast track and travels back up toward the atria while another part goes on to stimulate the ventricles. At the top of the AV node, the returning impulse "bridges" very slightly into the atrial tissue and turns back down the slow track, thus perpetuating the cycle (**C**). Of course, the returning impulse also sends an impulse across the atria, producing a retrograde P wave. This is a typical slow-fast reentry; the cycle may also be reversed with a fast-slow track.

nodal pathways that it's reproduced here as well as possible.) You'll note that there are two different, well-defined P-R intervals, one prolonged (0.46 second) and one normal (0.20 second). These two P-R intervals appear erratically with no apparent reason for the change.

Tracings like this were the first evidence of *dual AV nodal pathways*. The only way you can possibly explain the random change in P-R intervals is that there are two completely separate AV nodal pathways that are isolated from each other. In other words, when an impulse comes down one pathway, it doesn't affect the other. Invasive EP studies have shown that many individuals have dual AV nodal pathways, even though they don't show up in the surface ECG.

There's a slow pathway with a short refractory period, and a fast pathway with a long refractory period. Figure 4–2 shows what can happen. Normally, conduction comes down the fast pathway, but sometimes a beat will be conducted down the slow pathway—usually, this will be a premature atrial beat. Now there's the electric activity of the slow pathway still moving down the node when the fast pathway has fully recovered from its last transmission and is ready to conduct again. As one investigator put it, "The fast-track tissue manifests preferential retrograde conduction." Either way you say it, part of the impulse from the slow track enters the fast track and goes back up the AV node. Up at the top of the AV, very slightly into the atrial tissue, the impulse reenters the slow pathway and starts back down.

Thus, you have a reentry circuit right in the AV node. Of course, this reentry circuit throws off antegrade impulses that go on down into the ventricles and retrograde impulses that go back across the atria (Fig. 4–3). At other times, the activating impulse may come down the fast track and back up the slow track. Thus, you may have either a "slow-fast" or a "fast-slow" reentry circuit in the AV node.

Note how this process starts in Figure 4–3. The fifth beat is a premature atrial beat; typically, this starts the reentry circuit. For the first few beats, the retrograde P waves have changing relationships to the QRS complexes, depending on speed of conduction up and down. Toward the end of the strip, the relation of retrograde P to QRS settles down and becomes fixed. This is typical of the beginning of one of these AV nodal reentrant tachycardias (AVNRTs).

Figure 4–3.
Diagram of typical AV nodal reentrant tachycardia.

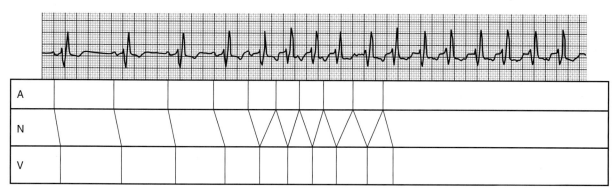

Figure 4–4.
AV nodal reentrant tachycardia, rate 214. Note retrograde P waves in bottom two leads.

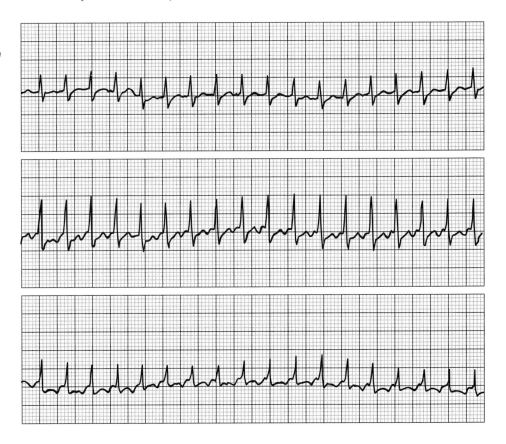

Figures 4–4, 4–5, and 4–6 are all examples of this type of arrhythmia. They constitute more than 90% of the supraventricular tachycardias you will see in the average emergency room or intensive care unit. The retrograde P waves may come just before, during, or after the QRS, depending on the relative speed of conduction back into the atria and forward into the ventricles. The rate will be rapid, in the range of 150 to 250.

Because this is a nodal rhythm, anything that depresses AV nodal conduction will turn off the reentry circuit and stop the tachycardia. Vagal stimulation, adenosine, digitalis, calcium blockers, beta blockers, and quinidine are all effective. It's logical to try vagal stimulation first by carotid sinus massage, the diving reflex, or the Valsalva maneuver. Adenosine is the next step: Between vagal stimulation and adenosine, you can terminate more than 90% of these tachycardias. Remember, these interventions stop the arrhythmia abruptly and completely. If the rate slows and then speeds again, you're not dealing with AVNRT. Look for another

Figure 4–5.
Onset of AV nodal reentrant tachycardia. Note that a premature atrial beat triggers the tachycardia (beat no. 4, top strip). Note also that there's some variation in the relation of P to QRS in the top strip while the rhythm "builds up." In the bottom strip, the relation of retrograde P to QRS becomes fixed. Instead of a P-R interval in these tachycardias, one sees an "R-P." There's a fairly long R-P here.

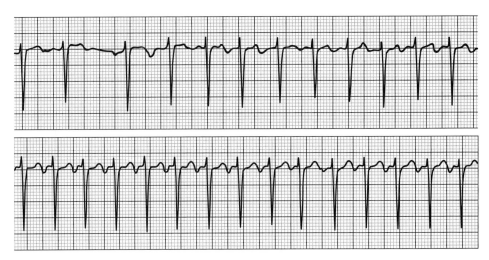

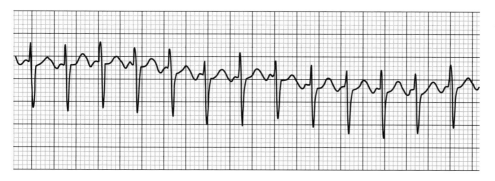

Figure 4–6.
Typical AV nodal reentrant
tachycardia, rate 187.

mechanism and another cause. AVNRT will almost always produce retrograde conduction across the atria. AV dissociation is very rare with AVNRT. AVNRT will never be the result of digitalis toxicity.

AV Nodal Reciprocating Tachycardia: "Preexcitation" Tachycardia

Figure 4–7 illustrates this simple mechanism. There's a bypass tract—some type of preexcitation. An impulse comes down the AV node and back up the bypass tract, forming a self-perpetuating circuit. It may also go around the other way, down the bypass tract and back up the AV node. (You'll read much more about this in the chapter on preexcitation, but it's introduced here to keep the record clear and complete.)

If the impulse comes down the bypass tract, the QRS will often have the typical deformity of Wolff-Parkinson-White conduction, so the diagnosis is simple (Fig. 4–8). If, on the other hand, the impulse comes down the AV node, the QRS will be normal, and it's difficult to decide if there's a bypass tract. One clue may be helpful: The impulse returning to the atria, back up the bypass tract, will naturally arrive at the atria *after* the antegrade impulse reaches the ventricles, so the retrograde P will come after the QRS. That should at least arouse your suspicion of a bypass tract (Fig. 4–9).

The rate will be the same as in AVNRT: The arrhythmia will begin and end abruptly. In other words, this is a true paroxysmal tachycardia.

Because the AV node forms one arc of the circuit, anything that depresses AV nodal conduction can end the arrhythmia, just as with AVNRT. Vagal stimulation, adenosine, and suppressive drugs will all be effective. In addition, drugs that depress conduction in the bypass tract (e.g., procainamide and quinidine) can end the arrhythmia.

Special note: You may have heard cautions about using AV nodal suppressant drugs like digitalis in the presence of preexcitation. That applies only when there's atrial fibrillation or flutter with a bypass tract. When the only arrhythmia is a simple paroxysmal tachycardia, you can depress either side of the circuit and stop the arrhythmia. Response to treatment will be abrupt, "all or nothing," just as with AVNRT.

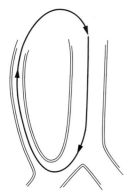

Figure 4–7.
Diagram of AV reciprocating cycle involving a bypass tract. In this case, the impulse comes down the AV node and goes back up the bypass tract. It can also go the other way.

Figure 4–8.
Reciprocating tachycardia with typical preexcitation deformity. The *top two strips* show intermittent WPW preexcitation with occasional normal beats. (The second and third beats in the top strip are normal.) The second beat in the top strip is normal, with a P-R of 0.22 second and a narrow QRS. Most of the other beats on the top two strips show a much shorter P-R (0.13 second), with a very wide QRS—a typical WPW deformity. In the bottom strip, there is a tachycardia in the same patient with a rate of 160 and the same wide QRS complexes, only modified a little by the rapid rate.

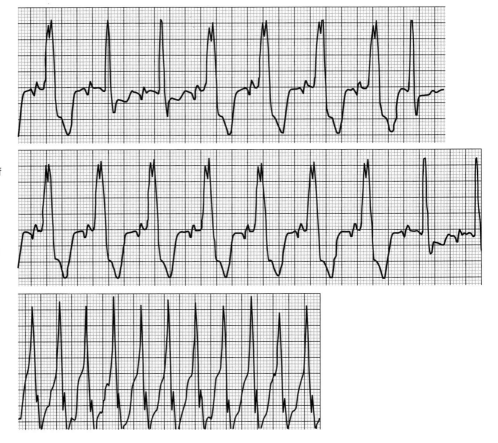

This arrhythmia, like AVNRT, will practically never be dissociated; the retrograde impulse practically always discharges the sinus node. This arrhythmia occurs spontaneously; it is not a digitalis-toxic arrhythmia. A good abbreviation for this arrhythmia would be AVPET: AV nodal preexcitation tachycardia. Nobody's proposed it yet, but it seems very reasonable, it's descriptive, and it's easy to pronounce. Why not?

Automatic or "Nonparoxysmal" Junctional Tachycardia

This is a simple type of arrhythmia; the only problem has been the inexcusably confused terminology.

Sometimes an automatic focus in the region of the AV junction begins to fire in the "accelerated" mode. The rate may be as low as 70 or as high as 130. You could properly call these either "accelerated junctional rhythm" or "automatic junctional tachycardia," depending on the rate (over or under 100). Instead, they're all lumped under the term *automatic junc-*

Figure 4–9.
Reciprocating tachycardia with "orthodromic" conduction, meaning that the impulse comes down the AV node and back up through the bypass tract. The retrograde P *following* the QRS suggests that this is really a reciprocating tachycardia.

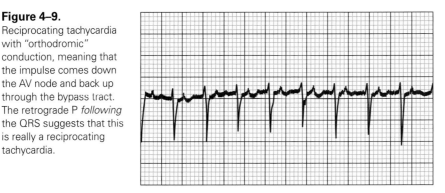

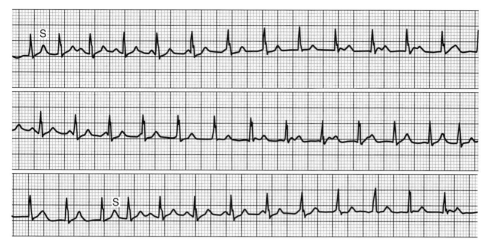

Figure 4–10.
Automatic junctional tachycardia dissociated from a sinus rhythm. The junctional tachycardia has a basic rate of 128. You can clearly see independent sinus P waves marching uninterrupted through the tachycardia. Every now and then, you see a QRS appearing early, which tells you that the sinus node has "captured" a beat (e.g., the second beat in the top strip: the sinus P wave is hidden in the preceding T). The sinus capture beats are labeled S. This kind of dissociation is very rare with AVNRT or AVPET, but is common with automatic junctional tachycardias—an important differential point!

tional tachycardia. How can you call something with a rate of 70 or 80 a "tachycardia"? Good question. The answer usually given is that you expect an automatic junctional rhythm to be slow, so a rate of 70 or more is a "relative" tachycardia!

The term *nonparoxysmal* is used because these arrhythmias don't have the abrupt, all-or-nothing beginning and end of the true paroxysmal tachycardias; they can begin and end more gradually.

Several features distinguish automatic junctional tachycardias from AVNRT and AVPET:

1. **Automatic junctional tachycardias are often dissociated from the sinus rhythm (Fig. 4–10). It's common to see dissociated sinus P waves "marching through" the junctional rhythm and occasionally capturing a beat.**

2. **The rate of these arrhythmias is much slower than the rate of true paroxysmal tachycardias (Figs. 4–11 and 4–12).**

3. **Onset may be gradual, and there are often no symptoms.**

4. **Automatic junctional tachycardias are very commonly caused by digitalis toxicity. The only treatment required is removal of the offending drug.**

Ectopic Atrial Tachycardia of Childhood

This is relatively rare. It's caused by the discharge of an ectopic focus in the atria. The AV node is only a passive conductor in this arrhythmia-unlike AVNRT; it has nothing to do

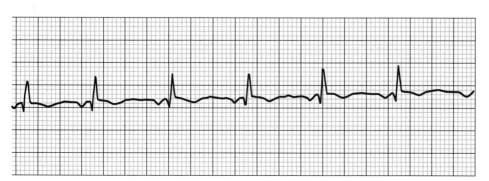

Figure 4–11.
Accelerated junctional rhythm, rate 88. This is also called an *automatic junctional tachycardia* even though the rate really isn't in the tachycardia range.

with the actual machinery. The actual mechanism may be a very small reentry circuit around an area in the atria or simply acceleration of an ectopic atrial focus.

The ECG is characterized by definite P waves with a consistent morphology, obviously different from the sinus P waves, and a P-R interval that is at least equal to the sinus P-R (Figs. 4–13, 4–14, and 4–15). The rate will usually range from 130 to 160—somewhat slower than AVNRT or AVPET.

This arrhythmia commonly appears early in life and tends to persist into adulthood. Although it isn't dangerous, it can be seriously disabling. Sometimes it can be controlled with drugs, but invasive treatment with ablation is often necessary.

Sinus Node Reentrant Tachycardia

This is probably the rarest of the group. It's simple to picture: There's an abrupt increase in rate, but the P waves look exactly like the normal sinus P waves (Fig. 4–16). There appears to be a kind of micro-reentry circuit involving the sinus node that starts and stops abruptly, like any reentrant tachycardia. The rate will be somewhat slower than the AVNRT-AVPET group, in the range of 130 to 160.

Figure 4–12.
Automatic junctional tachycardia, rate 102. The large spiky deflections that appear at the right-hand end of both strips are really dissociated sinus P waves; this patient happened to have massive atrial enlargement with bizarre P waves on the monitor, as recorded here. Again we see AV dissociation, common with this group of arrhythmias.

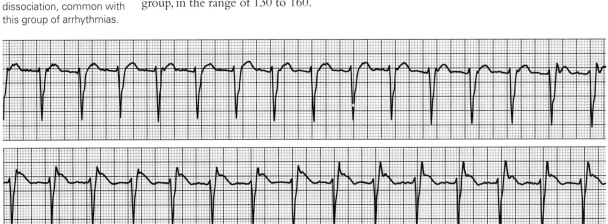

Figure 4–13.
Ectopic atrial tachycardia. Note well-defined but bizarre P waves with normal P-R interval.

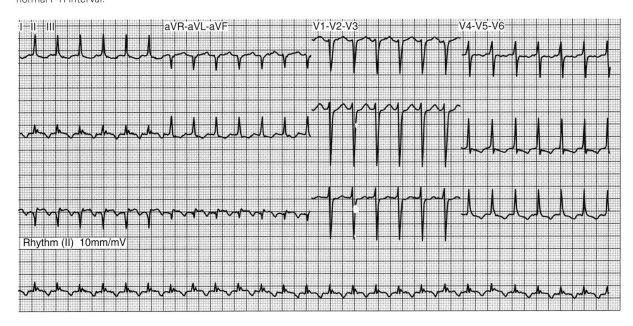

Rhythm (II) 10mm/mV

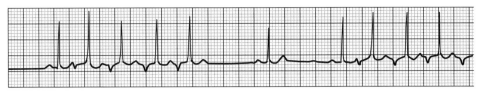

Figure 4–14.
Short runs of ectopic atrial tachycardia. Note the striking difference in morphology between the sinus P waves and the P waves of the ectopic focus.

Sinus node reentrant tachycardia starts and stops abruptly—that's how you distinguish it from a simple sinus tachycardia, which will always speed up and slow down gradually. Unless there's some coincidental disease in the AV node, the P-R interval during the tachycardia will be identical to the sinus P-R.

This, too, is a "nuisance" tachycardia, usually responsive to suppressive drugs. As far as anybody knows, it is not caused by digitalis toxicity, but the literature on the subject is scanty.

Multifocal Atrial Tachycardia

This is a tachycardia with a single, specific cause.

On the electrocardiogram, you see runs of atrial ectopic beats appearing in rapid succession with wildly differing P wave morphologies (Figs. 4–17 and 4–18). Remember that in Chapter 2 it was emphasized that each ectopic atrial focus produces a specific, characteristic P wave; that is, when you see P waves with differing shapes, it's obvious that a number of ectopic foci are discharging.

Figure 4–15.
End of a run of ectopic atrial tachycardia. The relatively slow rate (128) and the obvious difference between the ectopic P waves and the sinus P waves are characteristic.

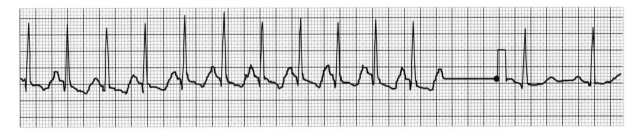

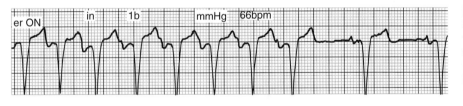

Figure 4–16.
Sinus node reentrant tachycardia: abrupt onset and end, P waves and P-R interval identical to sinus impulses.

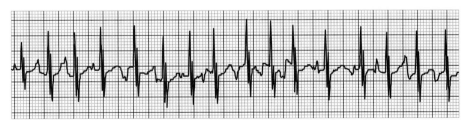

Figure 4–17.
Multifocal atrial tachycardia (*top strip*). Resumption of sinus rhythm interrupted by random atrial ectopic beats from multiple foci in the bottom strip after treatment with O$_2$ and magnesium.

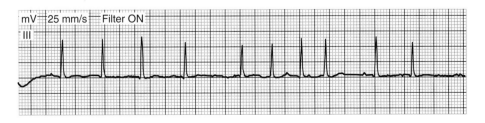

Figure 4–18.
Multifocal atrial tachycardia (*top strip*). Slowing of rate in bottom strip with multifocal single atrial, junctional, and ventricular ectopic beats, after treatment with O_2 and magnesium.

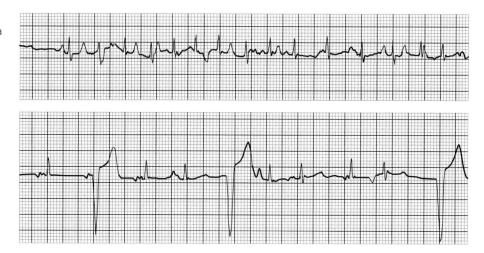

To diagnose multifocal atrial tachycardia (MAT), therefore, you must document rapid atrial ectopic beating from multiple foci. The diagnosis of MAT means that there are runs of three or more ectopic beats—single premature atrial beats, even though they come from multiple foci, are not the same thing. MAT practically always appears in short bursts of varying length, as in Figures 4–17 and 4–18. The result will usually be a completely irregular rhythm that could very easily be confused with atrial fibrillation. Look for the multiform P waves!

This is a hypoxic arrhythmia, and the treatment is proper oxygenation. Ordinary suppressive drugs like digitalis are not effective. In our institution, we have been using intravenous magnesium, which has given encouraging results with control in more than half of all cases. (This, of course, is still investigational.)

Paroxysmal Atrial Tachycardia with Block

This is an arrhythmia with a very specific clinical connotation. About 90% of the time, it is the result of digitalis toxicity. It differs in many respects from the tachyarrhythmias listed here and will be described where it belongs: in Chapter 16, Digitalis-Toxic Arrhythmias.

Five

Various Abnormalities of Intraventricular Conduction

You're already familiar with simple bundle-branch block. There are other forms of intraventricular conduction delay; recognizing them is sometimes critical. Mastery of all the variations of intraventricular conduction is an absolute prerequisite for anyone claiming competence in electrocardiogram (ECG) interpretation.

In this chapter, you will learn how to recognize six distinct entities:

1. **The normal septal Q wave. (The septal Q wave is important in some conduction defects; it's also a good idea to define it properly now so that you'll distinguish it from the pathologic Q waves of myocardial infarction.)**

2. **"Incomplete" bundle-branch block**

3. **Intermittent bundle-branch block**

4. **Normalizing fusion**

5. **The hemiblocks, or fascicular blocks, and bifascicular and trifascicular blocks**

6. **Nonspecific intraventricular conduction delay**

This may seem an intimidating list, but these are everyday workhorse skills. Normalizing fusion and intermittent bundle-branch block are not academic curiosities; they pop up in every busy emergency room and coronary care unit, and the electrocardiographer must be ready to recognize them.

The Septal Q Wave

When impulses pass from atria to ventricles, the left side of the septum is activated slightly before the right. Thus, a small left-to-right force is generated (Fig. 5–1). This will be recorded as an initial negative deflection in any lead out to the left of the septum—aVL, V5 to V6, or sometimes the inferior leads, II to III and aVF. This Q wave will be *narrow*; it will never be more than 0.02 second wide in a normal heart.

Figures 5–2, 5–3, and 5–4 are all variations of the normal septal Q. Remember, it's the *width* of the Q that tells you whether it's physiologic (septal) or pathologic (necrotic). We used to emphasize depth of Q, but careful pathologic correlations have shown it's the *width* that's the crucial element. (I've seen some really tragic mistakes when normal septal Qs were misread as pathologic Q waves—hence the emphasis on this topic here.)

"Incomplete" Bundle-Branch Block

Sometimes you'll see an ECG that looks exactly like left or right bundle-branch block with one difference: the QRS is a little narrower than it is in true bundle-branch block—0.10 or

Figure 5–1.
Genesis of the physiologic septal Q wave. The activating wave moves through the septum from left to right, producing a small initial negative force in leads to the left of the septum.

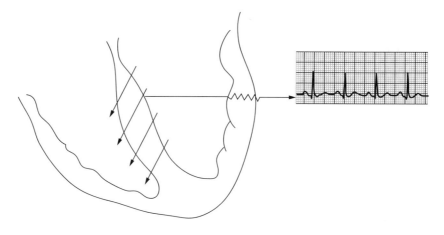

Figure 5–2.
Septal Q waves in lead I and aVL.

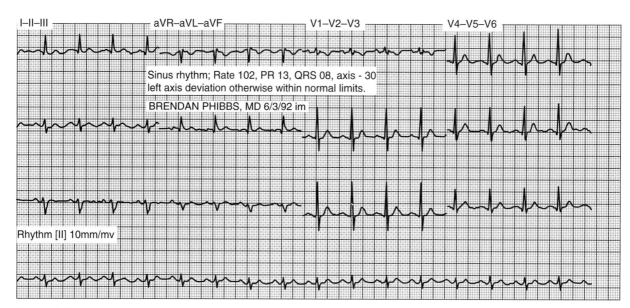

Sinus rhythm; Rate 102, PR 13, QRS 08, axis - 30 left axis deviation otherwise within normal limits.

BRENDAN PHIBBS, MD 6/3/92 im

Figure 5–3.
Septal Q waves in the inferior and anterior-lateral leads: II, III, aVF, and V5 to V6.

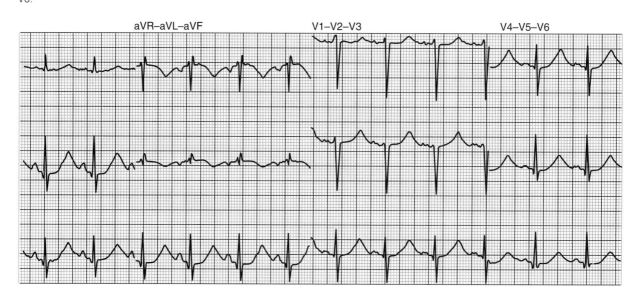

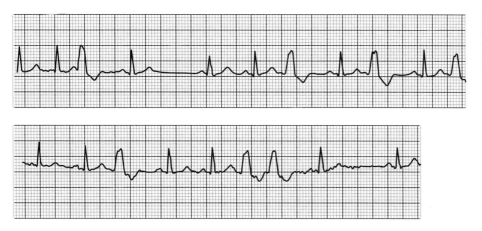

Figure 5–4.
Small septal Q waves in the sinus beats, not present in the VPCs.

0.11 second instead of 0.12 second (Figs. 5–5 and 5–6). Nobody knows exactly what this means. My own ECG has shown a progression from "incomplete" right bundle-branch block with a QRS of 0.10 to "complete" right bundle-branch block with a QRS of 0.12 over the past 8 years—the morphology remains precisely the same, but the QRS is slightly wider.

It has been postulated that in *incomplete* bundle-branch block, the malfunctioning bundle is actually conducting slowly, whereas *complete* bundle-branch block means that it doesn't conduct at all. Nobody is sure, and the whole topic would be nothing more than an ECG curiosity except for one critical difference: a change from incomplete to complete bundle-branch block can be critical in the diagnosis of myocardial infarction.

Look at Figures 5–7 and 5–8. Both have a left bundle-branch block configuration, but there are two important differences. First, the QRS complexes are narrower in Figure 5–7. Second, there is a septal Q in aVL in Figure 5–7 but not in Figure 5–8.

Think of the genesis of the septal Q as outlined previously and take another look at Figure 5–1. To have a septal Q, the normal activating wave has to come down the left side of the septum *first* and penetrate the septum from left to right. If the left bundle branch is blocked, that can't happen. The activating impulse has to come down the right bundle branch, and the septum has to be activated from right to left. There cannot possibly be a septal Q wave.

Thus, the classic diagnosis of left bundle-branch block must include the statement "no septal Q wave." Presumably, with the incomplete type of left bundle-branch block, there is penetration down the left side of the septum, albeit slow—hence, the presence of the septal Q.

Figure 5–5.
"Incomplete" left bundle-branch block. The deflection is negative in V1, but the QRS is only 0.11 second wide and there's a septal Q in aVL, indicating that there must be some conduction down the left side of the septum.

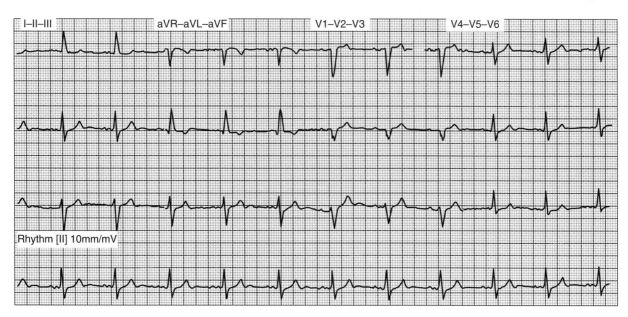

I–II–III   aVR–aVL–aVF   V1–V2–V3   V4–V5–V6

Rhythm [II] 10mm/mV

Figure 5–6.
"Incomplete" right bundle-branch block. The configuration is exactly like full-blown right bundle-branch block except that the QRS is clearly narrower—0.11 second.

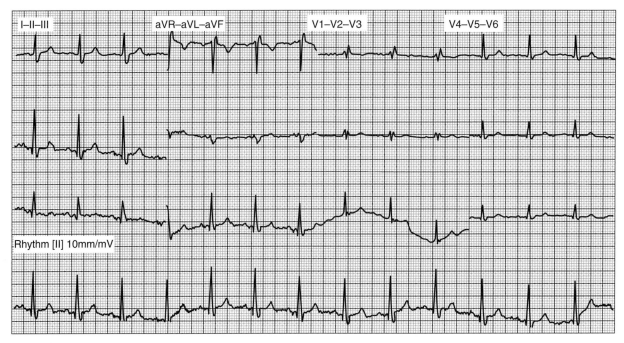

Figure 5–7.
Tracing on the day of admission for a suspected myocardial infarct. Incomplete left bundle-branch block pattern is obvious with septal Q in lead I and aVL.

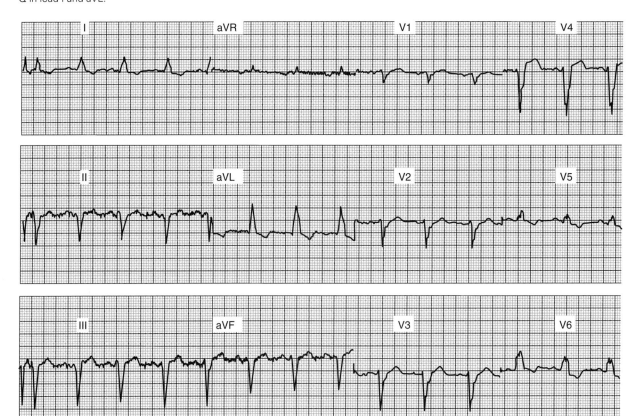

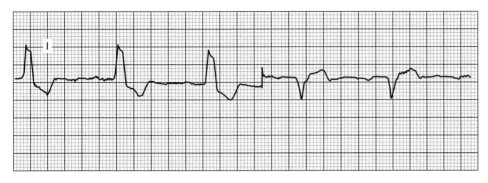

Figure 5–8.
Same patient, next day. The QRS is much wider (0.14 second), and the septal Q has disappeared. This was strong confirmatory evidence of acute ischemic change involving the septum.

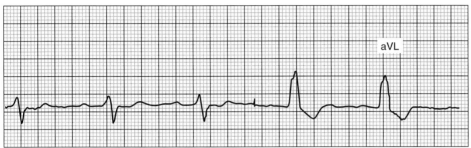

Why is this important? If there's an infarct involving the septum, the disappearance of a septal Q wave, with progression from incomplete to complete left bundle-branch block, may be the only ECG evidence of infarction. That was exactly the case in Figures 5–7 and 5–8.

Intermittent Bundle-Branch Block

Complete, permanent bundle-branch block means that some part of a bundle branch is totally dead in functional terms. Sometimes cells in a bundle branch are injured but not totally dead—they're still capable of functioning. Injured cells in a bundle branch will often take an abnormally long time to recover after each transmission. In other words, the refractory period of the bundle branch may be abnormally prolonged.

You may see a pattern of bundle-branch block only on alternate beats (Fig. 5–9). This can produce a confusing pattern, as in Figure 5–10. The trick here is to measure from the *beginning* of each QRS to the *beginning* of the next. That way the varying width of the QRS complexes won't confuse you. The QRS complexes in fact come exactly on time; the P wave of the narrow beat is hidden each time in the wide T wave caused by the bundle-branch block in the beat ahead of it.

Intermittent bundle-branch block can appear in more complex forms. In Figure 5–11, there are two wide beats followed by a narrow beat in a precise pattern. These are all sinus beats with a consistent P-R interval. This is 3:2 intermittent bundle-branch block. One normal conduction is followed by two beats with bundle-branch block. This can simply mean a very prolonged refractory period in the diseased bundle branch, or it may reflect more complex patterns with progressive partial penetrations of a bundle branch.

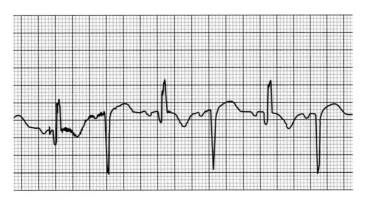

Figure 5–9.
Lead V1, 2:1 right bundle-branch block. The refractory period of the right bundle branch is so prolonged that it can conduct only every other beat.

Figure 5–10.
2:1 Bundle-branch block. To recognize what's happening, it's important to measure from the beginning of each QRS complex; in fact, they all measure out exactly despite the varying widths.

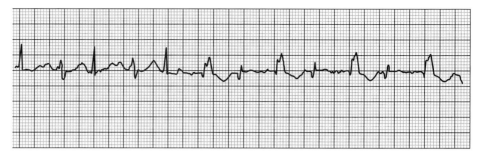

Normalizing Fusion

Remember ventricular fusion (in Chapter 2)? It's what happens when a ventricular ectopic beat starts across the ventricle and collides with an impulse coming down through the atrioventricular (AV) node, so that the ventricles are activated by two impulses. The resulting beat will be hybrid in shape, somewhere between the normal QRS and the wide QRS of the ventricular premature contraction (VPC). The P-R interval will always be *shorter than normal* because the VPC begins to be inscribed while the normal impulse is still up in the AV node.

Fusion beats tell you that the wide complexes without P waves that you see somewhere else in the tracing have to be VPCs because the only way two impulses can collide, or fuse, in the ventricles is for one impulse to start in the ventricles in the first place. When you see fusion beats during a wide-beat tachycardia, the diagnosis is ventricular tachycardia, with 100% accuracy. That's why fusion beats are important.

Here's an unusual kind of fusion you can see when bundle-branch block is present. Suppose a ventricular ectopic impulse fires in the blocked ventricle. Suppose also that by pure coincidence the VPC activates the *blocked* ventricle at the same instant that the normal impulse coming down from the AV node activates the other ventricle. Both ventricles will be activated at the same fraction of a second, and the QRS will be narrow. The bundle-branch block will disappear, for no apparent reason, for one beat (Fig. 5–12).

In other words, this is a kind of fusion that "normalizes" a bundle-branch block. The P-R interval of the "normalized" beat will be shorter than normal, just like any fusion beat. When you see a normal QRS interrupting a bundle-branch block for no apparent reason, it means there's a ventricular ectopic focus firing, normalizing the bundle-branch block. These normalized beats may be your only clue to ventricular ectopic firing in the presence of bundle-branch block; that's why it's important to recognize them (Figs. 5–13 and 5–14).

Fascicular Blocks, or Hemiblocks; Bifascicular and Trifascicular Blocks

The left bundle branch isn't the simple structure physicians used to think it was. About 25 years ago, investigators found that the left bundle branch has two distinct functional elements that conduct in different directions. If you dissect out the left bundle branch by special techniques, it looks like a fan with a long narrow handle—you can't make out any separate pathways or channels anatomically.

Figure 5–11.
3:2 Bundle-branch block. The refractory period is so prolonged that the malfunctioning bundle branch can conduct only on every third beat.

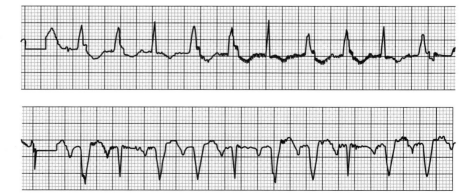

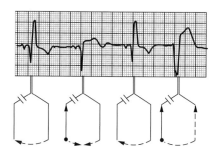

Figure 5–12.
Mechanism of normalizing fusion. When bundle-branch block is present, a ventricular ectopic beat may sometimes activate the blocked ventricle at the same instant that the other ventricle is activated normally, thus producing a normal, narrow QRS by accident.

Functionally, the story is totally different. The left bundle branch behaves as if it had two different functional elements, conducting in roughly opposite directions. These functional elements are called *fascicles*. The two fascicles are named according to the direction in which they conduct; thus, there is a posterior-superior, or leftward, fascicle and an anterior-inferior, or rightward, fascicle. The posterior-superior fascicle conducts upward and to the left at an angle of about −60 degrees (range, −40 to −90 degrees). The anterior-inferior fascicle conducts downward and to the right at an angle of about +100 degrees (range, +80 to +120 degrees) (Fig. 5–15).

When both fascicles are conducting normally, they balance each other out with a normal axis in the range of +30 degrees. When one fascicle fails because the cells are diseased or dead, the axis will swing far to the left or right, with unopposed conduction down the functioning fascicle. Thus, if the anterior fascicle fails, there will be unopposed leftward conduction, and the axis will lie between −40 and −90 degrees (Fig. 5–16).

Logical question: Can anything else swing the axis this far left? Not much. Left ventricular hypertrophy or a high diaphragm in a short, stocky person can produce an axis as far left as −30 degrees, but it won't go beyond that. A few rare degenerative diseases, like cardiac sarcoid, may deviate the axis far to the left, but even in these cases it's possible that degeneration of the anterior fascicle may be the cause. As a general working statement, it's fair to say that an extreme left axis as defined previously usually represents anterior fascicular block.

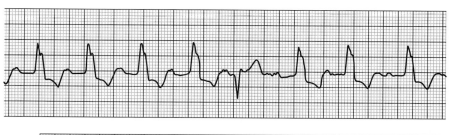

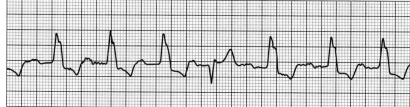

Figure 5–13.
Lead I. Normalizing fusion. In the middle of each strip, there's a narrow QRS preceded by a short P-R—a typical example of normalizing fusion.

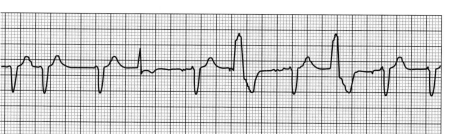

Figure 5–14.
Lead V1. Normalizing fusion in the setting of atrial fibrillation. Left bundle-branch block is present, and there's an ectopic focus firing in the left ventricle, producing the occasional wide beats. Beat four is narrow, obviously the result of normalizing fusion.

The common term for fascicular block is *hemiblock*. This isn't a very precise term because it implies that half of the bundle branch is blocked. In fact, the anterior fascicle is much smaller and more vulnerable than the posterior fascicle—possibly a quarter of the size. However, the term *hemiblock* is in common use, so it's acceptable. The conclusion from all this is that left anterior hemiblock is a relatively precise, positive diagnosis, based on axis.

It was formerly argued that there must be a small, or "septal," Q in I and aVL to establish the diagnosis of left anterior hemiblock, but this notion has been substantially discarded. It's

Figure 5–15.
Schematic representation of the direction of conduction of the two fascicles of the left bundle branch.

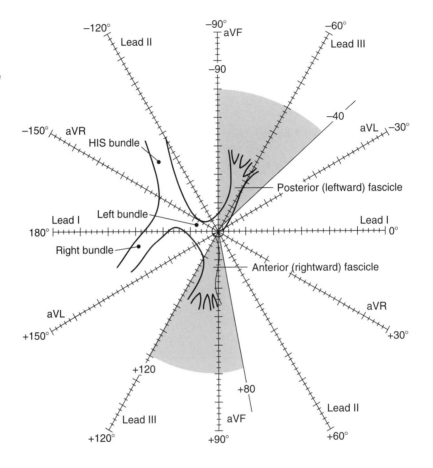

Figure 5–16.
Left anterior hemiblock with axis of −55 degrees. There is also intraventricular delay with a QRS of 0.10 to 0.11 second.

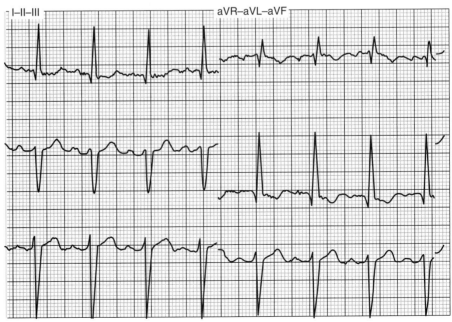

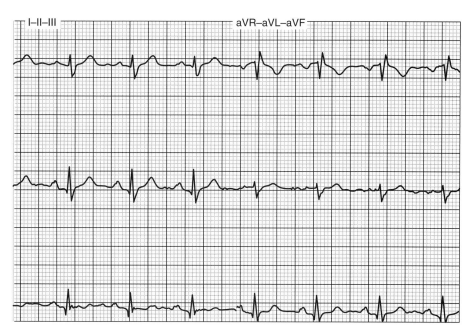

Figure 5–17.
Physiologic right axis deviation of +100 degrees in a tall, slender, young individual.

the axis that establishes the diagnosis. Left posterior hemiblock is trickier. Posterior hemiblock will produce an extreme right axis, in the range of +80 to +120 degrees, but so will many other conditions: right ventricular hypertrophy, pulmonary hypertension (acute or chronic), a tall slender habitus, or emphysema (Figs. 5–17 and 5–18).

Only when all other reasonable causes of an extreme right axis have been ruled out can you consider posterior hemiblock as a cause of right-axis deviation. Posterior hemiblock is therefore a diagnosis of exclusion.

Remember, you have to correct for age and body habitus when considering axis. It's normal for children and young people to have a right axis; on the other hand, if a slightly obese 65-year-old with otherwise normal heart and lungs turned up with a +90-degree axis, the only reasonable diagnosis would be posterior hemiblock. Posterior fascicular block is rare, presumably because the posterior fascicle is the larger of the two fascicles, with a more secure blood supply.

Special clinical significance: If a fascicular block of either variety appears abruptly in the course of an infarct, it may be a sign of acute ischemic change in the septum.

Fascicular blocks and AV conduction: In terms of AV conduction, fascicular blocks by themselves have no significance. In other words, the appearance of fascicular block does not present a significant risk for subsequent AV block. There's only one situation in which you'd be concerned about fascicular block and AV conduction, and that's when fascicular block is associ-

Figure 5–18.
Pathologic right axis deviation of +112 degrees appearing in a stocky, middle-aged individual early in the course of a myocardial infarction. Posterior hemiblock was the diagnosis of exclusion once a pulmonary embolus had been ruled out.

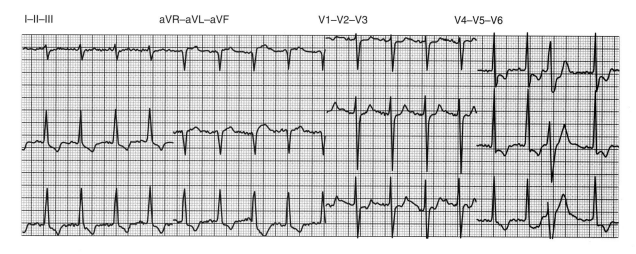

ated with right bundle-branch block. (Left fascicular block couldn't be associated with left bundle-branch block, obviously, because if the whole bundle branch is blocked, there is no possibility of conduction down one of the fascicles.) Figure 5–19 makes the problem clear.

If there is right bundle-branch block together with block of one fascicle of the left bundle, the ventricular component of AV conduction is reduced to one strand out of three—the one remaining conducting fascicle of the left bundle. At this point, the diagnosis is *bifascicular block*. Interruption or delay in this last remaining strand will produce some type of AV block.

How can you tell if one fascicle of the left bundle is blocked in the presence of right bundle-branch block? You do it by determining axis, just the way you do with ordinary hemiblock. Remember that you diagnose left anterior hemiblock by detecting extreme left axis deviation (−45 to −90 degrees). That's exactly how you go about it when right bundle-branch block is present, with one difference: you ignore the wide terminal wave that represents "backward" movement across the blocked ventricle.

You want to know what the axis is when the impulse is coming down the left bundle—that's being recorded during the initial part of the QRS. You simply measure the axis of the initial 0.06-second forces of the QRS. That's the axis that's recorded when the impulse is moving down the left bundle, and that's how you tell if one of the fascicles of the left bundle is blocked. Figure 5–20 shows how to do this.

When bifascicular block was first described, there was a widespread belief that if a patient presented with syncope and bifascicular block, it would be reasonable to investigate the possibility of intermittent AV block as a cause of the syncope. Studies over the past 20 years, however, have shown that bifascicular block isn't really much of a risk in terms of AV block. Bifascicular block is in fact fairly common, and the risk for progressing to AV block is low. Look at Figures 5–21 and 5–22 and practice this simple measurement.

Trifascicular block means that there's some kind of delay or failure in the one remaining fascicle. Thus, if you saw bifascicular block with a prolonged P-R interval, it would be possible that the delay might be in the one functioning fascicle, and *trifascicular block* would be the appropriate term (Fig. 5–23).

Figure 5–19.
Bifascicular block. The right bundle branch is blocked, as is the anterior fascicle of the left bundle. Conduction now depends exclusively on the posterior fascicle of the left bundle.

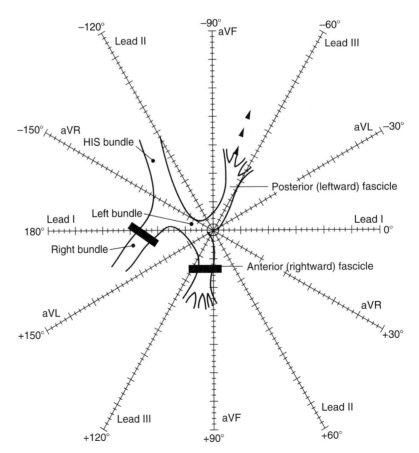

Nonspecific Intraventricular Conduction Delay

Sometimes you'll see widened QRS complexes that don't fit the definite pattern of any kind of bundle-branch block or fascicular block. The QRS will be 0.10 to 0.11 second wide, with no particular recognizable pattern. All you can use is the obvious term *nonspecific intraventricular conduction delay*, which is precisely what it is. There must be some slowing in the more distal arborizations of the bundle-branch system, but that's about all you can say. People used to play with terms like "local focal intraventricular block," but they don't mean much in terms of real pathophysiology. Appearance and disappearance of this kind of delay, of course, may be a clue to acute changes, ischemic or toxic, in the myocardium.

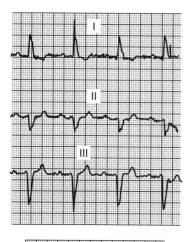

Figure 5–20.
Method of measuring axis in the presence of right bundle-branch block. Because you're trying to determine conduction in the left bundle, it's important to measure axis at the time the left bundle is being activated, in about the first 0.06 second of the QRS.

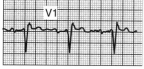

Figure 5–21.
Right bundle-branch block with left anterior hemiblock. Axis of initial 0.06 second is − 55 degrees.

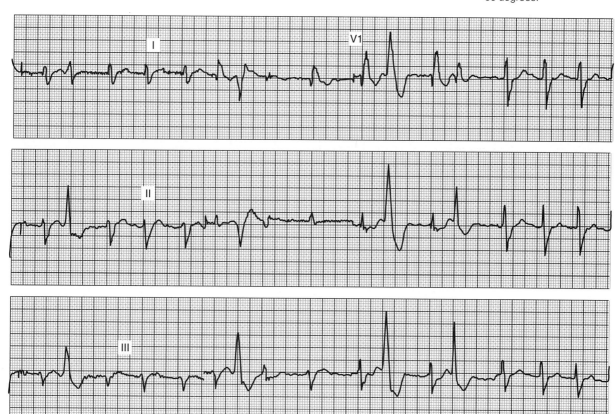

Figure 5–22.
Right bundle-branch block with left posterior hemiblock. Extreme right axis of initial forces is present (+118 degrees), and all other causes of right axis have been ruled out.

The term *peri-infarction block* has been used to describe the kind of nonspecific conduction delay shown in Figure 5–24. Intraventricular conduction had been normal previously; with the onset of a posterior-lateral infarct, the widened QRS appeared. It's tempting to call this a left anterior hemiblock, but note that lead II consists of a simple Q wave, whereas there are many smaller Q waves in other leads. It's probably inaccurate to try to estimate axis

| I–II–III | aVR–aVL–aVF | V1–V2–V3 | V4–V5–V6 |

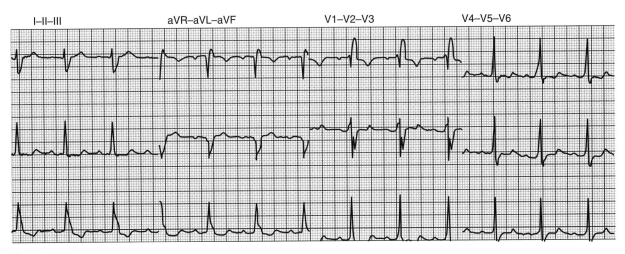

Figure 5–23.
Trifascicular block. Prolonged P-R in the presence of right bundle-branch block and left anterior hemiblock. This always raises the possibility that the P-R delay is in the one remaining conducting fascicle, that is, in the posterior fascicle of the left bundle. While this tracing was being recorded, the P-R interval prolonged dramatically, and a temporary pacemaker was inserted as the patient went into a high degree of AV block.

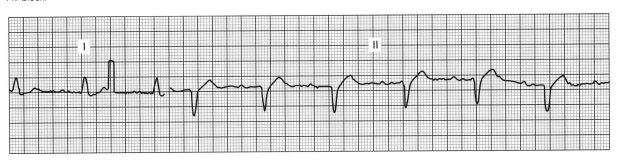

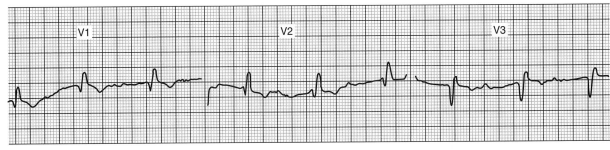

in the presence of pathologic Q waves, so the simple term *nonspecific intraventricular conduction delay* is a better descriptor. Some part of the fascicular tissues must obviously be involved to produce a pattern like this. Figures 5–24 and 5–25 are examples of this kind of nonspecific delay in intraventricular conduction.

Figure 5–24.
Intraventricular conduction delay in the setting of an acute posterior-lateral myocardial infarct. This kind of delay is sometimes referred to as *peri-infarction block*.

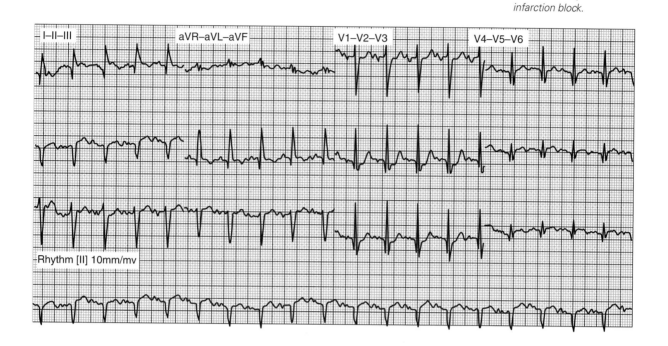

Figure 5–25.
Intraventricular conduction delay. The QRS complexes are wide, but they're narrower than in true bundle-branch block (0.10 to 0.11 second). There's some slurring of the QRS in several leads, a common finding in this setting.

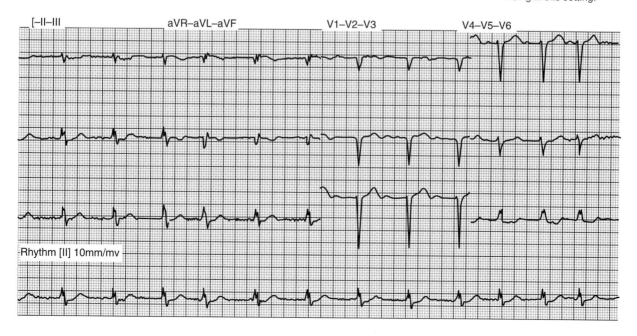

Six

More About Aberrancy

The competent electrocardiographer must be ready to recognize aberrant conduction in any of its forms. Combinations of wide beats, narrow beats, and beats with changing morphology may present life-and-death decisions. Learning the mechanism of the various types of aberrant conduction is an essential drill, reminiscent of the "gimme 50 pushups" we used to inflict on recruits in 1942.

In Chapter 5, you learned about simple "fixed," or permanent, aberrancy. This can present as bundle-branch block, fascicular (or bifascicular or trifascicular) block, and nonspecific intraventricular conduction delay.

Aberrancy is often transient. When it is, it will be the result of one of four mechanisms:

1. **Simple prolongation of refractory period with rate-dependent aberrancy**

2. **Ashman aberrancy**

3. **Bradycardia-dependent aberrancy**

4. **Random intermittent, or "non-rate-dependent," aberrancy**

Simple Prolongation of the Refractory Period with Rate-Dependent Aberrancy

In Figure 3–4, you saw a simple example of rate-dependent bundle-branch block. The same phenomenon can produce any of the other conduction defects listed previously. Thus, you may see rate-dependent fascicular blocks or rate-dependent intraventricular conduction delay (Fig. 6–1). The logic remains clear: There is normal conduction up to a certain rate, and the aberrant conduction appears at any higher rate.

Simple prolongation of refractory period can produce regular ratios of conduction, like the 2:1 or 3:1 bundle-branch block illustrated in Figures 5–7, 5–8, and 5–9. The concept remains the same: The refractory period is so prolonged that the structure can conduct only every other beat or every third beat.

Ashman Aberrancy

There's another common form of aberrancy, called *Ashman aberrancy* after the man who described it.

To understand Ashman aberrancy, you have to understand three simple facts:

1. **The refractory period of the tissues of the heart depends on the rate. The slower the rate, the longer the refractory period after each beat. As the rate speeds, the refractory period shortens (Fig. 6–2). (If you think about it, it has to, or the heart couldn't speed up very much.)**

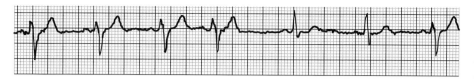

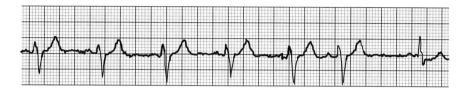

Figure 6–1.
Lead II. Rate-dependent intraventricular block—left anterior hemiblock. Throughout most of the tracing, the QRS complexes are 0.11 second wide and show a left axis of approximately –45 degrees. At the right-hand end of each strip, there is a pause after a premature atrial beat; after the pause, a narrow QRS is apparent (0.08 second) with a normal axis. This is an obvious case of rate-dependent block in the fascicular system.

2. **The refractory period of the heart is set one beat at a time. In other words, the refractory period after any beat depends on the distance between that beat and the beat ahead of it; the "rate," as far as any given beat is concerned, is the distance from the beat ahead of it. Therefore, if the distance between beats varies, the way it does in atrial fibrillation and other arrhythmias, the refractory period will also change from beat to beat.**

3. **This changing refractory period sets up conditions for Ashman aberrancy. Look at the bottom strip of Figure 6–2. Start with a long R-R interval. This means that there will be a long refractory period after the second beat of the pair. Now suppose the next beat comes early—there's a short R-R interval after a long one. The early beat will hit the refractory period set by the long R-R interval. Obviously, it will be blocked or aberrantly conducted. Thus, when you see a short R-R interval following a long one, look for aberrant conduction (Fig. 6–3).**

When there's a run of rapid beats, as there is in a paroxysmal supraventricular tachycardia, the second beat in the run is the one that's likely to show Ashman aberrancy because of the long R-R/short R-R relationship. The short R-R then "pulls in" the refractory period, and beats from then on are normally conducted. This is the "second beat in the run" phenomenon, typical of Ashman aberrancy (Fig. 6–4).

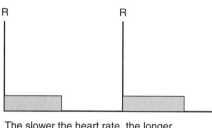

The slower the heart rate, the longer the refractory period in the conducting tissues

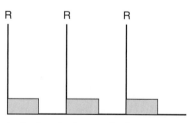

As the heart rate speeds, the refractory period shortens

Figure 6–2.
The mechanism of the Ashman phenomenon.

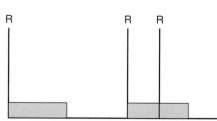

The Ashman phenomenon is the result of this rate-related change in the refractory period; when a short R-R follows a long R-R, the third beat encounters the refractory period set by the preceding long R-R and will be aberrantly conducted

Figure 6–3.
Ashman aberrancy in premature atrial beats. The premature beat provides the short R-R interval, which sets up the classic Ashman relationship.

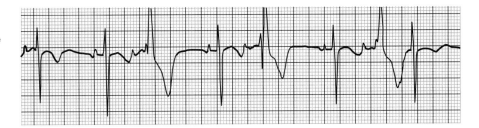

Figure 6–4.
Ashman aberrancy during paroxysms of atrial tachycardia. Each time there's a wide aberrant QRS, it comes when a short R-R interval follows a much longer one. The *two arrowheads* point to the third and fourth beats in a run of atrial tachycardia. Note that whereas the second beat in the run shows Ashman aberrancy, the subsequent beats have normalized because the continuing short R-R intervals have "pulled in" the refractory period.

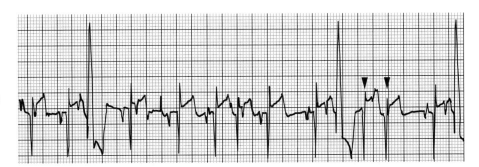

One of the common settings for Ashman aberrancy, of course, is atrial fibrillation, or flutter with varying atrioventricular (AV) conduction, because there are changing R-R intervals with every beat. This helps with the problem of wide beats appearing during either arrhythmia. Are they aberrantly conducted beats from the atria or are they ventricular premature contractions (VPCs)? If the wide beats appear when there's no Ashman ratio to explain them, they have to be VPCs (Fig. 6–5).

Moral: When you see wide beats during atrial fibrillation or flutter with varying AV conduction, look at the R-R interval of the two beats ahead of them. If there's not a long R-R interval ahead of the wide beats, you can't call the wide beats aberrant. They have to be VPCs.

Delayed Ashman Reset

If a tachycardia is very fast compared with the basic rate, it may take several seconds for all parts of the conducting system to reset the refractory period—that is, to shorten it. For this reason, you may see wide beats in a sustained run at the beginning of a tachycardia; then narrow beats appear at exactly the same rate. The fact that all the beats appear at the same rate means they're all coming from the same place, of course. It's simply the Ashman phenomenon prolonged for a few seconds. Precisely why this occurs has never been explained. It may

Figure 6–5.
Diagnosing ventricular ectopic beats by excluding any basis for aberrancy. You can't make out any Ashman relationship with the wide beats—in fact, they usually follow a long R-R interval instead of a short one. You can't invoke rate-dependent aberrancy either because the wide beats come at a much slower rate than many of the narrow beats. The wide beats therefore must be ventricular.

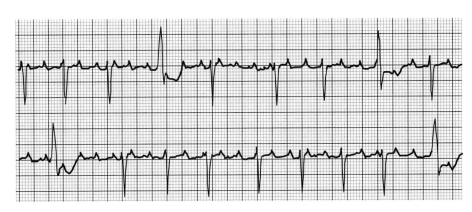

be because some parts of the ventricular conducting network aren't penetrated for the first few beats, and hence their refractory period isn't shortened (Figs. 6–6 and 6–7).

It's important to be aware of the possibility of delayed Ashman reset because it can produce wide-beat tachycardias that look exactly like ventricular tachycardia. Look for the normalized QRS complexes that appear at the same rate!

Special note: Rate-dependent aberrancy will produce a left bundle-branch configuration about 8 times out of 10. Ashman aberrancy will produce a right bundle-branch pattern about 8 times out of 10.

Phase 4, or Bradycardia-Dependent, Aberrancy

The idea of aberrancy that occurs because the impulse is coming too fast is simple. You can also see aberrancy when impulses come too slowly. Here's how it works:

Think of a conducting cell as an archer. Between beats, the bow is bent with the arrow drawn clear back. The cell is charged with *negative* energy, ready to release it. The energy is about −90 millivolts. It's potential energy, just like the bent bow. When the cell is activated, the energy is released, exactly like an arrow taking flight. The energy level in the cell goes down from −90 to about +10. After discharge, the cell is quiescent, passive—just like a bow after a shot. There's no potential energy. Then the cell recharges itself, like the archer drawing the bow for the next shot. It will recharge itself to about −90 millivolts.

Suppose our archer had to wait too long for the next shot. His arm gets tired, and he lets the bow go down to the half-drawn position. If he shoots from that position, it's going to be weak. The same thing can happen in conducting cells. Under certain conditions, *when there's a long time between beats*, the cells "leak" their charge, maybe to −50 millivolts. If they're stimulated at that low level of energy, they will fire weakly or maybe not at all.

The phase of cell activation between beats is called *phase 4*; that's when the cell should be at full charge, ready to fire. If the cells leak their charge during that period, it's called *phase 4 depolarization* or *bradycardia-dependent aberrancy*. Figures 6–8 and 6–9 are examples of this interesting and sometimes baffling phenomenon.

Random Intermittent, or "Non-Rate-Dependent," Aberrancy

This is the rarest form of aberrant conduction. In Figures 6–10 and 6–11, you see a bundle-branch pattern that appears and disappears at exactly the same rate as the normal beats. There's no Ashman phenomenon, no phase 4 mechanism, no rate change at all. The bundle-branch block simply appears and disappears in random fashion. This will always be the result of some intermittent acute change in the conducting tissues as a result of drug effect, electrolyte intoxication, or ischemia. When this type of random conduction defect appears, one should always check for a possible cause because it implies a changing, unstable condition in the conducting tissues.

Figure 6–6.
Delayed Ashman reset. The strip starts with a sinus rhythm with a rate of about 90. A supraventricular tachycardia with a rate of 187 appears. The first seven beats are wide (*arrowheads*), after which the tachycardia continues with narrow complexes at exactly the same rate. This is the same Ashman phenomenon except that it's delayed. When the rate is rapid, it often takes several seconds for the refractory period to "reset" to normal in all parts of the conducting system. If you saw only the first seven beats, it would be easy to confuse this with ventricular tachycardia. The fact that the narrow complexes continue to appear at exactly the same rate as the wide ones tells you they must all be coming from the same place: they're supraventricular.

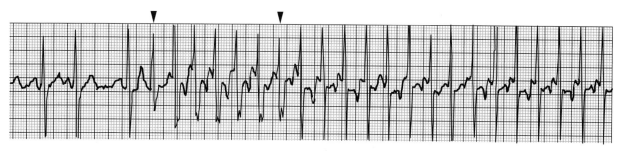

Figure 6–7.
Runs of supraventricular tachycardia with delayed Ashman reset, as in Fig. 6–6. In the top strip, there'd be no way to tell that the wide-beat tachycardia wasn't ventricular. In the bottom three strips, you see typical delayed Ashman reset with normalization of the QRS after several seconds. Note that the axis swings dramatically as the QRS complexes narrow, suggesting varying refractoriness in the fascicular system.

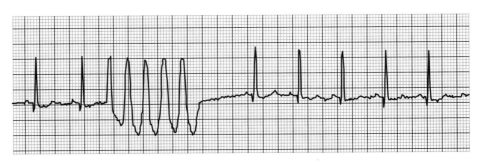

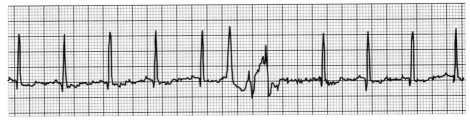

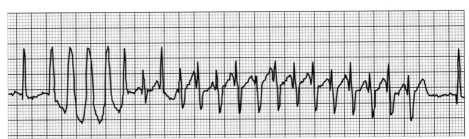

Figure 6–8.
Bradycardia-dependent bundle-branch block. In most of the leads, you see an obvious left bundle-branch block at a rate of 68. In leads V4, V5, and V6, there are normal narrow QRS complexes at a rate of 88. You can see the same thing in the rhythm strip at the bottom, with wide complexes at a slower rate and narrow complexes when the rate speeds.

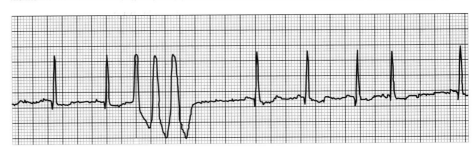

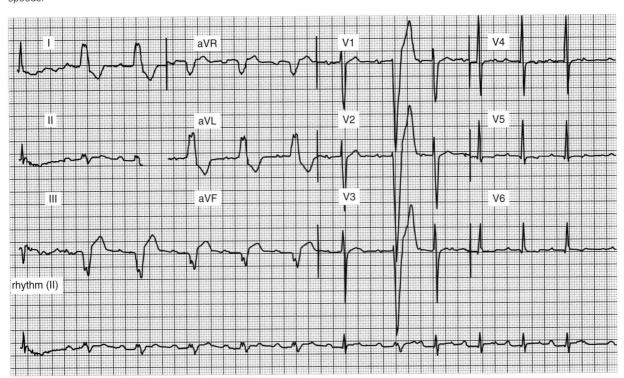

Figure 6–9.
Serial tracings. Marked sinus arrhythmia with one blocked premature atrial beat (at the right-hand end of the top strip). When the rate speeds to 88, the QRS is normal. Whenever it slows, a bundle-branch block is present. Typical bradycardia-dependent aberrancy is present.

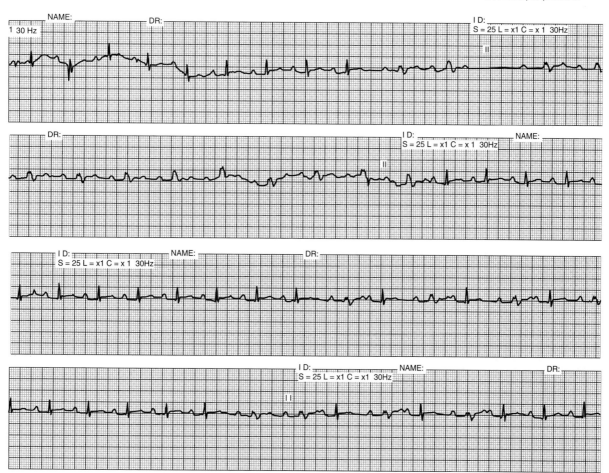

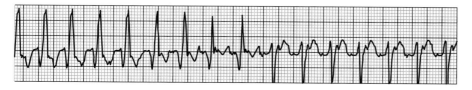

Figure 6–10.
Random, non-rate-dependent bundle-branch block. Lead V1, atrial tachycardia. Obvious right bundle-branch block pattern in the first portion of the tracing with normal intraventricular conduction in the second half. The rate is identical throughout, and there is obviously no change in rhythm.

Figure 6–11.
Random, non-rate-dependent aberrancy. Lead V1. Right bundle-branch block changing to normal QRS at the same rate (100). Note the interesting progression from complete to "incomplete" right bundle-branch block for one beat in the transition to normal intraventricular conduction.

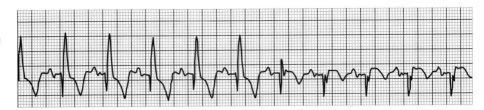

Self-Assessment I

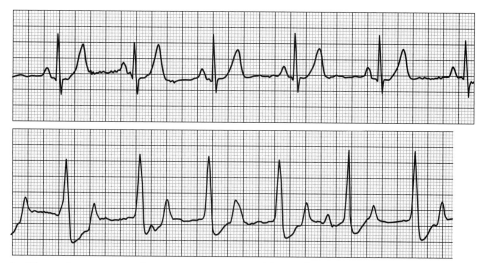

Figure SAI–1.

1. The patient came to the emergency room with an obvious anterior MI. He received thrombolytic therapy, and shortly thereafter this rhythm appeared.
   a. Diagnosis of wide-beat rhythm?
   b. Diagnosis of arrhythmia in the second strip?
   c. Is AV block present?
   d. Treatment?

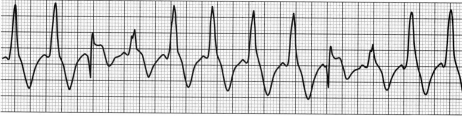

Figure SAI–2.

2. Wide-beat tachycardia.
   a. Where does it originate? How do you know?

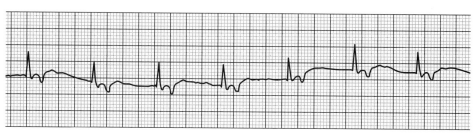

Figure SAI–3.

3. Narrow-beat bradycardia.
   a. Where does it originate?
   b. Why?

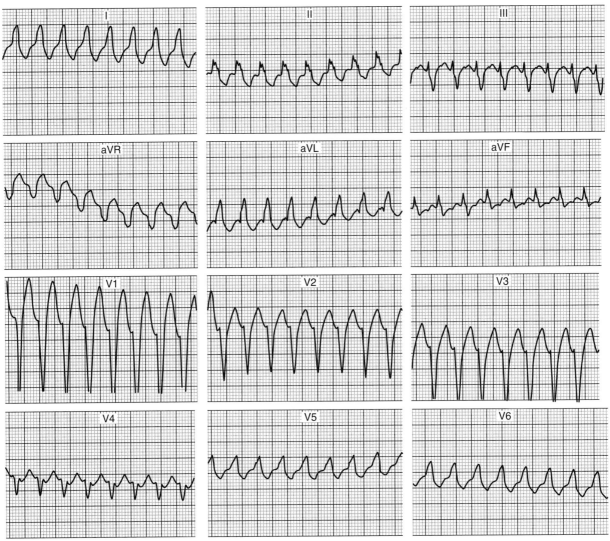

Figure SAI–4. 4. What are the diagnostic possibilities here?
        a. Can you distinguish between them?
        b. How will you treat this arrhythmia?

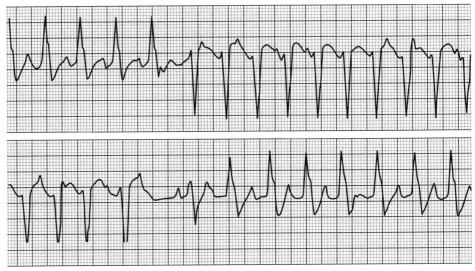

Figure SAI–5.
5. Wide-beat tachycardia with two differing morphologies, lead V1.
        a. Diagnosis of arrhythmia?
        b. How proved?
        c. This all appeared in the setting of an acute MI in a patient with a previously normal
           ECG. Significance? Prognosis?

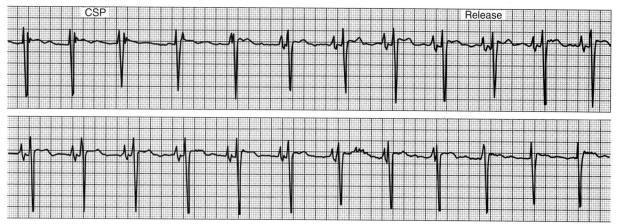

Figure SAI–6. 6. This rhythm appeared in a critically ill postoperative patient. (CSP refers to "carotid sinus pressure.")
   a. What's happening and why?
   b. Possible effect on hemodynamics?

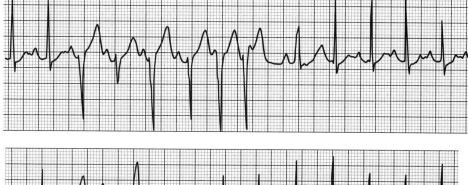

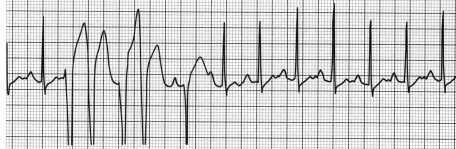

Figure SAI–7.

7. Wide beats, narrow beats, and intermediate beats.
   a. Diagnosis? Proof?

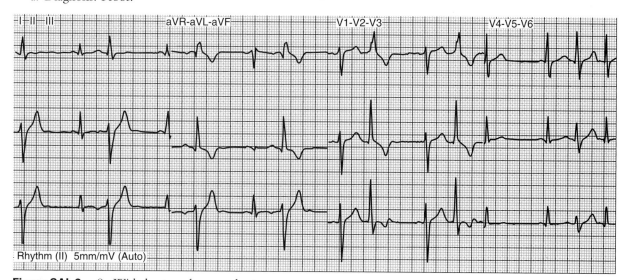

Figure SAI–8. 8. Wide beats and narrow beats.
   a. What are the wide beats?
   b. What's their pathophysiologic basis?

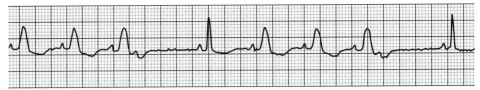

Figure SAI–9.

9. Wide beats and narrow beats.
   a. What are they, and why are they happening?

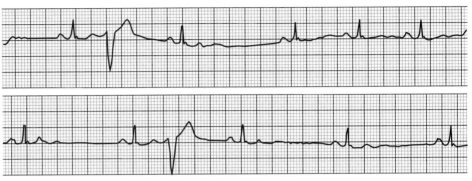

Figure SAI–10.

10. Wide beats, narrow beats, and abrupt pauses.
    a. Why the variation in QRS width?
    b. Why the abrupt pauses?

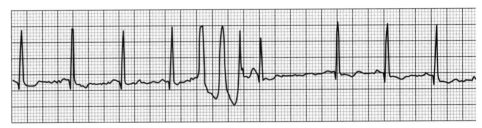

Figure SAI–11.

11. Sinus rhythm interrupted by a four-beat run of wide and narrow beats.
    a. What's the cause of the tachycardia?
    b. What's the pathophysiology of the changing QRS width?

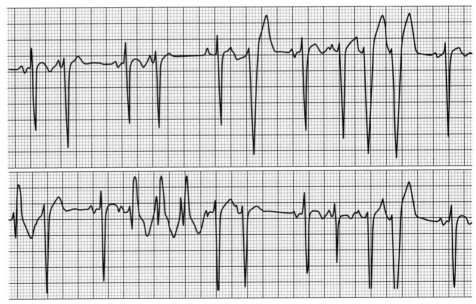

Figure SAI–12.

12. Somebody saw these wide beats in the emergency room and called for lidocaine.
    a. What's really going on?
    b. Pathophysiology of differing wide QRS morphology?

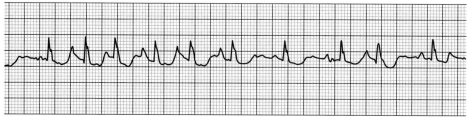

A

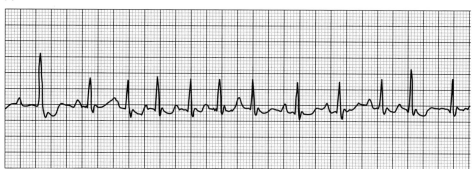

B

Figure SAI–13.

13. **A** and **B,** Both strips represent the same arrhythmia.
    a. Diagnosis?
    b. Cause?
    c. Treatment?

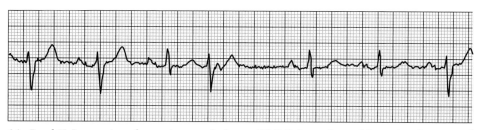

Figure SAI–14.

14. Lead II. Interesting change in morphology of QRS throughout this tracing. It appeared early in the course of an MI. (Hint: remember this is lead II; think *axis!*)
    a. Cause?
    b. Significance?

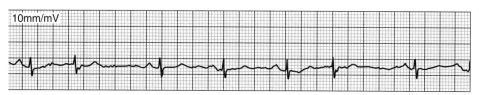

Figure SAI–15.

15. Arrhythmia? Cause of pause?

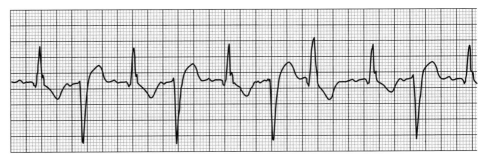

Figure SAI–16.

16. Dramatic change in QRS morphology.
    a. Cause?
    b. Significance?

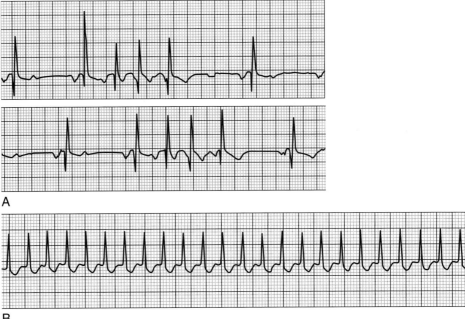

Figure SAI–17.

17. **A** and **B**, Two examples of supraventricular tachycardia: one in short paroxysms, one sustained.
    a. Cause in each?

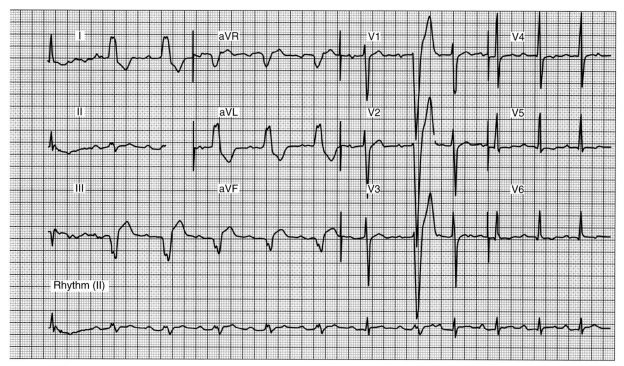

Figure SAI–18. 18. Wide beats, narrow beats. What's the basis for the difference?

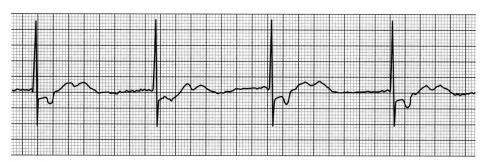

Figure SAI–19.

19. Rhythm?
    a. Why is it present? What's lacking?

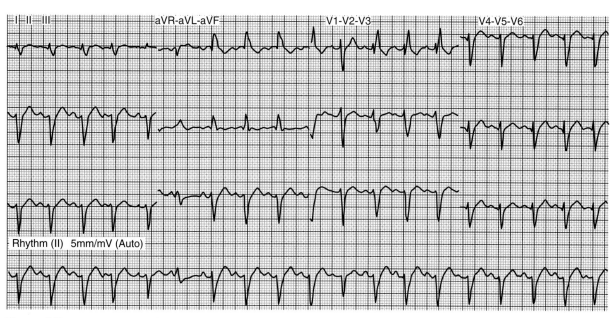

Figure SAI–20. 20. Easy. This tracing is recorded in an asymptomatic patient preoperatively.
        a. Diagnosis? Significance?
        b. Treatment, if any?

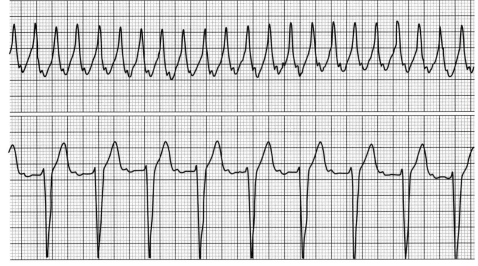

Figure SAI–21.

21. Both leads are V1. They're sequential.
    a. What's the wide-beat tachycardia in the top strip? Could it possibly be junctional with aberrancy?

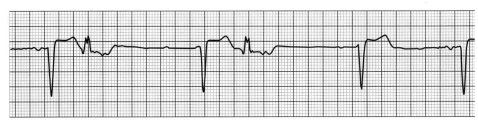

Figure SAI–22.

22. Note the abrupt slowing of rhythm.
    a. Cause?
    b. Treatment, if needed?

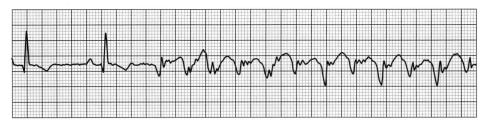

Figure SAI–23.

23. Here's a rare and dangerous bird. What do you note about the wide-beat tachycardia?

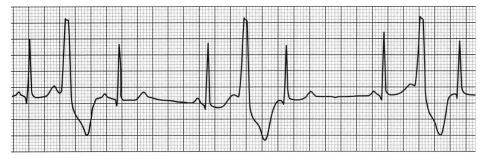

Figure SAI–24.

24. Comment on the wide beats. What's the mechanism that produces them?

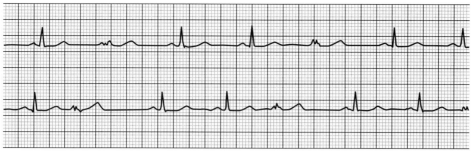

Figure SAI–25.

25. Comment on the wide beats. What's the mechanism that produces them?

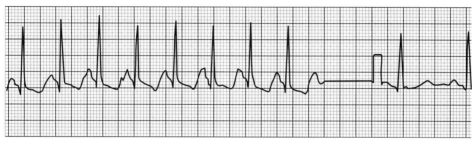

Figure SAI–26.

26. This rhythm appears in a 16-year-old who's been complaining of "fast palpitations" for years.
    a. Diagnosis?

Answers

1. The wide beats represent an accelerated idioventricular rhythm. Note fusion in the next-to-last beat in the bottom strip. The idioventricular rhythm "escapes" whenever the sinus rate falls below 60. In the bottom strip, there is complete AV dissociation but no—repeat *no*—AV block. This is simple interference-dissociation. No treatment needed.

2. Ventricular tachycardia. Note pairs of narrow beats. One is a complete capture beat, and the next is a fusion beat. Infallible diagnosis!

3. Accelerated junctional rhythm. Note prominent retrograde P waves. This retrograde conduction will of course suppress the sinus node unless it accelerates to a rate faster than the rate of the junctional focus.

4. Two possibilities: ventricular tachycardia or junctional tachycardia with bundle-branch block. You can't possibly make the distinction. *Treat as ventricular:* You may help, and you can't hurt.

5. The first four beats on the top strip are sinus beats with right bundle-branch block. This is followed by a wide-beat tachycardia with dissociated P waves; the same rhythm persists through the first four beats of the bottom strip. Dissociated P waves mean that the wide-beat tachycardia is almost certainly ventricular. Beat 5 in the bottom strip is a fusion beat: infallible diagnosis of ventricular tachycardia!

6. Accelerated idiojunctional rhythm in the first six beats. Carotid sinus stimulation suppresses the junctional focus and allows the sinus node to take over. In this critically ill patient, resumption of sinus rhythm with "atrial kick" was life-saving, so atropine was administered followed by atrial pacing. *Curious fact:* Carotid sinus stimulation affects junctional foci more than the sinus node.

7. Runs of ventricular tachycardia. In the bottom strip, you see four wide beats without P waves, followed by an obvious fusion beat. In the top strip, *all the ventricular beats are fused:* the sinus node happens to be going about as fast as the ventricular rhythm, so that there's fusion of every beat.

8. Premature atrial beats with Ashman aberrancy. Note the premature P waves tucked away in the preceding T waves.

9. Rate-dependent bundle-branch block with nonconducted premature atrial beats. Sometimes the pause after the PAC is long enough to allow normal intraventricular conduction to resume.

10. Frequent premature atrial beats with Ashman aberrancy. Look closely at the T wave ahead of the wide beats and you'll see that it's different from the T wave of the preceding beat. There has to be a P wave hidden in it. In the bottom strip, the premature atrial impulses are frequently blocked; note the T wave ahead of each pause and you'll note the different shape due to the P wave hidden in it. In this critically ill patient, the slowing was life-threatening; blocked PACs can be a dangerous "brake" on the sinus node.

11. Supraventricular tachycardia with delayed Ashman reset. The wide beats and the narrow beats come at precisely the same rate, so they must be coming from the same place—they're all supraventricular.

12. Runs of paroxysmal atrial tachycardia with Ashman and right bundle-branch patterns of aberrant conduction. Note again the phenomenon of delayed Ashman reset in the fourth, fifth, and sixth beats in the bottom strip.

13. Multifocal atrial tachycardia. Note dramatic changes in P wave morphology and rapid rate. This is always associated with chronic lung disease with hypoxemia. (In our institution, in addition to restoring oxygenation we've been using IV magnesium with about a 70% success rate.)

14. Rate-dependent left anterior hemiblock. Note that axis swings to about −60 degrees with the slightly wider beats; when the rate slows, the QRS complexes are narrow with a normal axis. Appearing acutely in an MI, this of course suggests an acute process involving the septum.

15. Two premature atrial beats with a long P-R. The premature P wave is hidden in the preceding T—look at the small notch on the T.

16. Alternating right and left bundle-branch block. This means that there's dysfunction of both bundle branches, with real danger of total failure of AV conduction. Intervention urgent!

17. **A**, Obvious AV nodal reentrant tachycardia. Note that each short paroxysm begins with a PAC with prolonged P-R. Note also the retrograde P waves with varying relation to QRS, typical of a reciprocating process. **B**, Paroxysmal supraventricular tachycardia. This could be AVNRT, or there could be a concealed bypass tract—you can't tell from this tracing alone.

18. The wide beats appear when the rate slows, the narrow beats when it speeds. Bradycardia-dependent aberrancy.

19. Junctional rhythm, rate about 38, with retrograde P waves. What's lacking? Sinus P waves, of course! There's no evidence of sinus node activity—hence the escape automatic rhythm functioning in its physiologic, life-saving mode.

20. Right bundle-branch block with left anterior hemiblock. We used to worry about asystole during anesthesia or surgery, but it turns out we didn't need to. No extraordinary measures are needed before or during surgery.

21. There's a wide-beat tachycardia with a right bundle-branch block configuration. This is followed by normal sinus rhythm with *left bundle-branch block*. The tachycardia must be ventricular; the alternative explanation of junctional tachycardia with right bundle-branch block is impossible. To have a pattern of right bundle-branch block, you have to have conduction down the left bundle branch. Because the left bundle branch doesn't conduct at all, this is impossible.

22. Two VPCs with retrograde conduction to the atria. The retrograde conduction discharges the sinus node and produces the pause that permits the escape of the junctional focus. If this pattern is repetitive with a slow rate that compromises hemodynamics, it's necessary to eliminate the cause—the VPCs.

23. Rare and dangerous form of ventricular tachycardia. Note the alternating amplitude of the wide complexes. This is ventricular tachycardia with electrical alternans, a very dangerous, near-terminal, digitalis-toxic rhythm.

24. VPCs. They're interpolated, meaning there's no postectopic pause. They're also *reentrant*—note the fixed coupling interval that continues for many repetitions.

25. VPCs, parasystolic. Note the wide variation in coupling to the preceding sinus beat. Note also that these beats appear at a fixed interectopic interval of about 480 milliseconds.

26. True ectopic atrial tachycardia. Note the well-defined P waves with different morphology from the sinus P. (This type of tachycardia is notoriously resistant to drug therapy; ablation as a means of treatment is very promising.)

Seven

AV Block: Where Is It Localized and What Do You Do About It?

Sites of AV Block

Start with the picture in Figure 7–1. In any consideration of atrioventricular (AV) block, you begin with the fact that the AV conducting system consists of two distinct, well-defined elements:

1. **The AV node–His bundle complex**
2. **The proximal portion of the bundle-branch system**

The cells in the AV node are different in structure and function from the cells down in the bundle branches. They discharge and recover differently. When they fail, the pattern of abnormal conduction is different, and so is the prognosis.

Thus, when AV block of any kind appears, it may be crucial to determine which element has failed. If you were a mad scientist and wanted to block conduction from atria to ventricles, the simplest way to do it would be to cut or poison the AV node. At this site, AV conduction—and often life itself—depends on a single strand of tissue. Down in the bundle-branch system, the task would be more complicated. If you cut only one bundle branch, you wouldn't interrupt conduction from atria to ventricles. You'd produce bundle-branch block, but as the reader already knows, AV conduction would continue down the other bundle with no delay. To interrupt conduction from atria to ventricles, you'd have to cut *both* bundle branches. Thus, only when both bundle branches are malfunctioning will you see failure of AV conduction in the bundle-branch system.

This may all seem obvious, but it's critical to some of the diagnoses you're going to learn to make in this chapter.

How to Localize Block and How to Classify It

The first step in logic is to determine the degree of AV block. AV block is rationally and usefully divided into first-, second-, and third-degree block. (A little while back, when invasive electrophysiologic studies were in first bloom, some cardiologists suggested that these three classic categories were obsolete; in fact, they have emerged as more useful than ever.)

In *first-degree block,* every atrial impulse reaches the ventricles but takes longer than normal getting there. The P-R interval is *fixed.* Anything over 0.20 second should be considered prolonged in the adult heart.

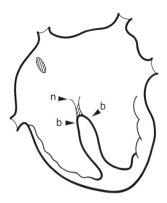

Figure 7–1.
The possible sites of AV block. Failure of AV conduction may be localized in the AV node (n) or in the proximal parts of the bundle branches (b). Note that AV conduction in this area will not be interrupted unless *both* bundle branches fail.

In *second-degree block,* some atrial impulses reach the ventricles, whereas others are blocked. Second-degree block may come in one of three forms:

1. **Type I, or Wenckebach, block. This is the most common form of second-degree block, and for practical purposes it's always located in the AV node.**

2. **2:1, or other "fixed ratio," block, such as 3:1 or 4:1. This may be localized in the AV node or in the bundle-branch system.**

3. **Type II, or Mobitz-II, block. This is always—repeat always—located in the bundle-branch system.**

Third-degree block means complete heart block with no transmission from atria to ventricles. It may be localized in the AV node or in the bundle-branch system.

Now try combining these items into specific diagnoses. Figures 7–2, 7–3, and 7–4 are all obvious examples of first-degree AV block. Where's the block? Look at the QRS complexes. They're *narrow.* A narrow QRS means that both bundle branches are functioning normally. The AV delay cannot possibly be located in the bundle-branch system; it must be up in the AV node.

Rule: When you see narrow QRS complexes, any failure of conduction must be located in the AV node. It cannot possibly be located in the bundle-branch system. (To imagine first-degree AV block with a narrow QRS localized in the bundle-branch system, you would

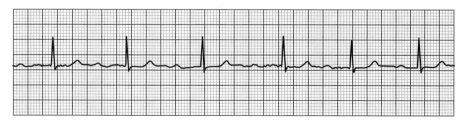

Figure 7–2.
First-degree AV nodal block, P-R 0.41 second.

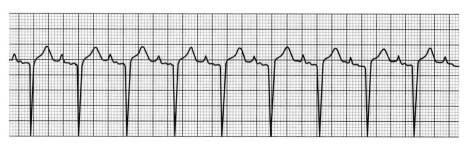

Figure 7–3.
First-degree AV nodal block, P-R 0.24 second.

Figure 7–4.
First-degree AV nodal block. In the top strip, the P is completely hidden in the T. In the bottom strip, the P can be seen as a notch coming off the peak of the T. P-R interval about 0.32 second.

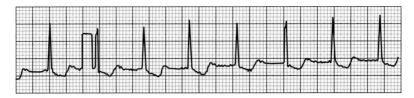

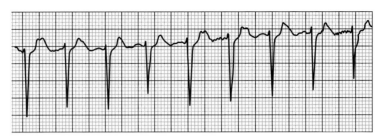

have to imagine absolutely identical delay, to the thousandth of a second, in the two separate bundle branches—an obviously absurd idea.)

Now consider Figure 7–5. Bundle-branch block is present, and there's a prolonged P-R interval. In this case, you can't tell where that delay is taking place. There's a single strand connecting atria and ventricles; it consists of the AV node and the one functioning bundle branch. The delay may be taking place anywhere along that strand—that is, in the AV node or in the bundle branch. You can't tell the difference from this tracing alone.

The difference here is not significant. First-degree AV block, no matter where it's local-ized or how prolonged the P-R, is never a threat to life, and no intervention is required.

Common error: Sometimes I hear residents commenting that "the P-R is too long to be conducted" when the P-R interval is in the range of 0.40 to 0.50 second. That, of course, is nonsense; prolonged P-R intervals of 0.60 second and even higher have been recorded. If you see a fixed P-R in a series of beats, you can be certain the atrial impulse is reaching the ventricles. It would be statistically impossible for two independent pacemakers to coincide within a hundredth of a second and produce a fixed, sustained P-R relation.

An occasional problem with first-degree block is illustrated in Figure 7–6. The P-R interval may be so prolonged that the P is hidden in the preceding T. You can see a "bump" on the T in the top strip that strongly suggests a P wave; to be certain, simply slow the rate by having the patient rest or by applying carotid sinus stimulation. When the rate slows, the P will move out of the T (see Fig. 7–6, bottom strip).

Figure 7–5.
First-degree AV block with left bundle-branch block. AV conduction now depends on a single functional strand consisting of the AV node and the right bundle branch (*arrowheads*). The delay in AV conduction could be taking place anywhere along that strand; you can't localize it from this tracing.

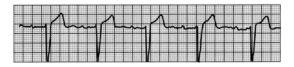

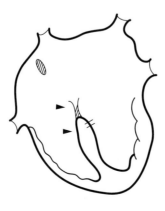

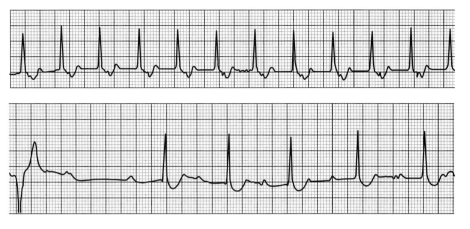

Figure 7–6.
First-degree AV nodal block unmasked by carotid sinus stimulation. In the top strip, you can't tell whether there's a P wave hidden in each T. By stimulating the carotid sinus, slowing the sinus and producing temporary AV nodal block, the clinician can unmask the hidden sinus P waves, making it clear that this is indeed a sinus rhythm with first-degree AV nodal block. P-R about 0.40 second.

The Three Types of Second-Degree Block

Type I, or Wenckebach, Block

There are five defining characteristics in type I block. They're all based on the character of AV nodal cells. These cells are activated by a slow inward current, and when they're diseased or intoxicated, they show *progressive fatigue,* ending in failure of conduction, with subsequent recovery.

The five specific characteristics of type I block are as follows:

1. **Progressive prolongation of P-R intervals. To document this, you have to see two or more consecutive P-R intervals, of course. This seems obvious, but it's surprising how often physicians lose sight of it.**

2. **Failure of conduction with a blocked P after maximum P-R prolongation.**

3. **Recovery with shortening of P-R interval after the blocked P wave.**

4. **A pause after the blocked P that is *less than the sum of the two beats before the blocked P.* This has to be the case because the P-R always shortens after the blocked P; naturally, this shortened P-R "pulls in" the QRS so that it comes relatively early—the pause has to be less than the sum of the two preceding beats.**

5. **R-P/P-R reciprocity. The sinus P waves keep coming at a fixed rate while the P-R prolongs. Obviously, each QRS is going to be "pushed out" closer to the next P (simple arithmetic!). Thus, there's a reciprocal relation between R-P and P-R. To put it another way, the closer each P wave comes to the preceding QRS, the more fatigued the AV nodal cells will be (because they've had less time to recover) and the longer the next P-R will be. Again, this seems obvious, but you'll use it to solve some complex problems.**

Figure 7–7 is an example of "typical" Wenckebach block. The maximum prolongation of P-R takes place in the second beat of the cycle with much smaller increments in subsequent beats. Where's the blocked P? Put your calipers on the P waves and you'll see that it's buried in the T wave of the last beat of the cycle. This is a common and sometimes confusing phenomenon. Look for all the other criteria of type I block.

If you measure the R-R interval carefully, you'll notice a curious phenomenon: Although the P-R interval grows longer, the R-R interval shortens a little. This is because the amount of prolongation of the P-R is less with each beat even though the total P-R is longer. The P-R intervals in Figure 7–7 start at 0.28 then jump to 0.32 in the second beat, 0.36 in the third, and 0.39 in the fourth. The R-R interval will actually shorten because the *degree of increase of the P-R is less* with each beat. Try it with a ruler and you'll see how it works.

Figure 7–7.
Typical Wenckebach block with progressive prolongation of P-R before the blocked P. (The blocked P is hidden in the T of the beat before the pause.) The pauses are always less than the sum of the two preceding beats because the P-R after the pause always shortens.

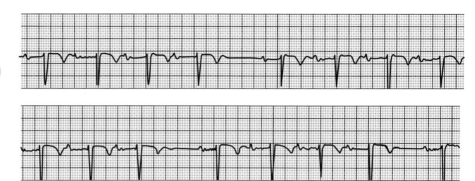

This is the "Wenckebach paradox" of shortening R–R when the P–R increases by diminishing increments. It's present in what is loosely termed "typical" Wenckebach block—maybe in 70% to 80% of all cases. If you remember this characteristic R–R shortening, it will help you recognize type I block in some unusual settings.

Figure 7–8 illustrates "atypical" Wenckebach block. There's minimal prolongation of P-R until the last beat of the cycle, when it prolongs abruptly. This tracing also illustrates a common complication of type I block. After the blocked P waves, there are junctional escape beats that at one point form a sustained idiojunctional rhythm.

Figure 7–9 shows 3:2 Wenckebach block, meaning that two beats are conducted while a third is blocked. Note that this forms a paired, or *bigeminal*, rhythm.

2:1, or "Fixed Ratio," Block

The tracing in Figure 7–10 takes the reader into the next pattern of conduction: "fixed ratio" block. Every other P wave is conducted with a fixed P-R interval, while the alternate

Figure 7–8.
"Atypical" Wenckebach block with maximum prolongation of P-R in the last conducted beats and many junctional escape beats (J). The junctional focus here, of course, is performing its normal "escape pacemaker" function.

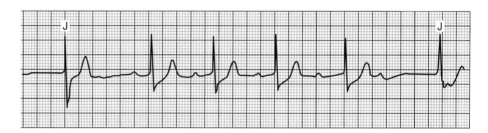

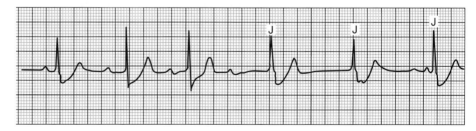

Figure 7–9.
3:2 Wenckebach block. The blocked P is seen as a notch in the T before the pause. Note that the 3:2 ratio of conduction produces a paired, or *bigeminal*, pulse.

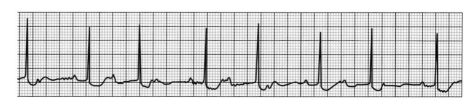

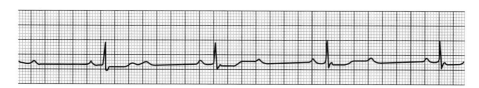

Figure 7–10.
2:1 AV nodal block. Note the fixed relation of P to QRS throughout.

P wave is blocked. You call this exactly what it is: 2:1 block; 2:1 block with a narrow QRS is of course located in the AV node.

Figure 7–11 illustrates both 2:1 and Wenckebach block in the AV node—a frequent combination. It's common to see 2:1 AV nodal block vary with Wenckebach periods because both types of block are really manifestations of the same AV nodal dysfunction.

2:1 AV Block with Bundle-Branch Block

Figure 7–11.
2:1 AV nodal block changing to a 3:2 Wenckebach cycle in the right-hand side of the strip. This is a common combination in AV nodal block.

This form of block (Fig. 7–12) is much more disturbing. Because one bundle branch is permanently blocked, the block of the alternate P waves might be taking place in the other bundle branch. In other words, this might represent *intermittent bilateral bundle-branch block*. It might also represent coincidental AV nodal block. You can't tell which from this tracing alone.

Figure 7–13 shows another example of "fixed ratio" block with bundle-branch block. In this case the ratio is 4:1. Note that the P-R interval of the conducted beats remains the same,

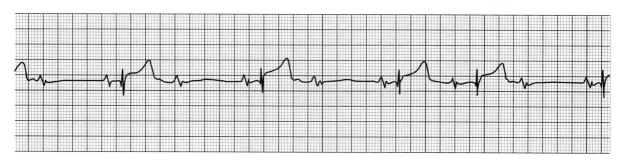

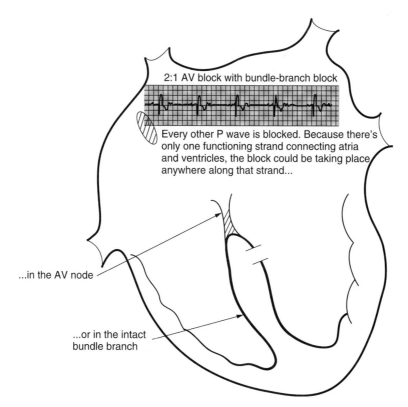

2:1 AV block with bundle-branch block

Every other P wave is blocked. Because there's only one functioning strand connecting atria and ventricles, the block could be taking place anywhere along that strand...

...in the AV node

...or in the intact bundle branch

Figure 7–12.
AV block with bundle-branch block. If the block is in the AV node, it's relatively benign. On the other hand, if it's in the bundle branch, there is *intermittent bilateral bundle-branch block*, a very dangerous situation. The need for pacing is urgent. You can't tell the difference from this ECG.

Figure 7–13.
4:1 AV block with bundle-branch block. Note the absolutely fixed relation of P to QRS throughout. Because you don't see two consecutive P-R intervals anywhere, you can't localize the block precisely. A rate this slow, however, will always produce central nervous system or cardiovascular symptoms, and intervention will be needed.

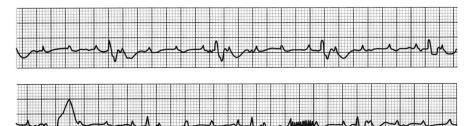

just as in 2:1 block. Again, the failure of conduction might reside in the AV node or in the one functioning bundle branch. There's no way to make the distinction from this tracing.

Rule: When you see 2:1 or other fixed ratio block with a narrow QRS, it means that the block is in the AV node. It's relatively benign and may be caused by drugs such as digitalis, beta blockers, or calcium blockers or by transient ischemia.

When you see fixed ratio block with a wide QRS, it raises the possibility that you're looking at intermittent bilateral bundle-branch block. This is potentially very dangerous. It will never be the result of such drugs as digitalis, although it can be the result of transient ischemia.

How do you make the distinction between block in the AV node and block in the other bundle branch? This introduces the third category of second-degree block: Mobitz type II.

Type II, or Mobitz-II, Block

In Figure 7–14, you see some periods of 2:1 block with a wide QRS (part of the QRS is almost hidden in the baseline, but it's really 0.12 second wide). You also see periods like the three beats in the middle, where there are two consecutive conducted beats followed by a blocked P—in other words, 3:2 block. Now you can diagnose the location of the block with absolute accuracy. During the period of 3:2 block, you see the following:

> 1. **Two consecutive conducted beats with the same P-R (no Wenckebach type of prolongation)**
>
> 2. **A blocked sinus impulse**
>
> 3. **A P-R interval in the first beat after the block with the same P-R interval as the beats before**
>
> 4. **A pause around the blocked P equal to exactly twice the sinus rate**

Figure 7–14.
Mobitz-II block with intermittent periods of 2:1 AV block. If all you saw were the two periods of 2:1 block in the left half of the strip, you couldn't localize the block, but the periods of 3:2 block on the right side tell you this block is localized in the one functioning bundle branch. Pacemaker!

You have made an absolute diagnosis of Mobitz-II block. That's all you have to see. What you're looking at is in fact intermittent bilateral bundle-branch block. You will see type II block only in the presence of preexisting bundle-branch block. It never takes place in the AV node.

During the periods of 2:1 conduction, of course, you couldn't be sure of the location of the block. Until you see two *consecutive* conducted beats, you can't be sure the 2:1 block won't slide into type I periods, as in Figure 7–11. Those two consecutive beats with a fixed P-R make the diagnosis for you; the other findings confirm it.

Type II block carries a very grave prognosis. The risk for catastrophic asystole is about 36% per year. Mobitz-II block is an absolute indication for permanent pacing. You don't wait

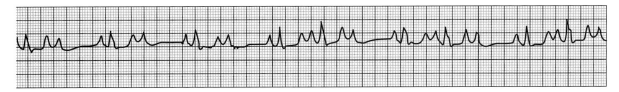

for symptoms because the first symptom is likely to be the last symptom that a patient ever experiences—especially if the asystole appears while the patient is driving a car!

Mobitz-II block is misunderstood more than any other abnormality of rhythm or conduction.

Figure 7–15 gives a diagrammatic representation of Mobitz-II block. Type II block is a result of the electrophysiologic characteristics of bundle-branch cells. They depend on the fast inward sodium current for activation, and when they fail, they fail abruptly. It's all-or-nothing conduction, just like rate-dependent bundle-branch block. This is in sharp contrast to AV nodal cells, which always show progressive fatigue and recovery.

Figure 7–16 is a typical example of type II block with a 3:2 ratio of conduction. Note the elements of type II block.

Figures 7–17 through 7–22 are examples of type I and type II block with wide and narrow QRS complexes. Try diagnosing each of them and compare your results with the legends.

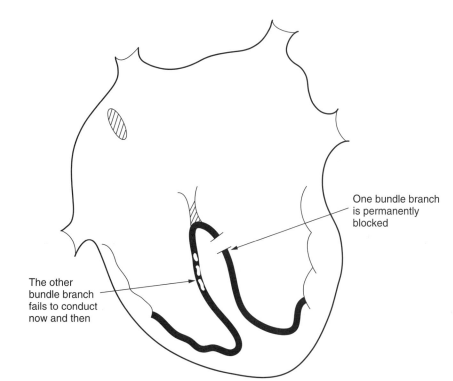

Figure 7–15.
Schematic representation of Mobitz-II block. Study this carefully. This is the most misunderstood phenomenon in electrocardiography and one of the most important. In Mobitz-II, the failure of conduction will always be abrupt. There is *no* warning prolongation of the P-R interval before the blocked P wave, and there is *no* shortening of the P-R interval in the first beat after the blocked P wave. Everything stays the same except that one or more P waves are suddenly not conducted. This kind of all-or-none conduction is seen only in the bundle branches, never in the AV node.

One bundle branch is permanently blocked

The other bundle branch fails to conduct now and then

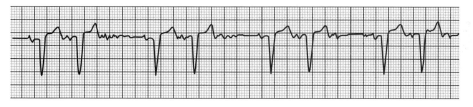

Figure 7–16.
3:2 Mobitz-II block. As always, bundle-branch block is present, the consecutive P-R intervals are constant, and the pauses are an exact double of the basic rate.

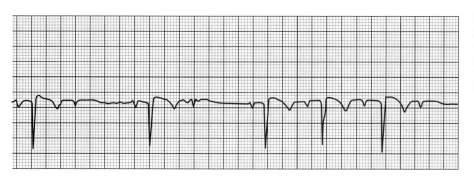

Figure 7–17.
2:1 AV nodal block with period of 4:3 Wenckebach block. Contrast this with the type II block in Fig. 7–16.

Figure 7–18.
Mobitz-II block produced by atrial pacing. The pacer spike precedes the P wave. All the features of type II block are present: the fixed P-R throughout and the pauses that equal a double sinus interval. (The QRS is really 0.12 second wide. This tracing has been reduced, and part of the QRS is hidden in the baseline.)

Complete Heart Block

The diagnosis of complete heart block is based on three elements:

1. **Complete AV dissociation with no capture beats; in other words, complete absence of AV conduction**

2. **A ventricular rate of 45 or less**

3. **A sufficient number of atrial impulses to probe all aspects of diastole**

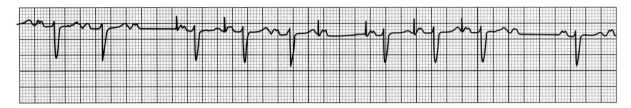

Figure 7–19.
Mobitz-II block in the setting of right bundle-branch block with left anterior hemiblock. The block is taking place in the posterior fascicle of the left bundle.

I

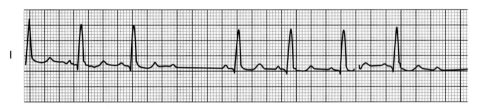

II

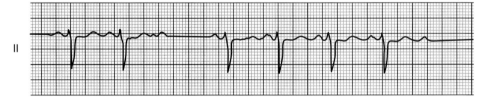

III

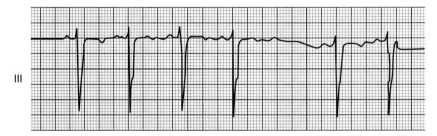

V1

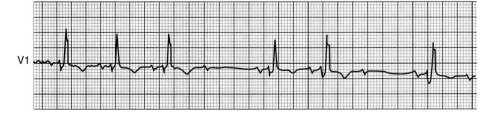

V2

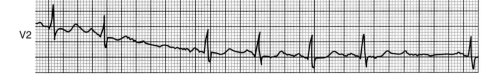

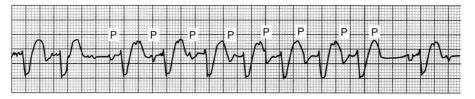

Figure 7–20.
Wenckebach block with bundle-branch block. It's perfectly possible to have AV nodal block in the presence of bundle-branch block, and that's what you see here. All the characteristics of Wenckebach block are present, and it would be exceedingly rare to see this happening down in the one functioning bundle branch. This was in fact digitalis-toxic AV nodal block.

Special note: The electrocardiogram (ECG) diagnosis of AV dissociation is based on two simple yes-or-no questions:

> 1. **Is there a changing relation of P to QRS? If yes:**
>
> 2. **Is the ventricular rhythm regular despite this changing P-R relationship? If yes:**

AV dissociation is present. Obviously the P waves and the QRS complexes have nothing to do with each other. Their relation is accidental, like a divorced couple passing in the street.

Figure 7–23 is a schematic illustration of complete AV block. In this patient, the block is localized in the AV node; note the narrow QRS. (I've had many staff ask me if AV nodal block can be complete, and of course the answer is "yes," just as illustrated here. AV nodal block can be complete and life-threatening.)

Note the term *AV dissociation.* Most physicians aren't very clear about what it means and what forms it comes in. It's time to stop and differentiate the two types of AV dissociation. One is common and harmless; the other is rare and dangerous. (After almost 50 years of teaching this subject, I know that AV dissociation ranks right up there with Mobitz-II block in the great misapprehension derby. This is not the fault of the medical profession at large; the language used to describe this simple phenomenon has been so complex and the definitions so vague that I'm reminded of the instructions with the E-Z assembly toys we all struggled with at 1 AM on Christmas morning.) Therefore, I now define AV dissociation and describe the two causes and types.

Definition: Complete AV dissociation means that the atrial and ventricular rhythms are separate and independent. The atria are driven by one pacemaker—usually the sinus node—while the ventricles are driven by an ectopic focus in the node or in the ventricles. The two rhythms have nothing to do with each other. They're divorced.

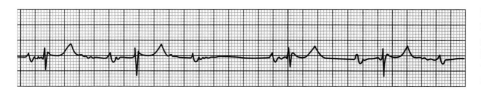

Figure 7–21.
3:2 Wenckebach block with sinus bradycardia. Regardless of the site of block, the effective rate is so slow that the patient will certainly experience symptoms, and some intervention will be needed. This case was not drug induced or transient, and permanent pacing was required.

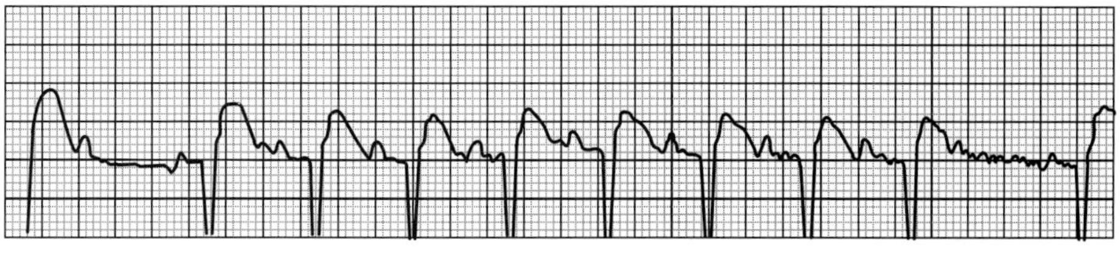

Figure 7–22.
Wenckebach block. Contrast this and Fig. 7–21 with Figs. 7–16, 7–17, 7–18, and 7–19, and the difference between type I and type II blocks becomes obvious.

Figure 7–23.
Complete AV nodal block. Ventricular rate 34. Complete AV dissociation; there are ample numbers of sinus P waves, but none come through to "capture" a beat. Conclusion: No conduction is possible.

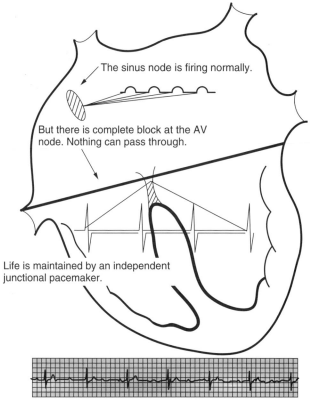

The sinus node is firing normally.

But there is complete block at the AV node. Nothing can pass through.

Life is maintained by an independent junctional pacemaker.

On the ECG there is a regular ventricular rhythm with random P waves that have no correlation with the QRS complexes.

Complete AV dissociation is not the same as complete AV block. In fact, about 99% of the time, it has nothing to do with AV block. A good example of the common type of AV dissociation is the kind you see in some cases of ventricular tachycardia (see Chapter 3). The ventricular tachycardia keeps bombarding the AV tissues so rapidly that they're refractory to any sinus impulse.

In this case, the AV dissociation is caused by the "interference" of the ectopic rhythm. The proper name for this kind of dissociation is *interference-dissociation*. You can see interference-dissociation any time an ectopic rhythm in the node or the ventricles fires rapidly enough to make the tissues refractory to the sinus impulses. In simple terms, the ectopic focus gets in the way of the sinus impulse. There's nothing wrong with the AV conducting tissues; there's no block (Fig. 7–24).

Figures 7–25 through 7–31 are all examples of interference-dissociation. Take some time with them and become thoroughly familiar with this harmless and much-misunderstood arrhythmia.

In Figure 7–25, there is a series of normal sinus beats interrupted by a junctional rhythm that fires a little more rapidly than the sinus node, forming the dissociated pattern of the last five beats.

In Figure 7–26, the predominant rhythm is an accelerated idioventricular rhythm dissociated from the sinus rhythm. The beats marked *C* represent capture by the sinus node when it fortuitously arrives at the AV node between ectopic beats. (Note the fusion beat marked *f*.)

In Figure 7–27, the dissociation is caused by a junctional rhythm firing a little faster than the sinus node, whereas in Figures 7–28 and 7–29, the dissociation is produced by an accelerated idioventricular rhythm discharging at almost the same rate as the sinus node. Figures 7–30 and 7–31 are again examples of interference-dissociation caused by a junctional rhythm discharging faster than the sinus node.

Study these well. They were all mistakenly diagnosed as AV block, and in several cases pacemakers were proposed!

Think of the AV conducting tissues as a door. The door's perfectly
normal; it can open and shut like any door with well-oiled hinges.

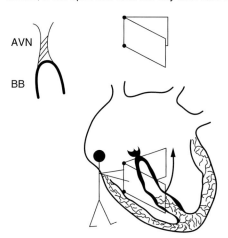

Figure 7–24.
Interference-dissociation.
The atrial and ventricular
rhythms are dissociated
because of the
"interference" of an
ectopic focus in the node
or the ventricles that fires
just fast enough to make
the AV tissues refractory
whenever a sinus impulse
arrives.

Think of yourself as the sinus impulse. Every time you try to pass
through the door a lunatic on the other side slams the door in your face.

The lunatic is an ectopic focus in the node or in the ventricles. It's firing
just fast enough to "slam the door"—that is, to make the AV tissues
refractory so that they can't conduct the sinus impulse.

Now you're ready for the definitive diagnosis of complete heart block. In Figure 7–32, you see complete AV dissociation. Next you see a ventricular rhythm of about 48. Finally, you note that there are P waves occurring all through diastole. There's plenty of time between those ectopic QRS complexes for an atrial impulse to come through and capture the rhythm if the AV system were capable of conducting. The slow rate of the rhythm driving the ventricles rules out any question of interference. The diagnosis is complete AV block. The narrow QRS tells you the block is in the AV node.

Figures 7–33 and 7–34 are both examples of complete AV nodal block. Examine each for the criteria listed earlier.

In Figures 7–35 and 7–36, you see complete heart block with wide ventricular complexes. There are two possibilities. First, the complete block may be the result of failure of both bundle branches; in other words, bilateral bundle-branch block. When the bundle-branch system fails, life can be maintained only by an idioventricular focus. Naturally, the ventricular complexes are wide, like these. This might also be the result of complete AV nodal block with bundle-branch block, which would account for the wide complexes. The only way you could make the distinction would be to see a previous ECG with normal intraventricular conduction.

Figure 7–25.
Interference-dissociation.
A normal sinus rhythm is
interrupted by a junctional
rhythm (sixth beat) that
fires a little faster than the
sinus node and keeps the
AV node refractory. The
P waves gradually
disappear into the QRS.

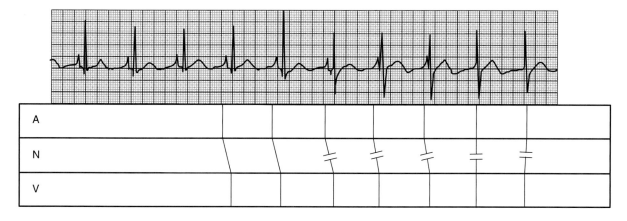

Figure 7–26.

Intermittent interference-dissociation. The first three beats are idioventricular beats. In the fourth beat, the sinus node "gets ahead" of the ectopic focus and captures the rhythm for three beats (C). The sinus rhythm and the accelerated idioventricular rhythm compete throughout the strip with periods of dissociation and periods of capture by the sinus node. During the idioventricular rhythm, the sinus P waves are buried in the QRS, but you can march them right out with the capture beats.

What's the difference whether the complete AV block is localized in the AV node or in the bundle-branch system? For one thing, block in the AV node is much more likely to be the result of drugs like digitalis, calcium blockers, or beta blockers. Digitalis and the calcium-blocking drugs have no effect on the bundle-branch system, and the effect of beta blockers, if any, is negligible.

Block in the AV node is also much more likely to be the result of transient ischemic insult, such as the AV nodal block that accompanies inferior myocardial infarction. This specific kind of AV block is always ultimately benign. It always disappears, and permanent pacing is never needed.

On the other hand, complete block in the bundle-branch system carries a much graver prognosis. It can be a result of high potassium levels or, rarely, of tricyclic drugs; but in most cases it represents intrinsic irreversible disease, and in such cases pacing is always indicated.

If transient toxic or ischemic effects have been ruled out and complete AV block is permanent, the distinction becomes academic because permanent complete block with ventricular rates this slow will always require pacing in any case.

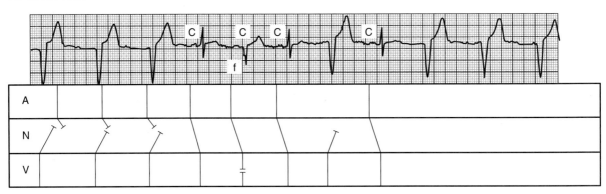

Figure 7–27.

Interference-dissociation caused by an accelerated junctional rhythm (*round black dots* in the diagram). The junctional rhythm is faster than the sinus rhythm (75 versus 63), so the junctional beats "interfere" with the sinus beats most of the time. There are occasional sinus capture beats (C) when the sinus impulse arrives at just the right time between ectopic beats.

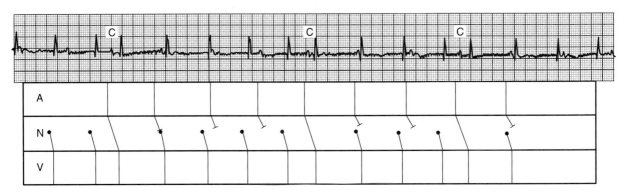

Before leaving this subject, be sure you understand the following:

1. **The five characteristics of type I block**

2. **The four characteristics of type II block**

3. **What fixed ratio block is**

4. **The essential difference between AV nodal tissue and bundle-branch tissue when conduction is impaired**

5. **How to diagnose AV dissociation**

6. **The two causes of AV dissociation**

7. **The three criteria for the diagnosis of complete heart block**

8. *Special note:* **Don't forget that a shortening R-R interval is typical of the common form of type I block. This phenomenon will help you recognize type I block when there are no P waves—for instance, with type I block around an automatic ectopic focus or with type I block in the lower node in the presence of a junctional rhythm.**

Figure 7–28.
Interference-dissociation caused by an accelerated idioventricular rhythm with a right bundle configuration (left side of strip). Beginning with the first beat marked C, the sinus node begins to capture the ventricles with progressive fusion (f) with the ectopic focus. The last two beats on the right show that there's really a left bundle-branch block.

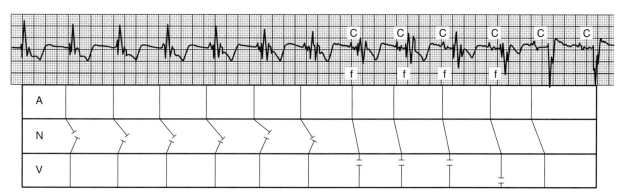

Figure 7–29.
Interference-dissociation caused by the discharge of an idioventricular pacemaker. The sinus impulses, labeled P, march through the idioventricular rhythm until they cycle out ahead of the ectopic focus and capture the rhythm.

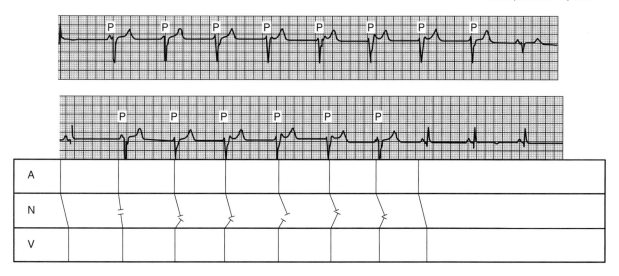

Figure 7–30.
Interference-dissociation caused by a combination of sinus bradycardia (rate 53) and an accelerated junctional rhythm (rate 62). Most of the beats are junctional, with an occasional sinus capture (C).

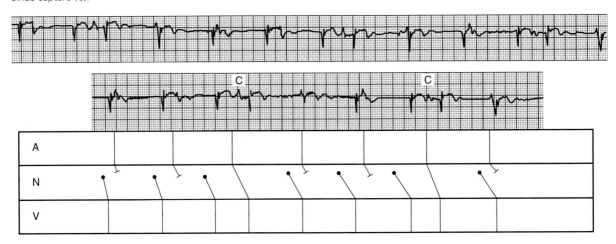

Figure 7–31.
Interference-dissociation caused by an accelerated junctional rhythm discharging at almost the same rate as the sinus node. In the middle part of the strip, the sinus and junctional rhythms are almost identical ("isorhythmic").

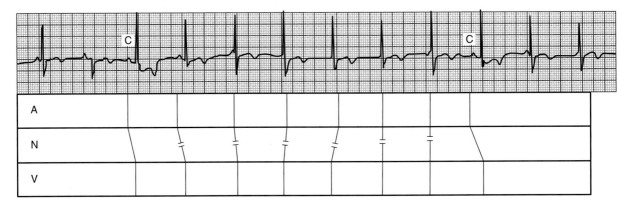

Figure 7–32.
Complete AV nodal block. There is complete AV dissociation with no capture beats, and the ventricular rhythm is set by a pacemaker in the junction with a rate of 45. There are P waves appearing all through diastole, far from the junctional beats, yet none are conducted—thus, the effect of "interference" is ruled out.

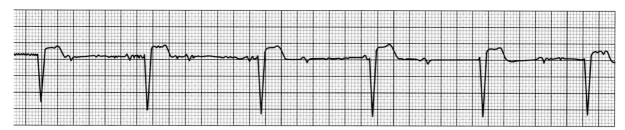

Figure 7–33.
Complete AV nodal block with a ventricular rate of 28. This is an example of life-threatening complete block in the AV node.

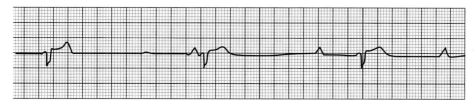

Figure 7–34.
Complete AV nodal block, ventricular rate 39. Note that all the criteria for complete AV block are present.

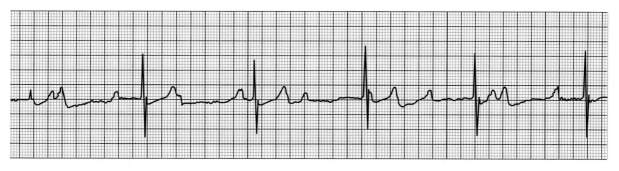

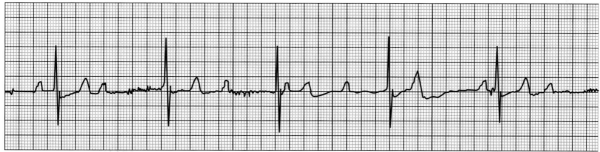

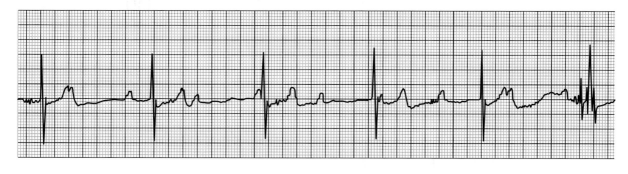

Figure 7–35.
Complete AV block in the bundle-branch system with an idioventricular rate of 32. This patient was a young woman who suffered from congenital primary fibrous degeneration of the myocardium. It is interesting to note that she attended high school and carried on a relatively normal life with this slow rate in the era before pacemakers. She finally died of congestive heart failure, not of asystole.

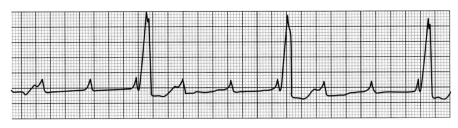

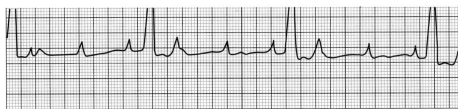

Figure 7–36.
Complete AV block, ventricular rate 39. The wide ventricular complexes could represent an idioventricular rhythm or a junctional rhythm with bundle-branch block. You couldn't tell the difference from this tracing. Because the block was shown to be permanent, not drug induced, the distinction became academic. Anyone with this degree of permanent block and this ventricular rate will need pacing, regardless of the site of the block.

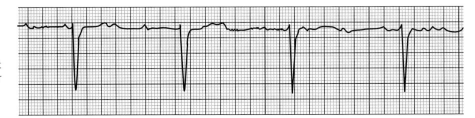

Eight

Diagnosis of Complex Forms of AV Block: Some Tricks, Some Booby Traps

High Degree of AV Block

The term *high-degree* is a good one for the kind of block illustrated in Figure 8–1. There are many blocked P waves with only occasional conducted beats. There's no fixed pattern of atrioventricular (AV) conduction in the top strip; the paired beats may represent random paired firing from a junctional focus. In the bottom strip, there's a consistent 4:1 ratio with a P-R of 0.52 second in the conducted beats. In other words, the term *high-degree block* is reserved for cases in which there are many blocked atrial impulses with occasional conducted beats, without any recognizable pattern of block.

Pseudoblock

The most common type of pseudoblock is illustrated in Figure 8–2. Here, there's a sinus rhythm with bundle-branch block. In the middle of all strips, there's an abrupt pause. Look carefully at the T waves of the beats before each pause—they're obviously different from all the other T waves. There's a small "spiky" deformity just at the end of these T waves that you don't see in most of the other beats. At the left-hand end of the bottom strip, you see a premature beat that's clearly supraventricular. In the T wave of the beat before this premature beat, you see the same deformity.

These are obviously premature atrial beats superimposed on the T waves. One is conducted, and the others aren't. Nonconducted, or "blocked," premature atrial beats are the most common cause of pause in a sinus rhythm. (We put quotation marks around the term *blocked* because the word *block* really implies subnormal conduction. There's nothing wrong with the conducting apparatus here; the problem is that the premature P comes too early for anything to be conducted.)

Rule: When you see an inexplicable abrupt pause, always look at the T wave ahead of the pause to see if there's a premature, nonconducted P wave hidden in it. Remember Jeremiah's rhetorical question: "Can the leopard change his spots?" Of course it doesn't, and in the same way, the T wave doesn't change his shape from beat to beat. When you see a change in the shape of a T wave, it practically always means there's a P hidden in it.

The nonconducted premature atrial impulse is wasted motion; it discharges the sinus node but it doesn't itself reach the ventricles—hence the pause. The nonconducted premature atrial contraction (PAC) acts as a "brake" on the sinus node.

The tracing in Figure 8–3 was actually misclassified as Mobitz-II block, and the patient was scheduled for a permanent pacemaker. The combination of right bundle-branch block and left anterior hemiblock certainly provides the right setting for Mobitz-II block, and there is in fact an abrupt pause in the sinus rhythm. At this point, you apply the rule and

Figure 8–1.
High degree of AV nodal block. Many blocked P waves in the top strip without any regular pattern of conduction. 4:1 Block in the bottom strip.

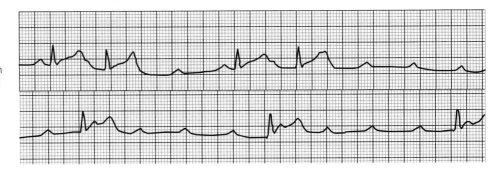

Figure 8–2.
Frequent nonconducted premature atrial beats. Occasional conducted premature atrial beats. Note the "glitch" in the T waves before the pause in each strip. These are obvious nonconducted P waves.

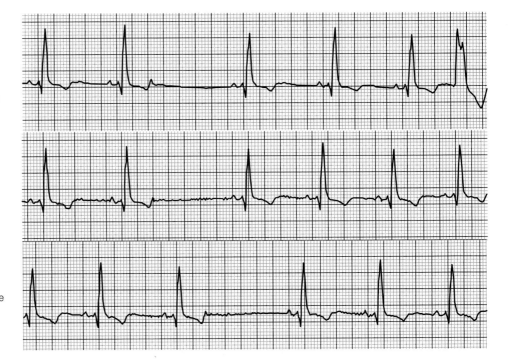

Figure 8–3.
A nonconducted premature atrial beat producing an abrupt pause in a patient with bifascicular block (right bundle-branch block with left anterior hemiblock).

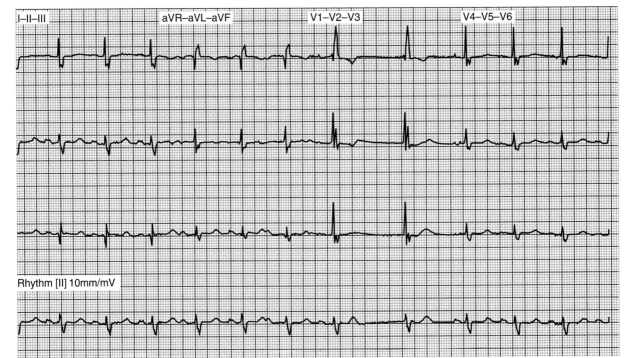

remember Jeremiah. The T wave of the beat ahead of the pause is clearly different in shape from all the other T waves. There has to be a P wave hidden in it—no other explanation. You're simply looking at a nonconducted premature atrial impulse. There's no significant failure of AV conduction. If you look at the second beat ahead of the pause, you'll notice that it comes early, with a prolonged P-R. Thus, there are two premature atrial beats, one conducted and one blocked. The patient doesn't need anything except reassurance.

Figure 8–4 is a tracing recorded early in the course of a myocardial infarct. Many wide QRS complexes appeared, some in runs, and there was the usual rush to lidocaine with the notion that the wide beats were ventricular.

To analyze this arrhythmia, look first at the fifth beat in the bottom strip. This shows what a normal sinus beat should look like. Now look at the first beats in each strip; each is followed by a premature atrial impulse. In the top strip, the premature atrial beat produces a sharp negative deflection in the T wave, and it's not conducted. In the bottom strip, the premature atrial beat produces a large upright P, and it is conducted with Ashman aberrancy. Look throughout both strips, and you'll see these premature atrial beats in the T waves; sometimes they're not conducted, but when they are, you see typical Ashman aberrancy—long R-R preceding short R-R. The final diagnosis is therefore "frequent premature atrial beats, some conducted aberrantly, some blocked." No ventricular ectopy, no need for lidocaine.

In Figure 8–5, the same phenomenon became life threatening. Early in the course of a severe myocardial infarction, some wide beats and some long pauses appeared. When the rate was 80, the blood pressure was barely maintained; during the pauses when the rate fell to the low 40s, the pressure plummeted, and the patient was quickly in distress. Every treatment but the right one was proposed: pacing (useless), atropine (useless), isoproterenol (lethal).

Again, look at the T waves ahead of the pauses. They're obviously different from the sinus T waves—there's a sharp, "spiky" element, very different from the flat, almost isoelectric sinus T. Blocked PACs are deforming the T waves; the nonconducted premature atrial

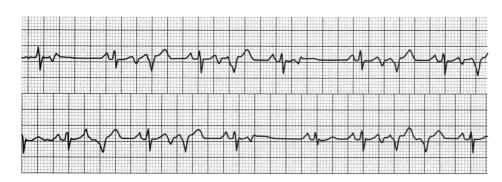

Figure 8–4.
Multiple premature atrial beats—some blocked, some conducted with Ashman aberrancy. Note how easy it would be to confuse this with ventricular ectopic discharge. See text for precise analysis.

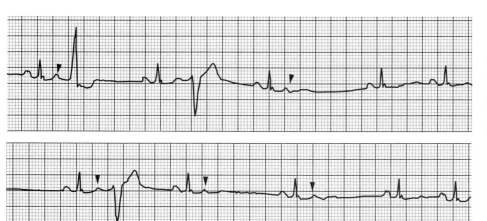

Figure 8–5.
Frequent premature atrial beats—some conducted with Ashman aberrancy, some blocked. The blocked PACs in this case produced a slowing of effective rate that jeopardized the patient's life.

impulses are producing the pauses. If you look at the T in front of the occasional wide beats, you also see a premature P deforming the T. These are conducted premature atrial beats, and the wide beats are simply another example of Ashman aberrancy.

If blocked PACs slow the heart rate critically, as they do here, what do you do? You treat the PACs, of course. You use drugs that suppress ectopic activity in the atria. Digitalis and quinidine are probably best; digitalis would be preferred in an acute situation because it can be given by vein. Blocked premature atrial beats cause the only bradyarrhythmia that is treated with suppressive drugs. The suppressive drug (digitalis) worked swiftly and completely in this case; the PACs disappeared, and the sinus rate of 80 was maintained.

(*Note:* When you make this diagnosis and prescribe this treatment, you'll be met by incredulous stares. This particular case was reviewed at the Arizona Heart Annual Scientific Session on two successive years by Drs. Bernard Lown and H. J. C. Marriott. One recommended digitalis, the other quinidine! Stick to your guns and ignore the possibly lethal recommendations of the uninformed.)

Figure 8–6 presents a case of very significant block made functionally much worse by the presence of ventricular premature contractions (VPCs). There's really a sinus tachycardia with a rate of 125. Many of the P waves are hidden in the QRS, as you'll see if you use the calipers. The AV block is complex.

Basically, these are Wenckebach periods, with 2:1 block at some points and many junctional ectopic beats. The wide QRS is cause for concern about possible Mobitz-II block, but there are no true type II patterns anywhere.

There are many long pauses when the effective rate drops to about 36. Note that these pauses always occur around a VPC. There's always a P wave just ahead of the VPC and one shortly after it. Neither atrial impulse can be conducted because of the interference of the VPC. The P wave just ahead of the VPC obviously doesn't get a chance to reach the ventricles, and the one after the VPC finds the AV conducting tissues refractory from the effect of the VPC on the bundle-branch tissues and the AV node.

Retrograde conduction of VPCs up the AV node is very common and often produces prolonged refractoriness with subsequent block of the sinus impulse. Always take this effect into consideration when you're analyzing AV block. Eradicating VPCs can often reduce the degree of block or eliminate it entirely.

Pseudo Mobitz-II Block: Concealed His Bundle Beats

If you see what looks like Mobitz-II block with narrow QRS complexes, take another look. It probably isn't Mobitz-II block. For practical purposes, Mobitz-II block is always found in the setting of preexisting bundle-branch block.

Figure 8–6.
High degree of AV block with long pauses around the frequent VPCs. The "interference" of the VPCs is actually exacerbating the effect of the block, with many long pauses.

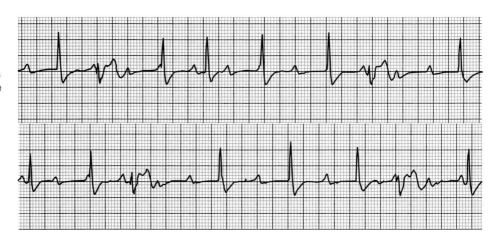

In Figure 8–7, the tracing certainly looks like type II block. There are fixed P–R intervals with occasional blocked sinus P waves. There's no change in the P–R after the blocked P. Why isn't this Mobitz-II block?

If you look elsewhere in the tracing, you'll see that many junctional premature beats are "sandwiched" between sinus beats, or to use a more scientific term, they are *interpolated*. (Although these beats may arise in the His bundle, I use the term *junctional* because it's more familiar and the effect is exactly the same.) There's no pause after them. That means that they were not conducted retrogradely across the atria; they didn't reset the sinus node. In other words, there is retrograde block to the junctional beats. Every now and then, there is also antegrade block. The ectopic focus in the junction or the His bundle fires and makes the tissue refractory, but you never see it. The only way you can tell it happened is that the next sinus impulse is mysteriously blocked.

Figure 8–8 is another example of the same phenomenon. There are obvious junctional beats (J). There are occasional blocked P waves, with the same P–R after the block as before. Note that the junctional beats labeled J are not conducted retrogradely; you know that because the next sinus P comes on time. Exactly when the next junctional beat should come, you see a blocked sinus P wave. This isn't real block; it's a form of interference caused by the discharge of the ectopic focus in the junction or the His bundle. This discharge is totally blocked, as illustrated in Figure 8–9.

Moral: When you see what looks like Mobitz-II block with a narrow QRS, look around for interpolated junctional beats. This isn't Mobitz-II block; it's as harmless as any random junctional (or His bundle) beats.

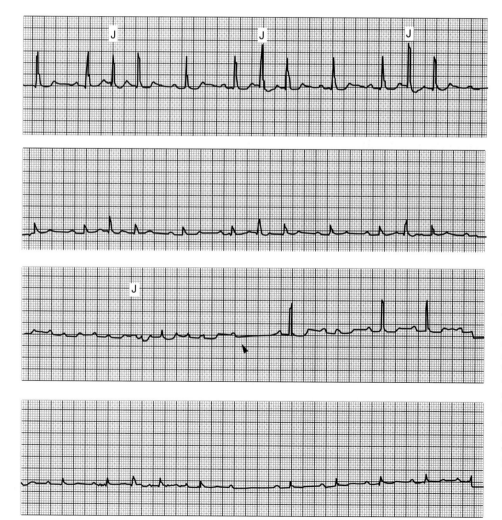

Figure 8–7.
Concealed His bundle beats producing a pseudo Mobitz-II phenomenon. This is a very old tracing that may look a bit fuzzy, but it's a classic example. In the top two strips, you see many junctional beats (J) interpolated between two sinus beats. These beats don't interrupt the sinus rhythm, which means they're not conducted back across the atria. There's retrograde block. In the third strip, right where the junctional beat should appear, you see a blocked P (*arrowhead*). It looks like Mobitz-II block because there's no Wenckebach prolongation of P-R ahead of the blocked P and no shortening of P-R after it. What's really happened is that the junctional focus wasn't conducted backward *or* forward. All it did was make the node refractory so that the P wave wasn't conducted. Harmless!

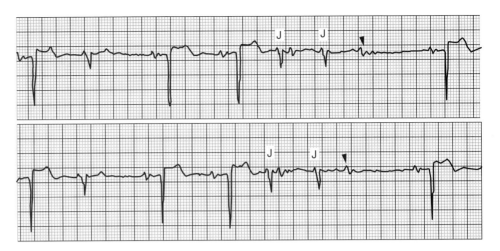

Figure 8–8.
Frequent concealed His bundle or junctional beats mimicking type II block. There are frequent junctional beats (J) often occurring in pairs. The sinus P waves march right through them, so you can tell that the junctional beats aren't conducted back across the atria. Exactly where the third junctional beat should occur, there's a blocked P (*arrowhead*).

Figure 8–9.
Diagram of the effect of completely concealed firing in the His bundle or in the region of the junction. The ectopic focus fires (*double arrowheads*); even though it isn't conducted anywhere, it leaves the tissue refractory. The P wave that comes just after this concealed firing is therefore not conducted. This can mimic Mobitz-II block, but in fact there isn't any block anywhere—there's only harmless interference. Junctional or His bundle beats, concealed or not, don't mean anything and don't require treatment.

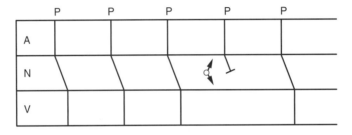

Langendorf-Pick Principle for the Diagnosis of Atypical Mobitz-II Block

Back to Wenckebach block for a moment. In Figure 8–10, you see a 3:2 Wenckebach block. Start with the first QRS of the pair in the middle of the strip. Notice the distance to the next P, or the R-P interval. It's about 0.44 second. Look at the distance from the second QRS to the following P. It's much shorter, of course—about 0.22 second. In other words, there's a reciprocal relation between the P-R and the R-P in Wenckebach block. "Of course!" you exclaim. "Since the P-R gets longer, it has to push the QRS out closer to each following P. After all, the P waves keep arriving right on time."

Think of the R-P as the rest period and the P-R as the working period. The longer a diseased AV node has to rest (R-P), the faster it conducts on the next transmission (P-R). When the rest period is shorter, the conduction will be slower. Down in the bundle-branch system, on the other hand, conduction is all or nothing. Consider rate-dependent bundle-branch block: the bundle branch is blocked or it isn't—nothing intermediate.

Now look at Figure 8–11. In the top strip, there's first-degree AV block with bundle-branch block. The P-R is 0.40 second. In the middle strip, the block is 3:1, and in the bottom strip it's 4:1. This patient was taking digitalis—is this digitalis-toxic AV nodal block, or is the block localized in the one functioning bundle branch?

You don't see two consecutive conducted beats anywhere, so your usual criteria for type I and type II block can't be used. What you do see, however, is a very wide change in the R-P interval. In the top strip, the R-P interval is 0.52 second. In the middle strip with 3:1

Figure 8–10.
Typical Wenckebach block with 3:2 ratio. The distance from the first QRS of each pair to the following P wave (R-P interval) is much longer than the distance from the second QRS to the third P wave of the cycle. In other words, there is a reciprocal relation between P-R and R-P. This is characteristic of AV nodal block.

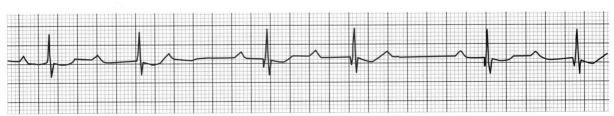

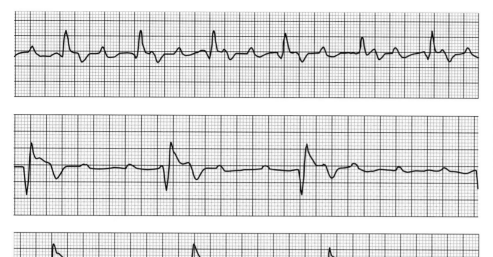

Figure 8–11.
The Langendorf-Pick phenomenon. Rapid increase in degree of AV block in a patient with preexisting bundle-branch block. Note that no matter how long the R-P becomes, the P-R remains exactly the same. This is a variant presentation of Mobitz-II block.

block, it's 1.64 seconds, and when the ratio goes to 4:1 (bottom strip), it's 2.6 seconds. R-P here means the interval from the R to the next conducted P. Ignore the blocked P waves. Despite this dramatic change in the R-P, the P-R remains absolutely fixed. The block has to be in the other bundle branch. It's a variant of Mobitz-II block.

With a degree of block this severe up in the AV node, you would inevitably see striking changes in the P-R interval to correspond with the changing R-P. The P-R with 2:1 block would be a lot longer than the P-R with 3:1 block, and so on. This is an absolute distinction. You can count on it.

Figure 8–12 shows another example of the same phenomenon. This is lead V1; there's right bundle-branch block, and there are many blocked P waves. In the top strip, there is one junctional escape beat and then the rhythm settles down to 2:1 block. In the middle strip, the ratio changes to 3:1 block; and in the bottom strip, the 3:1 block is interrupted by one episode of 2:1 block. When the ratio changes from 2:1 to 3:1, there's obviously a very large change in R-P—from 1.6 seconds to 2.48 seconds to be exact—but the P-R remains absolutely fixed. This is a variant of Mobitz-II block, and the patient needs a pacemaker without further ado.

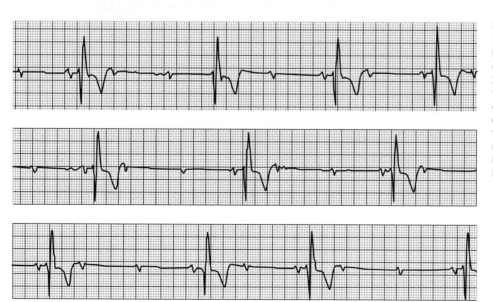

Figure 8–12.
Lead V1: right bundle-branch block. The ratio of conduction changes from 2:1 to 3:1 throughout the tracing, with corresponding drastic changes in R-P. Despite these changes, the P-R remains absolutely fixed. Mobitz-II conduction! Pacemaker!

Figure 8–13 shows the opposite picture. In the top strip, there's 3:1 block. In the middle strip, there's complete block; and in the bottom strip, the ratio shifts to 2:1 block with wide, aberrant ventricular complexes. The P-R with 3:1 block is 0.22 second, and the P-R in the bottom strip with 2:1 block is 0.39 second. See how dramatically the P-R changes in response to R-P change when the block is in the AV node? Even though there are wide QRS complexes, you can diagnose AV nodal block with complete confidence. All the patient needed was less digitalis!

Figure 8–14 shows R-P/P-R reciprocity in a little more complex setting (continuous strips). Basically, there's a dissociated junctional rhythm (J) with many blocked P waves. There are occasional capture beats (labeled *1, 2, 3,* and *4*). Look at the P-R intervals of the capture beats; they vary widely (beat 1, 0.28 second; beat 2, 0.32 second; beat 3, 0.36 second; beat 4, 0.40 second). Now look at the R-P intervals; they vary in an exact reciprocal pattern. The shorter the R-P, the longer the P-R of the capture beat, and vice versa. This is AV

Figure 8–13.
AV nodal block with changing P-R in response to changing R-P. *Top strip,* 3:1 block, P-R 0.21 second. *Bottom strip,* right-hand side, 2:1 block (with aberrant IV conduction), P-R 0.40 second. This is a variant of type I AV nodal block. The diagnosis is precise.

Figure 8–14.
R-P/P-R relation of AV nodal block manifested in the changing P-R of the capture beats (1, 2, 3, and 4). The P-R changes in precise reciprocal fashion with the R-P, thereby localizing the block in the AV node.

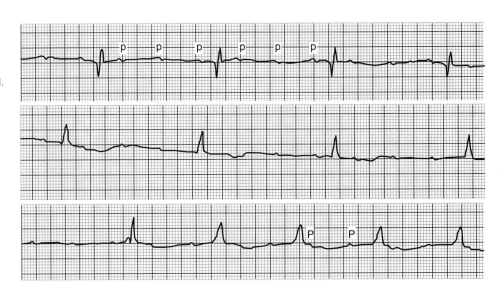

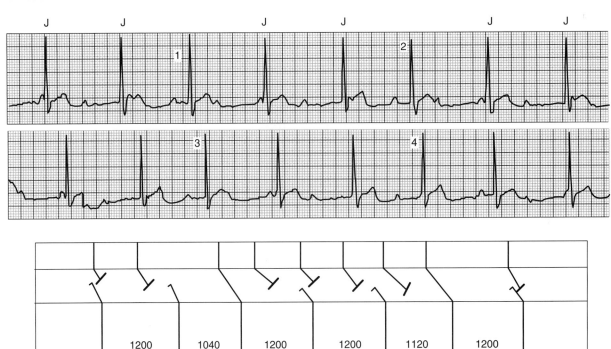

nodal behavior; all those P waves are being blocked in the AV node. (The narrow QRS is another give-away in this case, but even if the QRS complexes were wide, what you see here would give you an absolute diagnosis of AV nodal block.)

"Well fine," says the harassed cardiologist, "but what if you have just plain 2:1 block with bundle-branch block? How can you tell what's going on?" Figure 8–15 gives one answer. Use plenty of electrocardiogram (ECG) paper and wait for the ratio to change. Sometimes it changes spontaneously; more often, it changes when the sinus rate slows. Record an ECG during sleep, when the sinus rate normally slows. Slow the sinus rate with carotid sinus pressure. Simply have the patient lie quietly so that the heart rate slows.

This patient came into the intensive care unit with 2:1 block and bundle-branch block. The next day, this tracing was recorded as the patient lay quietly in the ECG department. The 2:1 block changes to first-degree in the top strip and back to 2:1 in the bottom strip. In the bottom strip, you see a classic Mobitz-II cycle as the ratio changes from first-degree to 2:1—fixed P-R intervals, blocked P, resumption of conduction with unchanged P-R.

Before leaving this topic, look at Figure 8–16. Which of these strips record Mobitz-II block? They were all diagnosed as possible Mobitz-II block. Stop here and analyze them yourself. In all five strips, bundle-branch block is present:

Strip A. Nonconducted premature atrial beat

Strip B. Sinoatrial block with abrupt dropping of one sinus P wave

Strip C. Typical Mobitz-II block

Strip D. 2:1 Block with bundle-branch block. Site of block cannot be determined; it could be in the AV node or in the other bundle branch.

Strip E. Mobitz-II block. The negative P waves are easily visible.

Intra-Hisian Block

This is a rare bird. When it became possible to record His bundle potentials, it was discovered that in some cases there is a "split" His potential. That is, there are two separate potentials recorded during passage through the His bundle—one proximal and one distal. Block can take place within the His bundle itself, between the proximal and distal potentials. This block can produce an atypical Wenckebach cycle or, as reported in one case, a true Mobitz-II phenomenon.

Mobitz-II block within the His bundle is excessively rare. In more than 50 years of studying ECGs, I've never seen a case. Intra-Hisian Wenckebach is probably more common. It's characterized by tiny increments in P-R interval, as shown in Figures 8–17 and 8–18. Note how small are the increases in P-R in these tracings compared with AV nodal Wenckebach. Sometimes the increases are so small you can hardly measure them, but they do progress to

Figure 8–15.
Solution to a perplexing clinical problem, namely 2:1 block with bundle-branch block. Where's the block? Answer: Run a lot of ECG paper looking for a change in the ratio of block!

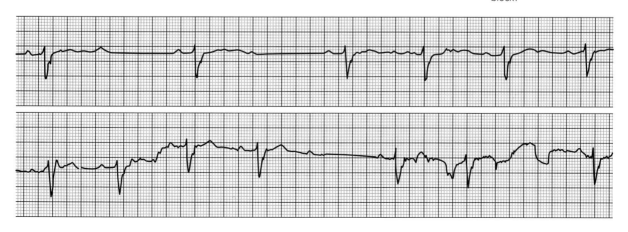

Figure 8–16.
Self-quiz (see text).

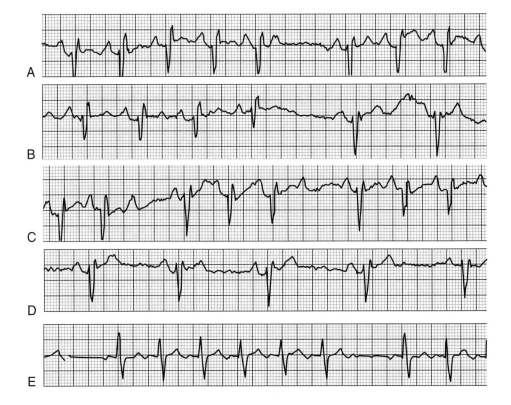

Figure 8–17.
Probable intra-Hisian block. Block within the His bundle itself may take the form of Wenckebach block with tiny increments of P-R, as here.

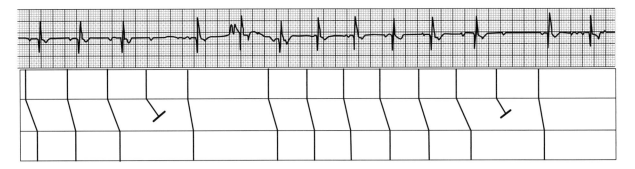

Figure 8–18.
Probable intra-Hisian Wenckebach block with tiny increments in P-R before the blocked P.

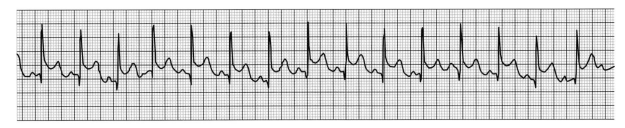

block of one impulse and subsequent recovery. Nobody has any idea of the significance or prognosis of this kind of block. Presumably pacing would be indicated only if the ventricular rate became so slow that it compromised central nervous system or cardiovascular function in some way.

P Wave Shortage

Beware the great P wave shortage (Fig. 8–19). Remember that one of the criteria for complete heart block is "enough atrial complexes to probe all aspects of diastole." In this strip, you start with complete AV dissociation in the first four beats. The ventricular rate is about 52. The last beat is a capture beat with a P-R of 0.23 second. Why the dissociation? *Measure the P-P interval and you find a sinus rate of 45.* That's the problem. The sinus rate is so slow, it lets an idioventricular rhythm escape with a rate a little faster than the sinus node. This sets up the pattern of dissociation that looks so alarming. There just aren't enough sinus impulses to test the system. When one does arrive at a reasonable time after the idiorhythm, it's conducted with nothing worse than first-degree AV block. The patient had sinus bradycardia caused by clonidine. There was nothing significant wrong with the AV conducting system at all.

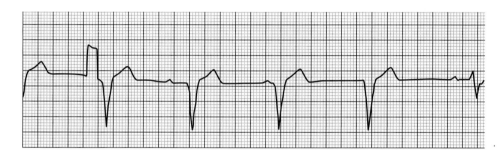

Figure 8–19.
Pseudoblock because of a slow sinus rate. There's an idioventricular rhythm with complete AV dissociation for the first beats. The reason for the idioventricular rhythm and the dissociation is simply the slow sinus rate.

Nine

Atrial Fibrillation

Atrial fibrillation is the most common of the major disorders of rhythm. Most of you already know what's happening in the atria during fibrillation—that the atria are traversed by myriad very fine, rapid, irregular impulses that bombard the atrioventricular (AV) node like sparks flying off a pinwheel (about 450 impulses per minute in an average case). The electrocardiogram (ECG) diagnosis of uncomplicated atrial fibrillation is remarkably simple:

1. **There are no recognizable P waves.**
2. **There are usually fine, fast fibrillary waves with no consistent morphology.**
3. **The ventricular rhythm is irregular.**

Note this last point: When the ventricles are responding to fibrillating atria, the ventricular rhythm will always be irregular—no exceptions.

(At this point, it's important to dispose of a semantic myth. Students are taught that an "irregular irregularity" is diagnostic of atrial fibrillation. By this time, the reader can probably think of three or four other arrhythmias that produce an "irregular irregularity," such as a pronounced sinus arrhythmia with a few premature beats, showers of ectopic beats from different foci, changing interplay of junctional and sinus rhythms, changing ratios of type I block, and so on. Before the end of the book you'll be able to think of 10 or more.)

There are several sources of confusion in the diagnosis of atrial fibrillation.

Character of the Fibrillary Waves

Typical fibrillary waves produce fine, fast deflections in the base line that vary in shape and timing from second to second (Fig. 9–1). Sometimes they're obvious, but sometimes they're so small they're not visible.

Figure 9–2 shows just how much these "f" waves can change. On the left-hand side, they're perfectly regular, like flutter waves for a little while, and then they dwindle away and disappear. These fibrillary waves must not be confused with flutter, which is a sustained, mathematically regular atrial mechanism. If there's the slightest variation in shape or spacing of the f waves, the diagnosis is fibrillation, even though the f waves may be large and nearly regular.

Figure 9–3 is an excellent example of *coarse atrial fibrillation*, or *flutter-fibrillation*. Note the large f waves at various parts of the tracing; they're almost regular for short periods. *One more time:* Do not confuse this with atrial flutter. The proper name is as above: coarse atrial fibrillation, or flutter-fibrillation. Prognosis and treatment are exactly the same as in any atrial fibrillation.

Figure 9–4 is a 12-lead tracing. Note that you can't even see fibrillary waves in any lead except V1, but here they're so coarse that they were mistakenly diagnosed as flutter. In fact, they're much too fast for flutter (about 450), and the morphology changes if you look at

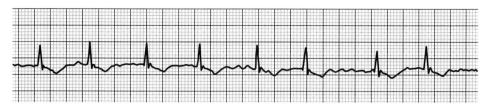

Figure 9–1.
Typical atrial fibrillation with characteristic f waves that appear and disappear. Note also the pseudo P wave before the second beat: it's really just an isolated f wave.

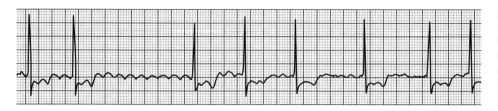

Figure 9–2.
Coarse atrial fibrillation, or flutter-fibrillation. The large, almost regular atrial complexes on the left side of the strip indicate a transient period of true flutter with an atrial rate of 300. They quickly dwindle into small fibrillary waves.

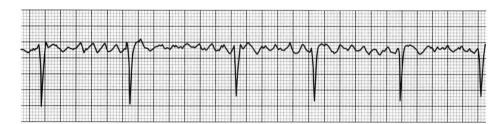

Figure 9–3.
Coarse atrial fibrillation. The complete variability in shape and timing of the atrial complexes rules out flutter.

Figure 9–4.
Flutter-fibrillation. Note that the atrial complexes are visible only in V1. They're too fast for flutter waves, which never exceed a rate of 300 in the adult. If you look closely, you can also see minute changes in morphology—another feature that rules out flutter.

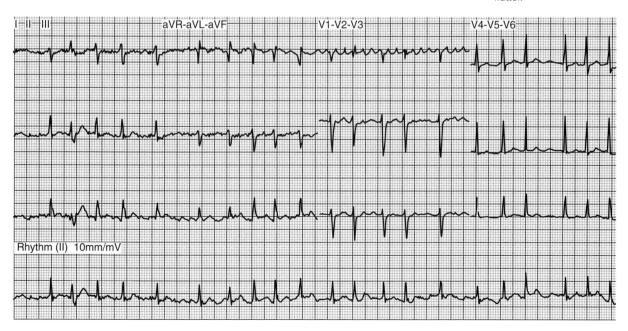

them minutely. Again, the diagnosis is coarse atrial flutter, or flutter-fibrillation, the latter an older but very descriptive term.

Figure 9–5 is another example of coarse fibrillation. (This particular phenomenon is described here at length because it's often confused with real flutter.)

What if you can't see any fibrillary waves, as in Figure 9–6? You can still make a diagnosis with about 99% accuracy. No P waves plus an irregular ventricular rhythm equals a presumptive diagnosis of atrial fibrillation.

Ectopic Beats

When the whole rhythm is irregular, it's often impossible to detect premature beating at the bedside. Obviously, you can't have atrial premature beats if the atria are fibrillating. It is possible to have junctional premature beats interrupting atrial fibrillation, but it's difficult to recognize them even on an ECG because the narrow junctional beats usually look exactly like the beats conducted from the fibrillating atria. There are two ways to recognize junctional ectopic beats during fibrillation; they're illustrated in Figure 9–7.

First, the junctional beats may be aberrantly conducted, like the ones here (typical Ashman aberrancy). Second, and even more important, note that the two aberrant beats come much closer to the beats ahead of them than any two consecutive beats coming down

Figure 9–5.
Flutter-fibrillation in a child. Note the coarse, almost regular atrial complexes that appear briefly on the left side of the tracing. This often confuses observers, but the proper diagnosis is coarse fibrillation, or flutter-fibrillation.

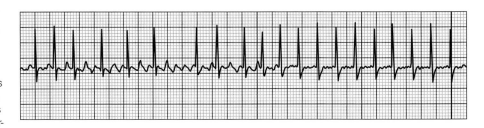

Figure 9–6.
Atrial fibrillation with one VPC. The fibrillary waves are so small they're invisible, but the absence of P waves and the totally irregular spacing of QRS gives the diagnosis.

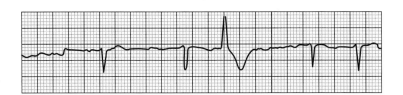

Figure 9–7.
Atrial fibrillation with two aberrantly conducted junctional beats. The two junctional beats are close to the preceding conducted beats. Inspection of the R-R intervals in the rest of the strip tells you that the AV node couldn't conduct that fast. The beats have to be reentrant junctional ectopic beats.

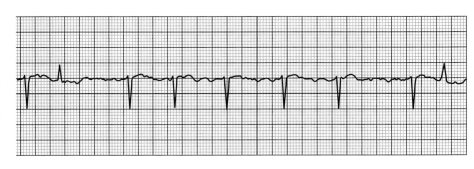

from the fibrillating atria. In other words, it's obvious from looking at the rest of the tracing that the AV node couldn't conduct this fast. These early beats have to be the result of a reentrant ectopic focus.

The important ectopic beats are ventricular, of course. During an acute myocardial infarct, they may be harbingers of fatal arrhythmias. They may also be an important early sign of digitalis toxicity (see Chapter 16).

In Figure 9–8, you see typical wide ventricular ectopic beats interrupting atrial fibrillation. How can you tell they're not aberrantly conducted impulses from the fibrillating atria? Apply the same criteria you did with the junctional beats. In the first place, the distance from the wide beats to the preceding conducted beat is shorter than any R–R anywhere else in the tracing. It's obvious the AV node couldn't conduct that fast, so these beats can't be the result of aberrant conduction from the atria. Furthermore, remember the rule about reentrant ectopic beats: they come at a relatively constant distance from the conducted beats that precede them (within a few hundredths of a second). This *constant coupling* to the preceding beats also rules out random conduction from the fibrillating atria.

Figure 9–9 is an example of a ventricular premature contraction (VPC) interrupting atrial fibrillation. This wide beat might also be junctional with aberrancy. How do you make the distinction? *Simple:* Look to see if there's any basis for aberrancy. In Figure 9–9, the wide beat comes after a relatively long pause, so you rule out rate-related aberrancy. There is also no Ashman relationship, so there's simply no reason for aberrant conduction. The beat has to be ventricular.

Rule: You know the three causes of aberrant conduction. Don't diagnose aberrancy unless you see one of them.

These wide beats are VPCs. In the setting of an acute myocardial infarction (MI), reach for the lidocaine!

Ventricular Rhythm Turns Regular

Of course this might mean that a normal sinus rhythm is now present. On the other hand, consider Figure 9–10. The regular rhythm might come from an idioventricular rhythm like this one, firing just fast enough to "take over" from the fibrillary impulses for a time. The idioventricular rhythm is discharging at a rate of 90, and of course it's regular. While the

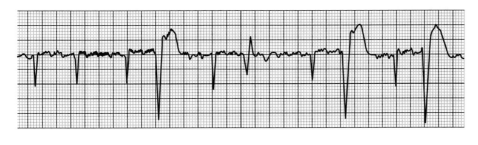

Figure 9–8.
Atrial fibrillation with ventricular ectopic beats. The short, consistent coupling interval of the wide beats to the preceding narrow beats rules out any possibility that the wide beats are the result of random aberrant conduction from the fibrillating atria.

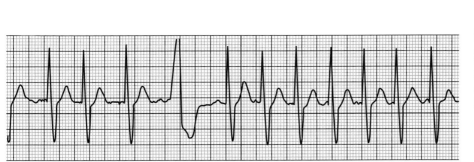

Figure 9–9.
Atrial fibrillation with one VPC. There's no possible basis for aberrant conduction, so the wide beat has to be ventricular.

idioventricular rhythm is present, there is complete AV dissociation. None of the fibrillary impulses reach the ventricles. There's no block—remember, this is interference-dissociation caused by the discharge of an ectopic focus.

Rule: When the ventricular rhythm becomes regular during atrial fibrillation, it may be the result of complete AV dissociation with a junctional or ventricular rhythm driving the ventricles.

Figure 9–11 shows another example of an accelerated idioventricular rhythm interrupting atrial fibrillation.

The interplay between the idiorhythms and the fibrillary impulses can produce some complex patterns, as in Figure 9–12. The beats labeled *I* arise in the junction, whereas the beats labeled *C* are conducted from the fibrillating atria. *Moral:* When you're examining a patient with known atrial fibrillation, listen carefully for any periods of regular beating. If there's the slightest question, record an ECG. Accelerated idiorhythms in the normal range are harmless; on the other hand, if they are slow, it's time to start thinking about heart block.

Look again at Figure 9–12, for example. The rate of the idiorhythm is slow—about 58. There's plenty of time between ectopic beats for impulses from the fibrillating atria to come through the AV node if it were functioning normally, but obviously it isn't—the idiorhythm controls the ventricles for long periods at a slow rate. There must therefore be a considerable degree of AV block. It's not complete because there are periods when the fibrillary impulses do reach the ventricles. This is therefore a type of second-degree AV block in the

Figure 9–10.
Atrial fibrillation with intermittent accelerated idioventricular rhythm. Note the fusion beat (F).

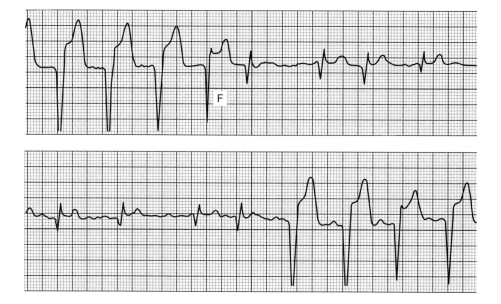

Figure 9–11.
Atrial fibrillation interrupted by an accelerated idioventricular rhythm.

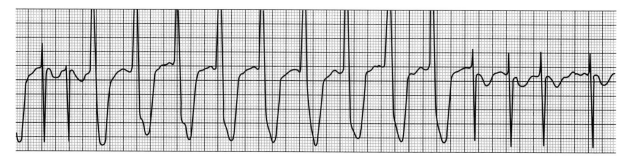

presence of atrial fibrillation. Some impulses reach the ventricles, whereas others don't, even though they have plenty of time to do so. Because there are no P waves to measure from, this is as precise as you can be.

AV block in the presence of atrial fibrillation is very important because almost all patients with atrial fibrillation are taking some kind of medication that depresses AV nodal conduction. You must be alert to the possibility of significant heart block and detect it before it becomes life threatening. Because there are no P waves, you have to use simple logic, as described earlier.

Criteria for AV Block in the Presence of Atrial Fibrillation

> 1. **A slow but irregular heart rate (Fig. 9–13). Remember that the fibrillating atria are bombarding the AV node about 425 to 450 times a minute. If all the impulses reached the ventricles, of course, the patient would die quickly. Two things keep this from happening: the refractory period of the AV nodal tissue and the phenomenon of concealed conduction.**

The effect of the refractory period on speed of conduction is obvious. The cells can't conduct until they recover from the previous transmission. Concealed conduction in this setting simply means partial penetration of the AV node by many impulses, with resulting fatigue of the nodal cells and a slower rate of conduction. A healthy AV node should conduct fibrillating impulses at a very rapid rate—up to 170 to 180. In older patients, it's common to see slower conduction with normal ventricular rates.

Figure 9–12.
Atrial fibrillation interrupted frequently by short runs of an accelerated idiojunctional rhythm. The idiojunctional beats (I) form a complex pattern with the conducted beats from the fibrillating atria (C). The slow rate of the junctional rhythm (58) means that there must be some degree of AV nodal block.

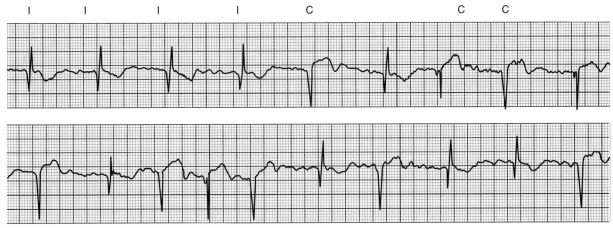

Figure 9–13.
Atrial fibrillation with slow ventricular rate varying from 43 to 68. The slow rate indicates a substantial degree of AV block; the irregular response indicates that it is not complete.

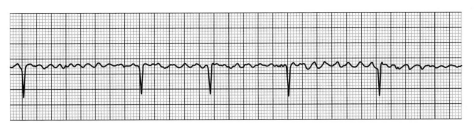

Figure 9–14.
Atrial fibrillation with complete AV block. All the criteria for complete block are present: complete AV dissociation without capture beats, slow ventricular rate (42), and ample atrial complexes to probe the conducting system.

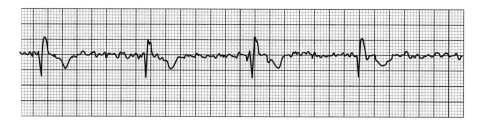

In Figure 9–13, however, some of the R–R intervals are equivalent to a rate of 38, and the average rate is about 60. There must be a significant degree of AV block, although it's not complete.

> 2. **Periods of AV dissociation with a slow idiorhythm—in the range of 55 to 65. As in Figure 9–12, this means a high degree of block, less than complete.**
>
> 3. **Complete AV dissociation with a rate of 45 or less (Fig. 9–14). The rate is perfectly regular, and there are no episodes of conduction from the fibrillating atria. The diagnosis is complete heart block. You use the same criteria you use for any complete heart block: complete AV dissociation with no capture beats, a slow ventricular rate, and enough atrial impulses to test the system all through diastole. (In atrial fibrillation there's a surplus of atrial impulses to do the testing!)**

Atrial Fibrillation and Paroxysmal Tachycardia

When the rate becomes rapid and perfectly regular, in the range 140 to 240, paroxysmal tachycardia is interrupting the atrial fibrillation. The tachycardia may be junctional or ventricular.

Figure 9–15 is an example of junctional tachycardia; right bundle-branch block was present chronically. After periods of typical random conduction from the fibrillating atria, a regular rhythm appears for several seconds at a time. The rate is 150.

Figure 9–15.
Atrial fibrillation interrupted by runs of paroxysmal junctional tachycardia (right bundle-branch block).

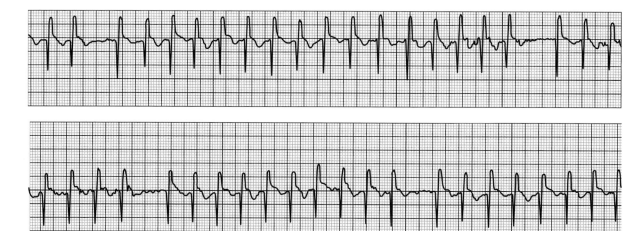

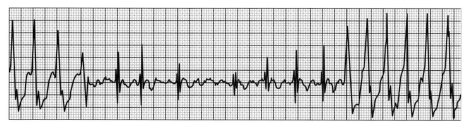

Figure 9–16.
Atrial fibrillation interrupted by paroxysms of ventricular tachycardia. Note the striking progressive fusion beats and the end and the beginning of each episode of ventricular tachycardia.

Rule: A rapid junctional rhythm in the high-normal to tachycardia range is the most common sustained digitalis-toxic tachyarrhythmia. When you see this type of arrhythmia in a digitalized patient, always assume digitalis toxicity (see Chapter 16).

If a wide-complex tachycardia appears, it may be ventricular or junctional with aberrancy. Sometimes it's possible to make the distinction by using the same criteria you learned in Chapter 3:

> 1. **Look for fusion beats. When the atria are fibrillating, there are so many impulses coming through the AV node that there are many chances for fusion. In Figure 9–16, you can see the beginning and end of two paroxysms of ventricular tachycardia. The narrow beats in the middle of the strip represent the normal pattern of conduction. There is striking progressive fusion with the ventricular beats at the beginning and end of each run of tachycardia.**

Figure 9–17 is another example. In Figure 9–17A, you see a simple wide-beat tachycardia. From this strip alone, you can't make the distinction between junctional and ventricular

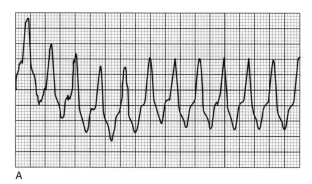

A

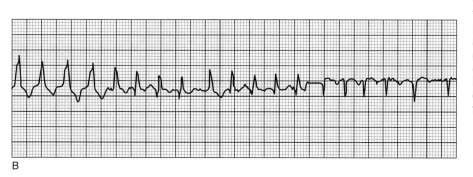

B

Figure 9–17.
Atrial fibrillation interrupted by a paroxysm of ventricular tachycardia.
A, A wide-beat tachycardia is shown that might be ventricular or junctional with aberrancy.
B, Progressive fusion is seen between the impulses from the ventricular tachycardia and those conducted down from the fibrillating atria. The very rapid rate of the narrow beats also rules out any possibility of rate-dependent aberrancy as an explanation for the wide beats. (At the right-hand end of **B**, the lead changes to aVR.)

origin. In Figure 9–17B, there are many obvious fusion beats as the rhythm changes to atrial fibrillation.

> **2. Look for a rate basis for aberrancy. Do the wide beats appear at a rapid rate and disappear when the rate slows? Figure 9–17B gives an answer here as well. The narrow conducted beats appear at a rate *more rapid* than the wide L beats. Forget aberrancy!**

Atrial Fibrillation with Rate-Dependent Bundle-Branch Block

Atrial fibrillation with fixed bundle-branch block is no problem. As in Figure 9–18, there are the typical wide QRS complexes appearing irregularly, without P waves. The QRS complexes do not change even when the rate varies.

Rate-dependent bundle-branch block can produce patterns that might be confused with paroxysms of ventricular tachycardia, but the distinction is simple. In Figure 9–19, there are periods of wide-beat tachycardia interrupted by occasional normally conducted beats. In the pauses, there are obvious f waves. The wide-beat rhythm is totally irregular, with some R-R intervals twice as wide as others. The rate in ventricular tachycardia can vary a little, but never that much. Whenever the rate slows below a certain point, the QRS is normal. This is obviously rate-dependent bundle-branch block and not ventricular tachycardia.

Clinical note: When you're considering the possibility of rate-dependent bundle-branch block, slow the ventricular rate by carotid massage or adenosine. You'll have the answer in seconds.

Figure 9–18.
Stable right bundle-branch block with atrial fibrillation. Note the characteristic wide variation in R-R, as in any atrial fibrillation.

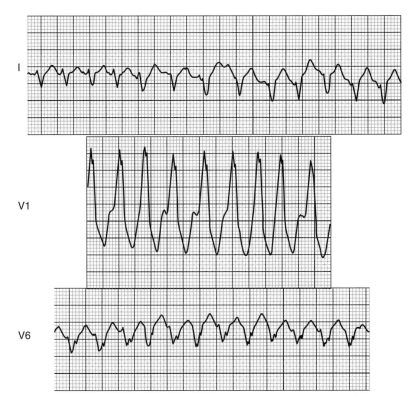

What Fibrillary Waves Look Like Inside the Atria

When you're localizing a transvenous pacemaker electrocardiographically, you have to know what fibrillary waves look like inside the atria. Figure 9–20 records the change from ordinary surface f waves to the giant "spiky" inscriptions recorded when the electrode is in the right atrium. The atrial deflections are huge, much larger than the ventricular complexes, and they're sharp and narrow. MA refers to atrial impulses recorded from the mid right atrium. HRA refers to impulses recorded when the electrode was withdrawn to the high right atrium at the junction with the superior vena cava.

Figure 9–19.
Atrial fibrillation with rate-dependent bundle-branch block. Whenever the rate slows, as in the bottom strip, the QRS narrows. Note also the very wide variation in R-R intervals, characteristic of conduction from fibrillating atria.

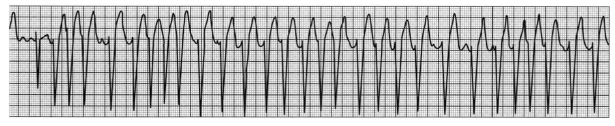

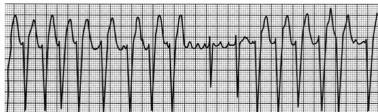

Figure 9–20.
Intra-atrial recording of atrial fibrillation. Note the progressive enlargement of the F waves as the electrode moves through the superior vena cava and into the right atrium. Complexes arising in the high right atrium (HRA) are large and irregularly sawtooth shaped; complexes arising in the midatrium (MA) are huge, narrow spikes.

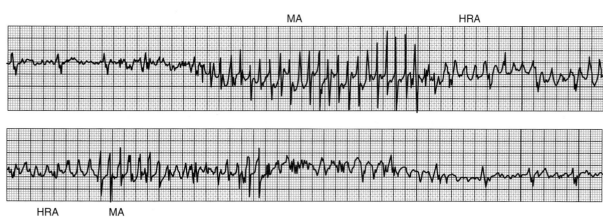

Ten

Atrial Flutter

The salient point to pin in your memory about atrial flutter is that the atrial rhythm is absolutely regular. Atrial flutter is a remarkable mechanism; the complexes it produces are precise in timing and shape within a hundredth of a millimeter and a hundredth of a second. If there is the slightest variation in the atrial complexes, the rhythm isn't flutter.

You make the diagnosis of atrial flutter by recognizing flutter waves in the ECG. (It's alleged that you can recognize flutter waves in the jugular venous pulse, but this is so rare that it's no more than a pious hope. You can probably see jugular flutter waves only about 1 time out of 10.)

The first thing you notice about typical flutter waves is that there's no flat, isoelectric period between them. The end of one wave is the beginning of the next; this produces the classic sawtooth configuration (Fig. 10–1). It also reflects the continuous atrial activity of flutter. The atrial rate here is 300; with the usual 2:1 conduction, the ventricular rate is 150. In Figure 10–2, the flutter rate is much slower—about 188. The precise reproduction and timing of each flutter wave is obvious. In the bottom strip, carotid sinus pressure was applied so that the flutter waves are isolated, with only two ventricular responses in the whole strip. Note also the different appearance of flutter waves in the different leads.

Figure 10–3 is another example of 2:1 flutter. One negative sawtooth is about 0.16 second ahead of the QRS, whereas the other comes just after the QRS. Place the tips of your calipers on these two negative deflections, and you'll see that they march out perfectly with a rate of 215.

In Figure 10–4, you see an important variant in flutter. The ratio of conduction changes from 2:1 to 3:1 and 4:1 in various parts of the strip. The ventricular response is therefore completely irregular, and at the bedside, it couldn't be distinguished from atrial fibrillation.

One third of all cases of atrial flutter manifest changing ratios of conduction to the ventricles with an irregular ventricular rhythm. (A few years ago while I was lecturing on this topic, a physician stood up and maintained with some heat that if the ratio of conduction changes, "you have to call it fibrillation!" Nothing could be further from the truth. The accident of conduction down the atrioventricular [AV] node has nothing to do with what's happening in the atria.)

Where do you see flutter waves? They tend to be isolated. Usually you see them in only one lead system—II, III, and aVF as a rule. In Figure 10–5, the flutter waves are obvious in II, III, and aVF, but you'd have a hard time recognizing them anywhere else. There's a small "glitch" just after the peak of the T in these leads that represents the nonconducted flutter wave; if you look closely, you can see the same deflection in V4, V5, and V6.

Sometimes flutter waves are visible in only one lead. Figure 10–6 is a dramatic example of this phenomenon. There are large, unmistakable flutter waves in V1, but you can't find anything in the other leads that you could positively identify as a flutter wave. In the limb leads, there's not a clue.

Two Tips for Identifying Flutter Waves

Figure 10–7 illustrates a typical 2:1 flutter. Note two characteristics of the flutter waves:

> 1. **The alternate flutter wave intersects the QRS *above* the baseline. When you see this consistently through a strip, you're dealing with flutter—flutter waves are the only atrial complexes that do this.**
>
> 2. **You can draw an imaginary line from the top of the flutter wave just before the QRS down through the ventricular complex and see the flutter wave emerge on the other side.**

Watch for these two unique characteristics of flutter waves.

Because the diagnosis of flutter rests on your visual recognition of flutter waves, here are some examples of the different forms they can take.

In Figure 10–8, the flutter waves are really hard to see. At the right side of the tracing, you can see very small, perfect "spikes" as indicated by the arrowheads. They're most obvious when the ratio shifts to 3:1. In the pause between QRS complexes, the tiny flutter waves are clearly visible, with a rate of 300. Once you've identified them, you can follow them all the way through the tracing with a pair of calipers.

Figure 10–9 illustrates another variation. You see typical flutter waves in II, III, and aVF, but if you look at V1, you see what flutter waves usually look like in the right precordium. They're commonly small, discrete, upright waves not at all like the sawtooth waves you see in the limb leads.

If you look at the examples so far, you can see that the atrial rate in flutter can range from as high as 300 down to 210 or 215. In the adult heart, the atrial rate practically never exceeds 300.

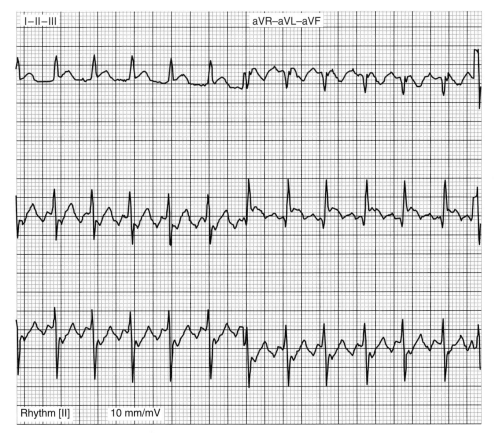

Figure 10–1.
Typical flutter waves in the limb leads. Note how prominent the flutter waves are in II, III, and aVF, whereas you can't see them in I and aVL.

Figure 10–2.
Relatively slow flutter waves in the limb leads. The period of carotid sinus pressure in lead 3 gives you a chance to see the isolated flutter waves. Note the mathematical regularity.

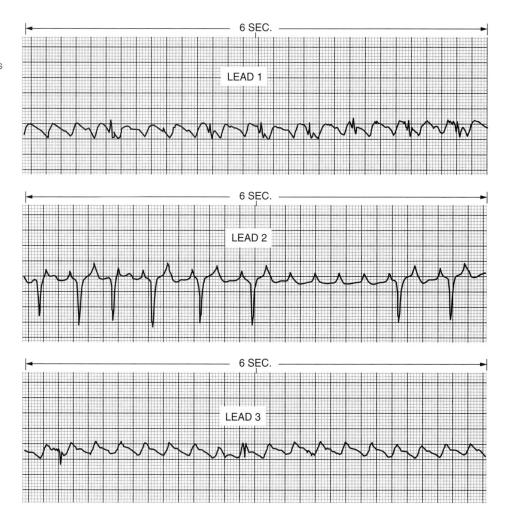

Figure 10–3.
2:1 Flutter.

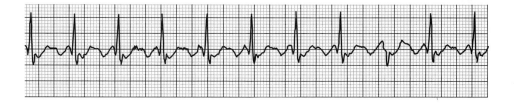

Figure 10–4.
Flutter with varying ratios of conduction to the ventricles. Note grossly irregular ventricular rhythm.

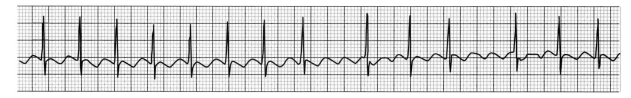

Figure 10–5.
Prominent flutter waves in
II, III, and aVF. The flutter
waves are practically
invisible in the other leads.
(You can see tiny
deflections in V4–V6.)

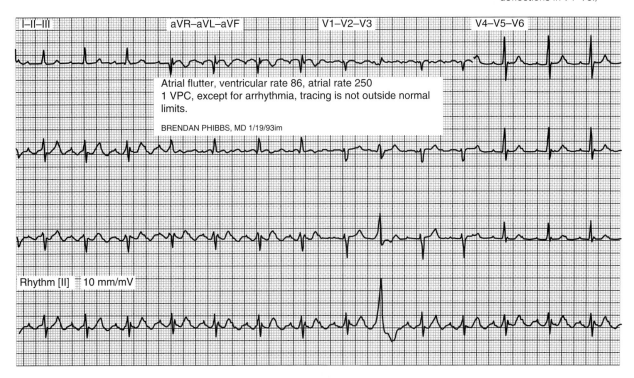

Atrial flutter, ventricular rate 86, atrial rate 250
1 VPC, except for arrhythmia, tracing is not outside normal
limits.

BRENDAN PHIBBS, MD 1/19/93im

Figure 10–6.
Isolated flutter waves in V1
only. They're absolutely
invisible everywhere else.
Be sure to look at all leads
before you rule out flutter!

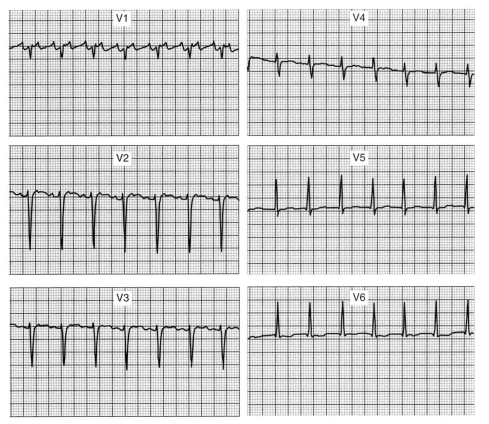

Figure 10–7.
A simple trick for recognizing flutter waves is to follow a flutter wave through the QRS complex.

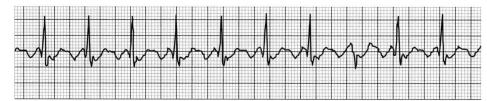

Figure 10–8.
Tiny but definite flutter waves (*arrowheads*) that become really visible only when the ratio of conduction shifts.

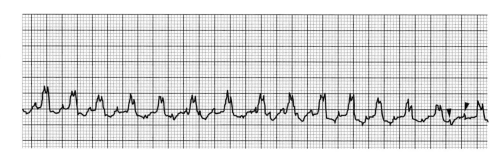

Figure 10–9.
Comparison of flutter waves in inferior leads (II, III, aVF) and V1. In V1, flutter waves often appear as small, discrete atrial complexes, resembling rapidly inscribed P waves. In this case, the atrial rate would reveal the diagnosis even if you couldn't see the obvious flutter waves in the inferior leads.

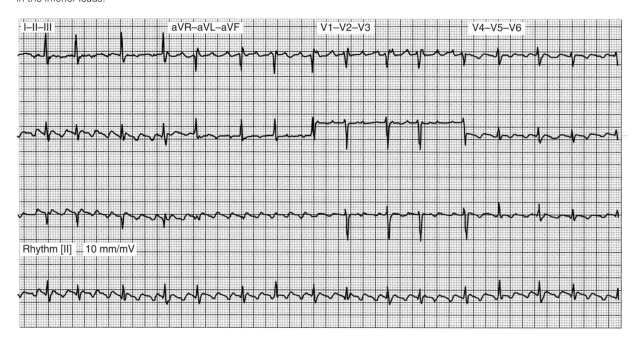

Vagal Stimulation in the Diagnosis of Flutter

Sometimes it's absolutely impossible to diagnose flutter until you cause a block in the AV node that lets you see the isolated flutter waves. Figure 10–10 is an excellent example. Looking at the right-hand side of the strip only, you couldn't possibly make the diagnosis. Carotid sinus stimulation blocked transmission through the AV node and made the flutter obvious.

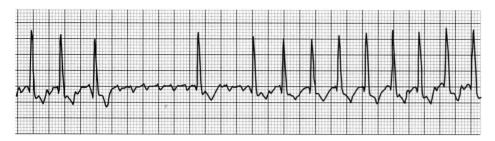

Figure 10–10.
Unmasking of atrial flutter by carotid sinus stimulation. It would not be possible to make a diagnosis from the right-hand part of the strip.

Figures 10–11, 10–12, and 10–13 are examples of obscure flutter unmasked by carotid sinus stimulation. Now that adenosine is available, temporary blockade of the AV node is even easier and safer. Use this maneuver whenever you see a baffling supraventricular rhythm like the ones illustrated here.

To diagnose block in the presence of atrial flutter, you need only to substitute flutter waves for sinus P waves, and the problem becomes simple. In Figure 10–14, you see a slow, regular ventricular rhythm with a rate of 43. Now look carefully at the flutter waves ahead of each QRS. *Note that there's a changing relation of flutter wave to QRS.* That's analogous to seeing a changing P-R when the sinus node is discharging. Despite the changing flutter–R relation, the ventricular rhythm is absolutely regular. The diagnosis is therefore complete AV dissociation. The ventricular rhythm arises in the AV junction, and the flutter waves never penetrate to the ventricles. Because the ventricular rate is 43, all the criteria for complete heart block are present.

In Figure 10–15, there is obviously a high degree of block, but it's not complete. The ventricular rhythm is irregular, and if you look closely, there are minute changes in the relation of flutter waves to QRS complexes.

Figure 10–16 is an example of complete block in the presence of atrial flutter. There are two idioventricular foci discharging at different rates. The ventricular rhythm is regular for short periods (the first four beats on the top strip and the last four on the right-hand side of the bottom strip). During these periods of regular ventricular firing, the relation of flutter wave to QRS changes in a totally random manner. There is therefore complete heart block with two idioventricular pacemakers discharging.

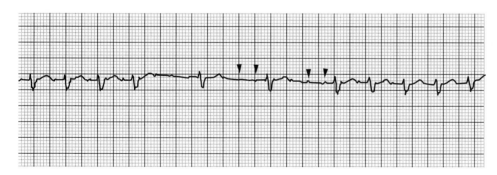

Figure 10–11.
Unmasking of atrial flutter by carotid sinus stimulation. The flutter waves are tiny (*arrowheads*) but absolutely regular. Without AV nodal blockade, diagnosis would be impossible.

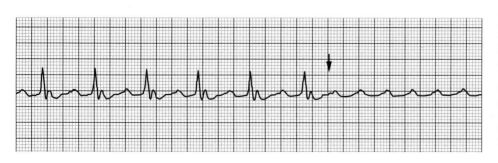

Figure 10–12.
Unmasking of atrial flutter by carotid sinus stimulation (*arrow*). The left side of the strip looks remarkably like a normal sinus rhythm! (Thank your resident deity for adenosine in cases like this.)

Figure 10–13.
A baffling arrhythmia that
was unmasked only by
carotid sinus stimulation
while V3-R was being
recorded. *Always* use AV
nodal blockade, and *always*
record numerous different
leads when tracking down
obscure flutter.

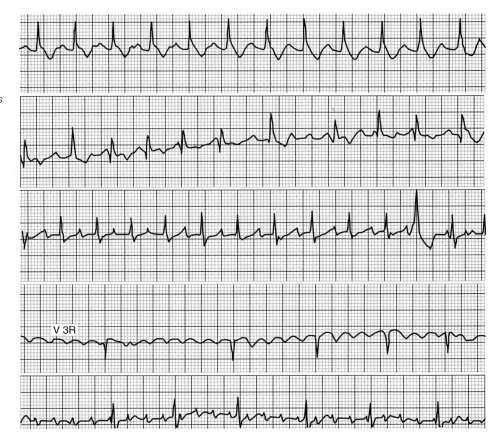

Figure 10–14.
Complete AV nodal block
in the presence of flutter.
Instead of a changing P-R
relation, look for a
changing flutter–R in the
presence of a regular
ventricular rhythm to
establish the diagnosis of
dissociation.

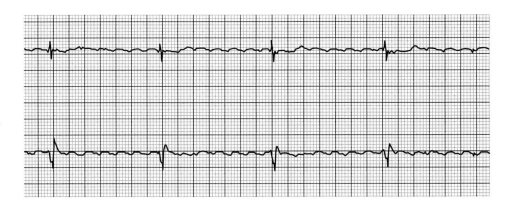

Figure 10–15.
High degree of AV nodal
block in the presence of
atrial flutter. The changing
R-R interval tells you the
block probably isn't
complete.

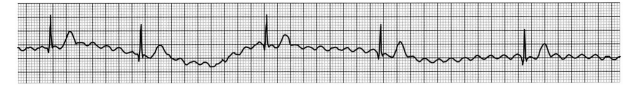

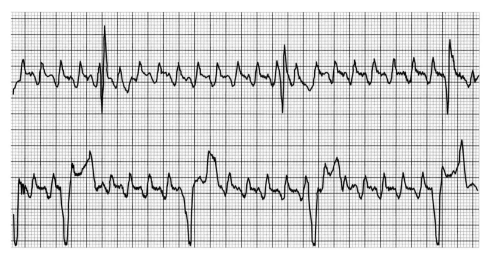

Figure 10–16.
Complete AV block in the presence of atrial flutter. Multiple idioventricular pacemakers.

Figure 10–17 is an example of simple complete block with a ventricular rate of 26. Look carefully at the flutter–QRS relation, and you'll see that it changes throughout the strip, thus confirming complete AV dissociation.

Wenckebach Block in the Presence of Atrial Flutter

In Figure 10–18, there is a definite paired, or bigeminal, rhythm with obvious flutter waves. The diagram below the strip explains what's happening. In ordinary 2:1 flutter, one flutter wave is conducted and one isn't. The flutter wave that isn't conducted doesn't penetrate the AV node at all. In other words, in flutter, there is always one level of block between the atria

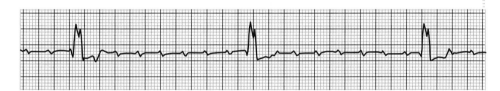

Figure 10–17.
Atrial flutter with complete AV block. Note the changing flutter–R relationship with the regular slow ventricular rhythm.

Figure 10–18.
Two-level block with atrial flutter. Wenckebach block to the alternate flutter impulses.

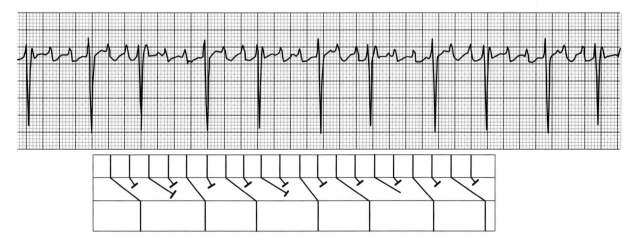

and the AV node. Many times, there will be some kind of block to the impulse that does go down the AV node, thus there's a second level of block.

The trick to recognizing this is to ignore the alternate flutter waves that don't penetrate the AV node at all and concentrate on the ones that do. In other words, look for a pattern of block on the alternate flutter wave, as illustrated in Figure 10–18. Ignore the nonconducted flutter waves and look at the alternate ones that penetrate the AV node. Here there's an absolutely regular pattern of progressive prolongation of flutter–QRS until the third alternate flutter wave is blocked. Like any 3:2 block, this gives a paired, or bigeminal, rhythm.

1:1 Flutter and How to Avoid It

It's fortunate that every flutter wave doesn't reach the ventricles; the heart would usually race itself to death if they did. There are two conditions when 1:1 flutter can occur.

1-A Drugs

Quinidine and procainamide can both produce 1:1 flutter, especially quinidine. There are two reasons for this:

> 1. **Both quinidine and procainamide are mildly vagolytic; by enhancing sympathetic drive, they accelerate conduction through the AV node. This is actually a minor effect.**
>
> 2. **Both drugs slow the flutter rate in the atria. A flutter that's been firing at 300 may slow to 210 to 215. At this rate, it's possible for every wave to penetrate the AV node and pull the ventricular rate up to the atrial rate. The results may be catastrophic.**

Rule: Never give a 1-A drug for flutter until there's adequate blockade of the AV node by digitalis or other drugs to prevent 1:1 conduction.

Figure 10–19 is an example of 1:1 flutter caused by administration of quinidine without digitalis. Atrial and ventricular rates are both 250. At this point, of course, the patient was critical, and only rapid AV nodal blockade saved his life.

Exercise

The patient who complains to you about pounding of the heart during exercise may be describing this phenomenon.

In Figure 10–20, you see what happened during a treadmill test. From a sinus rate of 118, the patient suddenly went into a very rapid tachycardia with a rate of 215. There was no way of knowing what this rhythm was until there was transient slowing as a result of carotid sinus stimulation (Fig. 10–21). Here you can clearly see flutter waves (F). If you measure the flutter rate, you'll see that it's 21—exactly the same as the ventricular rate on the right-hand side of the tracing. This is *exercise-induced 1:1 flutter.* The surge of catecholamines that accompanies exercise enhances AV conduction and allows every flutter wave to reach the ventricles. Keep this possibility in mind when people tell you they "feel as if their heart is racing" during tennis or bicycling!

Treatment of Atrial Flutter

We progress! There is a whole new body of very useful information about the mechanism of flutter, and with this information has come a prospect of permanent cure.

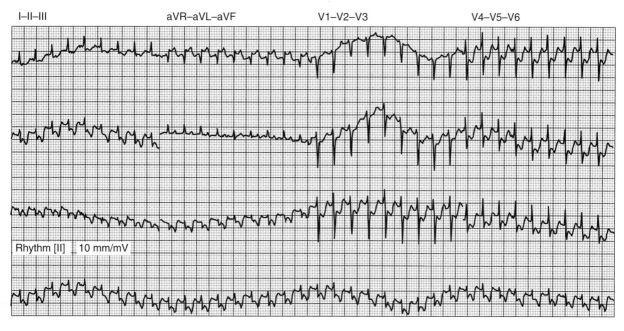

Figure 10–19.
1:1 Atrial flutter caused by administration of quinidine without digitalis or other source of AV nodal blockade.

I–II–III   aVR–aVL–aVF   V1–V2–V3   V4–V5–V6

Rhythm [II]   10 mm/mV

Figure 10–20.
Tracing recorded during treadmill exercises. After three sinus beats, a tachycardia appears that settles down to a steady rate of 215.

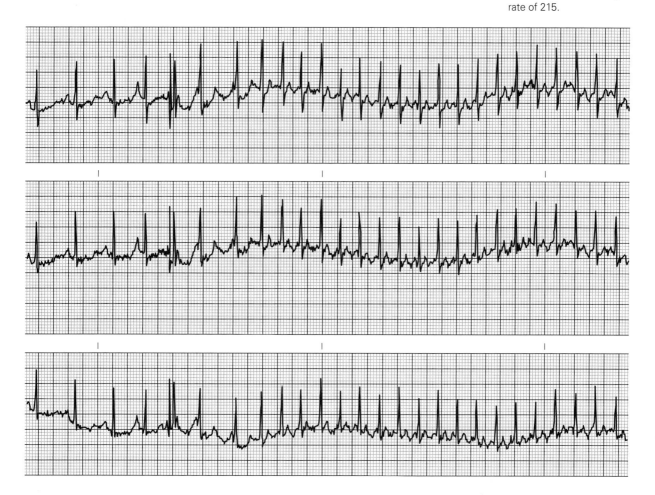

Figure 10–21.
With carotid sinus stimulation and slowing of the rate, obvious flutter waves can be seen (F). The rate of the flutter waves is exactly the same as the ventricular rate: 215. This is exercise-induced 1:1 flutter.

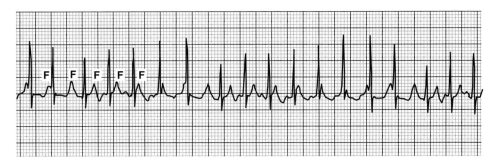

Flutter may be a transient complication of some acute process such as congestive heart failure or myocardial infarction. In this setting, drug treatment or cardioversion will usually be successful with little prospect of recurrence.

BUT... if atrial flutter is sustained or recurrent, *ablation* may provide a permanent cure. The possibility of ablation should always be investigated.

How does ablation work? It is now clear that flutter is a true circus mechanism—a continuous, self-perpetuating loop in some part of the atria.

Look at Figure 10–2, leads 1 and 3. Notice the classic sawtooth flutter waves with deep negative components. This type of flutter is very likely to be caused by a counterclockwise loop in the right atrium. An essential part of this loop is the isthmus between the inferior vena cava and the tricuspid valve. If that isthmus is interrupted, the flutter stops.

Other loops may involve the left atrium and the interatrial septum (see Fig. 10–5).

Flutter that depends on an isthmus like this is called *isthmus-dependent flutter* and, according to the direction of the loop, may be called *counterclockwise isthmus dependent* (CCWID) or *clockwise isthmus dependent* (CWID). (It's always good for the clinician to understand the jargon of the laboratory.)

In the great majority of cases, ablation is successful.

Moral: When atrial flutter is sustained, refractory, or recurrent, always refer to the EP lab for study and possible ablation!

Self-Assessment II

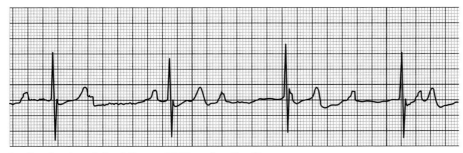

Figure SAII–1.

1. Conduction defect? Degree? Where localized?

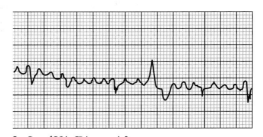

Figure SAII–2.

2. Lead V1. Diagnosis?

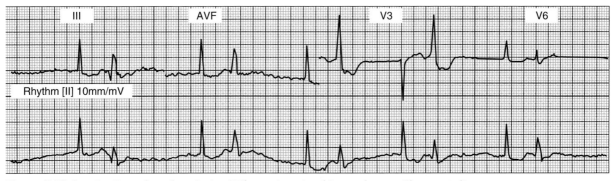

Figure SAII–3. 3. Complete description? The patient is taking unknown "heart medi-cine." Probable diagnosis?

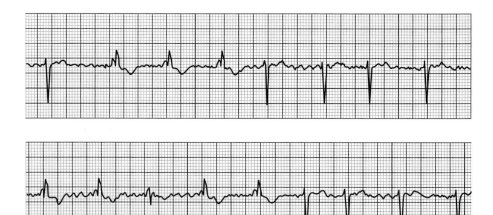

Figure SAII–4.

4. Complete description? Significance of wide beats? Treatment, if any?

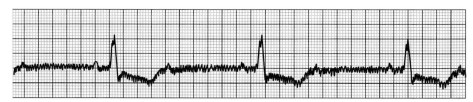

Figure SAII–5.

5. Conduction defect? Can you localize it? Possibilities and significance?

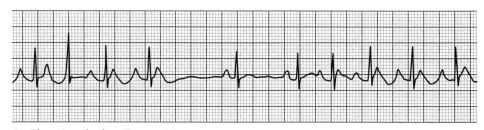

Figure SAII–6.

6. Changing rhythm. Diagnosis?

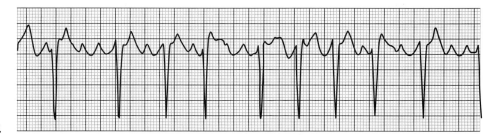

Figure SAII–7.

7. Rapid irregular ventricular rhythm. Diagnosis?

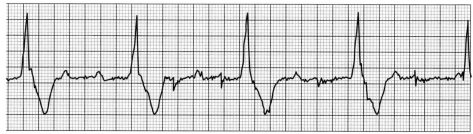

Figure SAII–8.

8. Conduction defect? Possible sites? Significance? Treatment, if any?

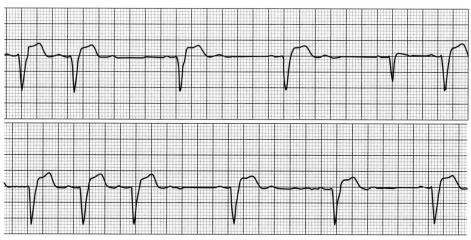

Figure SAII–9.

9. Changing rate and rhythm, changing QRS width. Cause? Significance?

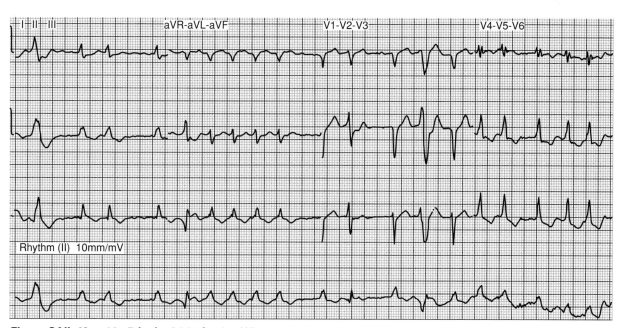

Figure SAII–10.   10. Rhythm? Mechanism(s)?

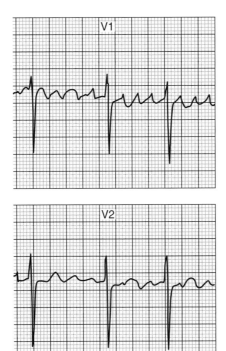

Figure SAII–11.

11. Rhythm?

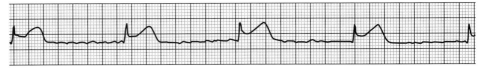

Figure SAII–12.

12. Rhythm? State of AV conduction?

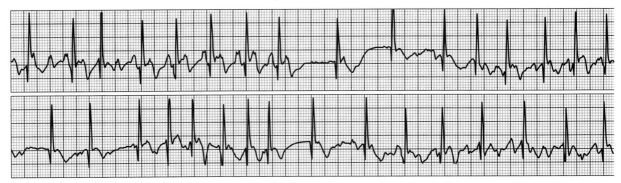

Figure SAII–13.   13. Grossly irregular rhythm. Diagnosis?

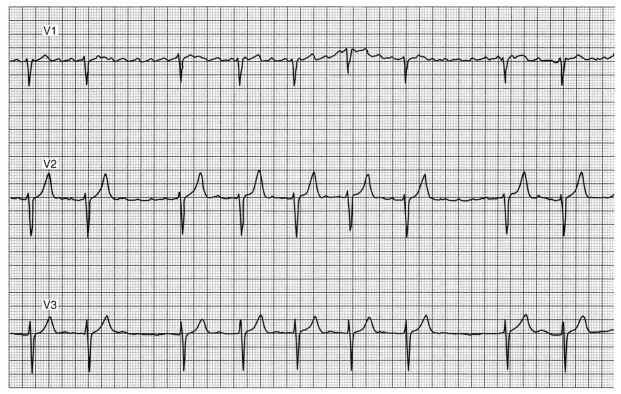

Figure SAII–14.   14.   Basic rhythm. Cause of pauses?

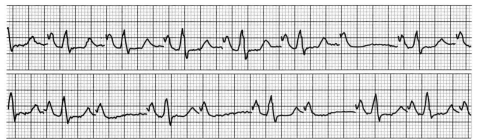

Figure SAII–15.

15.   You have a pacing wire in the right atrium, pacing at a rate of 77. The following pattern
      appears. Significance? Treatment, if any?

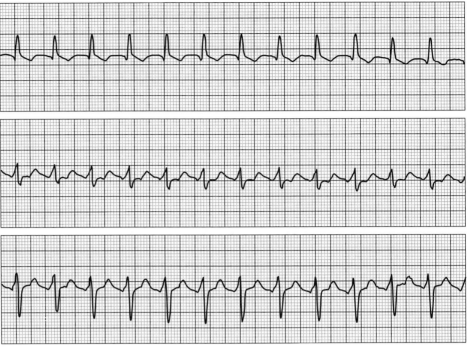

Figure SAII–16.

16. The patient is distressed but the pulse is regular, rate 115. What's really going on? How can you tell?

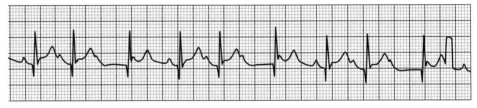

Figure SAII–17.

17. Irregular irregularity of the pulse. Cause?

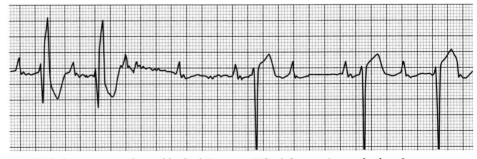

Figure SAII–18.

18. Wide beats, narrow beats, blocked P waves. What's happening and where?

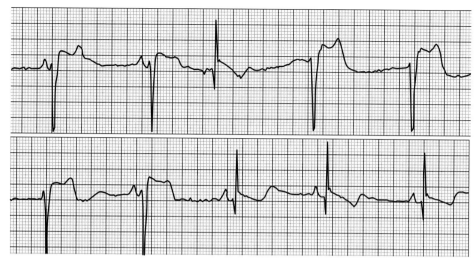

Figure SAII–19.

19. State of AV conduction? Block or no block? What's going on during the first seven beats, and what does it mean?

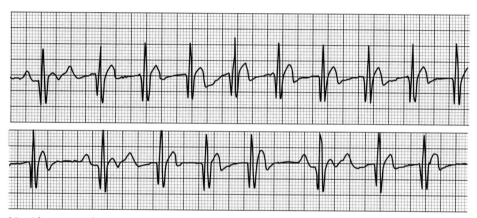

Figure SAII–20.

20. Almost-regular rate with occasional pauses. Diagnosis? Anatomic site of problem?

Answers

1. Complete AV block, localized in the AV node. Note all the criteria for complete block.
2. Coarse atrial fibrillation. Even though the fibrillary waves are large and regular for short periods, they're much too fast for flutter, and their rate and shape change if you look closely. Atrial rate in flutter will never be faster than 300 in the adult heart.
3. Atrial fibrillation with a high degree of heart block. The conducted beats are slightly irregular, indicating that the block isn't complete. Reentrant VPCs are present. Digitalis toxicity!
4. Atrial fibrillation interrupted by runs of accelerated idioventricular rhythm. This is benign and should cause the cardiologist only to look for long pauses in conduction that lead to the escape of the ventricular focus.
5. 2:1 AV block with bundle-branch block. The block could be localized in the AV node or in the other bundle branch, which could make it a variant of type II block. You can't make the distinction from this tracing alone.
6. Paroxysms of atrial flutter with two sinus beats.
7. Atrial flutter. Note the typical "sawtooth" atrial complexes in the wider R-R intervals in the middle of the strip.

8. Complete AV block. The wide complexes of the dissociated ventricular rhythm raise two possibilities: this could be AV nodal block with a junctional rhythm and bundle-branch block, *or* it could be bilateral bundle-branch block with an idioventricular rhythm—much more serious!

9. Mobitz-II block. Fixed P-R in two or more consecutive beats before the blocked P, same P-R after the blocked P as before, bundle-branch block. Typical. Additional feature: rate-dependent bundle-branch block. Pacemaker!

10. Atrial fibrillation, bundle-branch block, runs of junctional tachycardia producing the regular wide-beat rhythm. Occasional ventricular ectopic beats.

11. Again, very coarse flutter or flutter-fibrillation. Don't confuse this with true flutter. The changing morphology of the atrial complexes is the tip-off.

12. Atrial fibrillation with complete AV nodal block.

13. Paroxysms of atrial flutter with junctional rhythm between paroxysms.

14. Tricky. Atrial flutter with runs of completely dissociated junctional rhythm. Note regular ventricular rhythm with totally random relation of flutter waves to QRS—this is the same as a regular ventricular rhythm with a changing P-R: it equals dissociation. High degree of AV block, but the ventricular rate is too rapid to permit diagnosis of complete AV block. (Tracing courtesy of Dr. Frank Marcus.)

15. Mobitz-II block revealed during atrial pacing. Bundle-branch block with all the criteria for Mobitz-II block. Pacemaker!

16. 2:1 Atrial flutter. Note typical sawtooth configuration between ventricular complexes.

17. Wenckebach block. Three conducted beats with extreme prolongation of the last P-R; the blocked P is half hidden in the last QRS of the cycle. The QRS following the very prolonged P-R may in fact be a junctional escape beat, so that there would be two non-conducted P waves in each cycle.

18. V1. The first two beats show a typical Wenckebach progression with block of the third P wave. Right bundle-branch block is present; the pause after the blocked P reveals that the bundle-branch block is rate dependent. The fourth P wave is also blocked, and Wenckebach periods resume on the right-hand side of the strip. Diagnosis: AV nodal block with rate-dependent bundle-branch block.

19. The first, second, fourth, and fifth beats in the top strip and the first two beats in the bottom strip are clearly dissociated from the sinus P waves. Beat 3 in the top strip and the last three beats in the bottom strip are sinus beats. Thus, there is a basic sinus rhythm with periods of dissociation caused by the discharge of an idioventricular pacemaker. Is block present? Of course not, the sinus beats tell you that! *The reason for the intermittent dissociation is the slow sinus rate—about 42—which permits "escape" of the idioventricular focus.* Remember the last commandment in the diagnosis of complete heart block: "enough atrial impulses to probe all aspects of diastole."

20. Long Wenckebach runs with very gradual prolongation of P-R. The large deflection following the QRS is a P wave, and you can see it moving minutely closer to the preceding QRS with each beat until one P wave is finally blocked.

Eleven

Preexcitation

Preexcitation pathways, or bypass tracts, are strands of conducting tissue that have the capacity to bypass part or all of the atrioventricular (AV) conducting system. Let's start with two general statements:

> 1. **Bypass tracts can conduct very rapidly—more than 300 beats per minute in many cases.**
>
> 2. **Bypass tracts have no innervation. They are not affected by the sympathetic or parasympathetic systems or by drugs that work through those systems.**

There are three general classes of bypass tracts; if you understand how they're connected, you can reason out the electrocardiogram (ECG) configuration with each.

Wolff-Parkinson-White Conduction

Wolff-Parkinson-White (WPW) conduction was the first type of bypass tract to be described anatomically and electrocardiographically.

A bypass tract called the Kent bundle is located out in the AV groove, relatively far from the AV node (Fig. 11–1). The bypass tract completely "short-circuits" the AV node; because bypass tissue conducts rapidly, the P-R is short—less than 0.12 second in the adult heart. Thus, the short P-R interval is the first element in recognition of WPW preexcitation.

The bypass tract inserts in the bundle-branch system below the bifurcation of the bundle branches. This eccentric activation causes a deformity, or "slurring," of the initial part of the QRS as part of the impulse moves backward up toward the common bundle while the rest moves normally forward (see Fig. 11–1). This combination of events produces the typical slurred R wave or "delta-R" first described in WPW conduction. The slurring can also be a negative deflection, depending on what lead you're looking at, so the best term is *delta wave*.

The delta wave is a slowly inscribed deflection; it reflects the relatively slow retrograde force moving back up toward the common bundle. Often this wave collides with the normal antegrade impulse coming down through the AV node so that there's a kind of fusion. The delta wave may be larger or smaller, depending on where the fusion takes place. If the retrograde impulse travels all the way to the common bundle and "over the top" into the other side, the deflection is called the "full" preexcitation pattern.

Figure 11–2 is a typical example of WPW preexcitation. The short P-R and the delta wave are obvious, but from this strip alone, you can't localize the preexcitation.

The first attempt at anatomic localization of a bypass tract was relatively simple. If the bypass tract inserts in the *left* bundle, V1 will look like *right* bundle-branch block, except that the QRS will usually be narrower. There will be a typical delta-R wave leading into a broad R (Fig. 11–3). This was called type A WPW for the rather naïve reason that V1 looks like

Figure 11–1.
Anatomy of a Wolff-Parkinson-White bypass tract. AVN, atrioventricular node; "A" and "B," bypass tracts; HIS, His bundle.

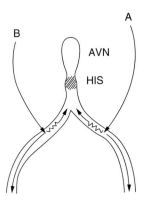

Figure 11–2.
Typical WPW preexcitation. Arrow indicates delta wave.

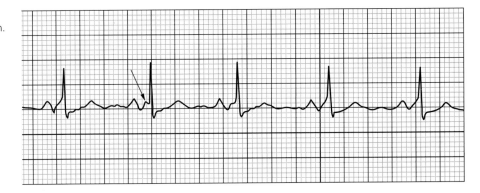

Figure 11–3.
Type A WPW. The wide, slurred initial part of the R wave is obvious across the precordial leads and in leads II, III, and aVF.

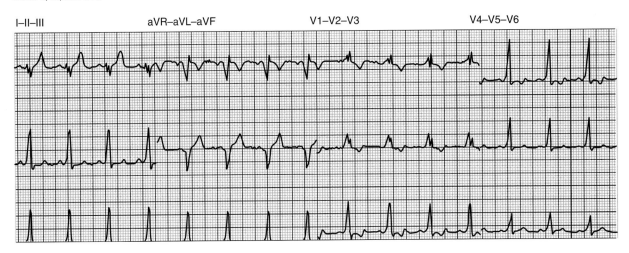

an "A." (The reason that preexcitation into the left bundle produces a right bundle-branch block pattern is elementary. When right bundle-branch block is present, the order of activation is first left ventricle, then right ventricle. When the left bundle is preexcited, of course, the same sequence follows: left ventricle first, right ventricle second.)

If the Kent bundle attaches to the right bundle, V1 will look like left bundle-branch block. The delta wave will be directed downward. The QRS won't usually be as wide as in left bundle-branch block, but it will consist of a broad S wave (Fig. 11–4). This is called type B WPW.

This elementary differentiation still has some validity. Modern studies have shown that when type A is present, the bypass tract often lies in the left posteroseptal area, whereas when type B is present, the connection lies anteriorly and rightward.

With the help of mapping techniques, it has become clear that the picture is much more complicated than everyone thought. In fact, at least 10 possible sites for AV bypass tracts have been identified, but the common feature in all is the short P-R interval with deformity of the first part of the QRS. At least 90% of the cases you will see will fit into the type A or type B category, and that's about as far as the clinical electrocardiographer needs to go. There have been attempts to localize the bypass tract more precisely by the orientation of the delta force, but they are relevant only if ablation is contemplated, at which point precise intracardiac mapping is necessary in any case. What the clinical electrocardiographer needs to recognize is preexcitation per se.

Lown-Ganong-Levine Preexcitation

Lown-Ganong-Levine (LGL) preexcitation may in fact be the most common form of pre-excitation. There's a short P-R interval with a *normal* QRS. How can this happen? Consider Figure 11–5A and B.

Remember that you can have a normal QRS only if the impulse comes from above, down the normal bundle-branch tract. In LGL preexcitation, that's exactly what happens. A special kind of bypass tract, called a *James fiber* (after Thomas James, the discoverer), connects the atria to the His bundle. There's a short P-R because the AV node has been bypassed, but conduction down through the ventricles is normal. The whole diagnosis depends on recognizing the short P-R interval (see Fig. 11–5B). That's why the magic minimum number of 0.12 second for normal AV conduction has to be burned into the electrocardiographer's brain. Some recent investigators have suggested that a short P-R may be simply a normal variant, but a P-R like the one in Figure 11–5B cannot be the result of anything but LGL preexcitation—always assuming you've made sure those are normal sinus P waves and have thus ruled out a junctional rhythm.

Figure 11–4.
Type B WPW. Note the wide, downward deflection in V1 with slurring of the initial part of the complex. The slurring is the delta wave, here seen as a negative deflection. The delta wave is clearly visible in leads I and II and V3 to V6.

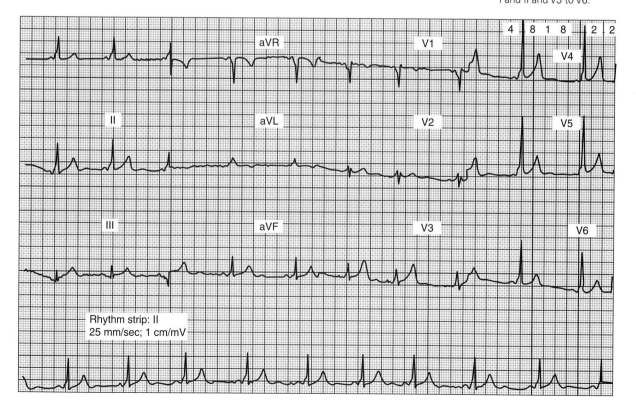

Rhythm strip: II
25 mm/sec; 1 cm/mV

Figure 11–5.
LGL type of preexcitation. **A**, The bypass tract, probably a James fiber, connects the atria to the His bundle. The activating impulse follows a normal course down through the bundle-branch system. As a result, there is a short P-R interval, and the QRS is normal. **B**, The P-R is about 0.09 second, and the QRS is 0.08 second.

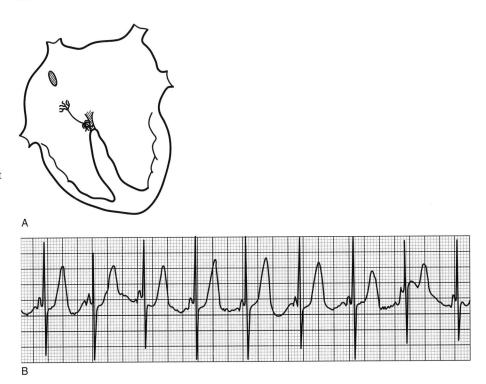

A

B

Mahaim Fiber Preexcitation

Figure 11–6 illustrates another type of preexcitation, caused by small "jump" or "short-circuit" fibers described by Mahaim. They may connect the AV node or the His bundle directly to the bundle-branch system. In either case, there will be a typical delta wave and usually some degree of P-R shortening. If a Mahaim fiber originates low in the His, however, the P-R may be within the limits of normal, and the only hint of preexcitation will be the delta wave. In this case, you could only suspect preexcitation, but you couldn't prove it from the surface ECG.

Why Is Preexcitation Important?

Preexcitation and Arrhythmias

With a bypass tract, there is a perfect setup for a "circus" movement. An impulse can come down the bypass tract and back up the AV node, around and around in a self-perpetuating circuit. It can also go the other way around, down the AV node and back up the bypass tract (Fig. 11–7A and B). In either case, there will be a *paroxysmal supraventricular tachycardia*. Patients with bypass tracts may have recurrent paroxysms of supraventricular tachycardia because they have the anatomic setup for it.

Figure 11–6.
Mahaim fibers. As indicated, these are usually short tracts that can lead from the AV node (AVN) or the His bundle (HIS) to some part of the bundle-branch system.

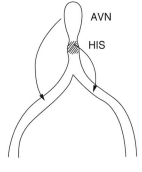

AVN

HIS

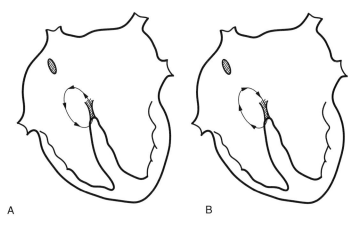

Figure 11–7.
Mechanisms of paroxysmal tachycardia. **A,** Antidromic bypass tract. Circuit is down the bypass tract and back through the AV node. The QRS will be abnormal with a typical delta wave. **B,** Orthodromic bypass tract. Circuit is down the AV node and back through the bypass tract. The QRS will be normal.

If there is WPW preexcitation, you can tell which way the impulse is traveling by looking at the ECG. If the impulse is coming down the bypass tract, there will be a typical deformed QRS with a delta wave (Fig. 11–8). If the impulse comes down the AV node, the QRS will be normal. Just by looking at the ECG during the tachycardia, you can't tell that there was a bypass tract (Fig. 11–9).

With the LGL type of preexcitation, the QRS complexes are normal, and the tachycardia will look like any other paroxysmal supraventricular tachycardia.

Moral: When a patient has recurrent paroxysmal tachycardia, you have to consider preexcitation whether the QRS complexes show a delta-R or not.

Bypass Tracts with Atrial Fibrillation

(This book is primarily about diagnosis, not treatment, but in this specific setting, the two are so closely intertwined that they have to be considered together.)

The slow conduction of the AV is often lifesaving. That's especially true in atrial fibrillation, as we pointed out in Chapter 9. The AV node protects the ventricles from being bombarded 425 times a minute by the impulses from the fibrillating atria. When there's a bypass tract, that protection is weakened. The bypass tract can conduct very rapidly, up to

V1–V2–V3

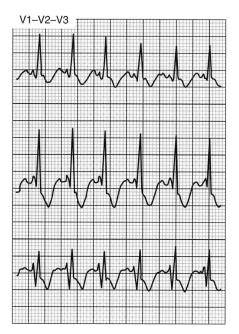

Figure 11–8.
Paroxysmal tachycardia in a patient with type A preexcitation. The activating impulse is coming down the bypass tract, producing the wide, deformed QRS.

Figure 11–9.
Paroxysmal tachycardia in a patient with type B WPW. The activating impulse is coming down the AV node, producing a normal QRS. Just by looking at this tracing, you can't tell there was a bypass tract.

300 times a minute. The heart would race itself to death if this happened for very long. The only reason it doesn't is that some impulses come down the AV node and make the ventricular tissues refractory to the impulses from the bypass tract. Thus, there is a kind of "competition" between the AV node and the bypass tract: the AV node acts as a "brake" on the bypass tract and keeps it from driving the ventricles into a disaster (Fig. 11–10).

How can you tell there's preexcitation when the patient is fibrillating? After all, there are no P waves to measure from. There are two clues. First, there may be typical delta waves with

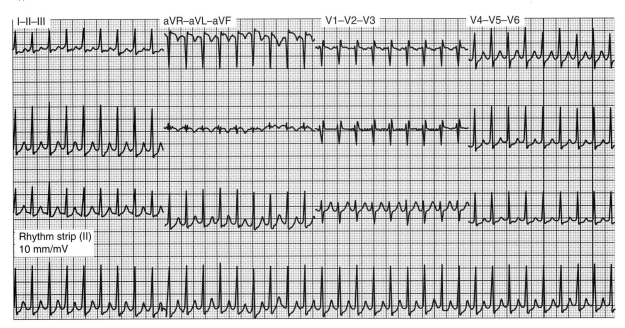

Figure 11–10.
Atrial fibrillation in the presence of a bypass tract. Note dual pathways from atria to ventricles, one down the AV nodal path and one down the bypass tract. The impulses that come down the AV node will make the conducting tissues refractory to some of the impulses from the bypass tract. Thus, the AV node acts as a brake on the bypass tract, which could otherwise drive the heart at a rate that might well be fatal. Drugs like digitalis and verapamil that depress conduction through the AV node without affecting the bypass tract can be lethal in this situation.

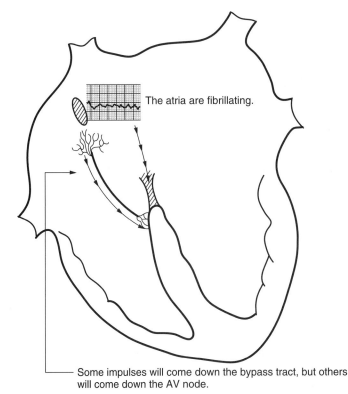

The atria are fibrillating.

Some impulses will come down the bypass tract, but others will come down the AV node.

deformed QRS complexes (Fig. 11–11). Second, you can get a pretty good idea from the rate. *Bypass tracts conduct rapidly.* They conduct faster than the AV node could possibly conduct.

1. **If you see R-R intervals equal to a rate of 300 (one large square apart), you can be certain there's a bypass tract.**

2. **If you see R-R intervals equal to a rate of 280 or more, you can make the diagnosis of a bypass tract with about 99% confidence.**

3. **If you see many R-R intervals equal to a rate of more than 250, you should be very suspicious of a bypass tract (Fig. 11–12; see also Fig. 11–11).**

Detecting a bypass tract in the presence of atrial fibrillation can be of life-and-death importance. Why? Simple. The first drug you think of when you treat atrial fibrillation is digitalis. Digitalis slows conduction through the AV node but has no effect on bypass tracts. If you depress AV nodal conduction with digitalis, you remove the "brake," and the bypass tract can run wild. The heart rate can race into a catastrophe.

The same thing is true of verapamil, beta-blocking drugs, and many calcium-blocking drugs. They depress the AV node without affecting the bypass tract. With any of these drugs, the resulting rapid rate can produce congestive heart failure or a fatal arrhythmia.

The only safe drugs to use in this setting are quinidine and procainamide. They both depress conduction through the bypass tract. They are the only safe drugs that do. The 1-C

Figure 11–11.
Atrial fibrillation with type A WPW. Besides the wide, slurred QRS complexes, the preexcitation is obvious in the rate. Note the R-R interval indicated by an arrow; it's equivalent to a rate of 300.

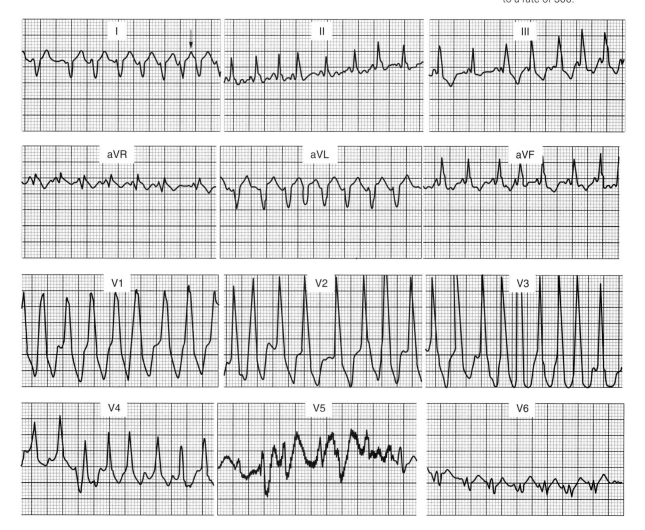

drugs encainide and flecainide are excellent for depressing bypass tract conduction, but they're so dangerous that encainide isn't even on the market anymore. Flecainide could be used in an otherwise healthy patient, but it's excessively dangerous if there's any depression of AV function.

Moral: Whenever you confront a new case of atrial fibrillation, look for the signs of pre-excitation—the delta-R or the rapid rate (or both). If there is any suspicion of preexcitation, don't use digitalis or verapamil until you have carried out a simple test that will tell you with 100% accuracy whether preexcitation is present or not.

Test? What test? This test can be carried out in any emergency room or clinic where there's an ECG machine. It's based on the fact that bypass tracts have no nerve supply. If you stimulate the vagus, you may slow conduction through the AV node, but you won't affect the bypass tract.

1. **Stimulate the vagus by carotid massage. If the rate slows, there's no bypass tract. If the rate speeds, a bypass tract is present. Think about it for a moment and you'll see how it works.**

2. **If carotid sinus stimulation is ineffective, administer adenosine. Adenosine slows AV nodal conduction but has no effect on bypass tissue. Use the same logic as above.**

In either case, be sure to keep a rhythm strip running all the time and watch for changes in rate.

Note: Administration of adenosine during atrial fibrillation to rule out a bypass tract is an excellent and very specific maneuver, but it's not harmless. During the 6 seconds or so of AV nodal blockade that is induced by adenosine, the bypass tract can drive the ventricles into fibrillation; this has already been recorded in two case reports when the patients were only saved by prompt defibrillation. When administering adenosine to rule out preexcitation during atrial fibrillation, always have a defibrillator on standby!

Bypass Tracts and "Artificial" QRS Deformity

The odd initial force, or delta wave, can show up in some leads as a negative deflection, or Q wave. People with perfectly normal hearts may be told they've had a myocardial infarct when all they have is preexcitation (Figs. 11–13 and 11–14).

Figure 11–12.
Examples of atrial fibrillation with preexcitation. The QRS complexes are normal, but the very rapid rate is the clue. Many R-R intervals are equivalent to rates over 250, which makes preexcitation probable. LGL preexcitation was in fact present in these cases.

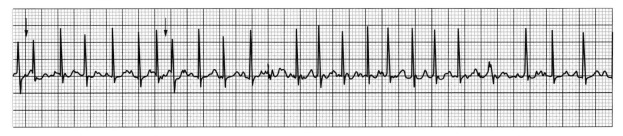

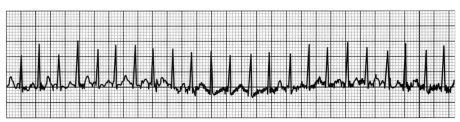

The bypass tract may attach so far down the bundle branch that it produces a full-blown bundle-branch block pattern (Fig. 11–15).

What do you do if you find preexcitation in a routine ECG? Another simple answer. If the patient is asymptomatic, you don't do anything. You inform the patient that this congenital "short circuit" is present because the knowledge might be helpful if tachycardia or fibrillation appeared. Beyond that you do nothing. You don't frighten the patient, because the chances of a serious complication are 1:40,000 in an otherwise normal individual! (Some enthusiasts recently recommended that all patients with preexcitation undergo exhaustive invasive testing. They were roundly rebuked by competent authorities, and certainly there are no data to support such an approach. Don't subject patients to stress, fear, pain, and expense for an anomaly that will probably never mean a thing.) Figures 11–16, 11–17, 11–18, 11–19, and 11–20 are typical examples of preexcitation in various settings.

Figure 11–13.
"Pathologic" Q waves in aVF are really upside-down delta waves. The clue is the presence of obvious delta waves in other leads.

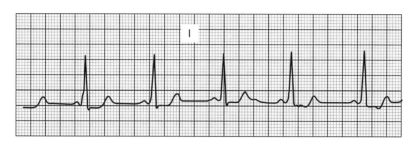

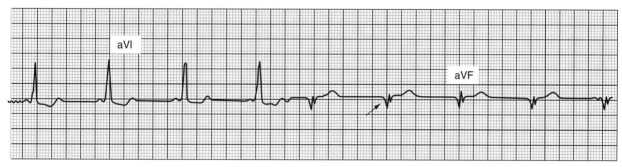

Figure 11–14.
"Pathologic" Q wave in aVL. (This is another one of those leads you'll learn about in Chapter 17, Myocardial Infarction). The obvious delta R waves in II, III, and aVF reveal that this supposed Q wave is simply an inverted delta wave.

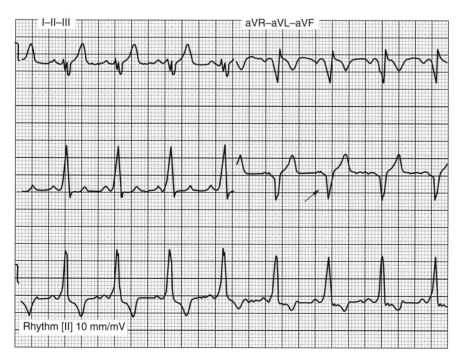

Rhythm [II] 10 mm/mV

Figure 11–15.
Intermittent WPW preexcitation producing a pattern like bundle-branch block. The obvious clue is the short P-R interval of the wide beats. The bypass tract must insert far down the bundle branch to produce this kind of pattern.

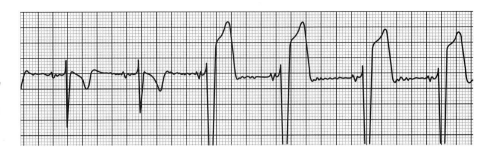

Figure 11–16.
Intermittent WPW. The wide QRS complexes represent WPW preexcitation; the narrow beats with inverted P waves are actually ectopic atrial beats with normal conduction.

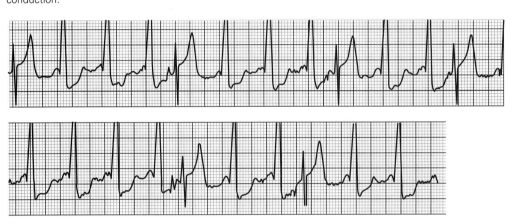

Figure 11–17.
Intermittent WPW with occasional normally conducted beats. This would be very easy to confuse with bundle-branch block, but the short P-R is the clue to the diagnosis, as well as the appearance of occasional normally conducted beats.

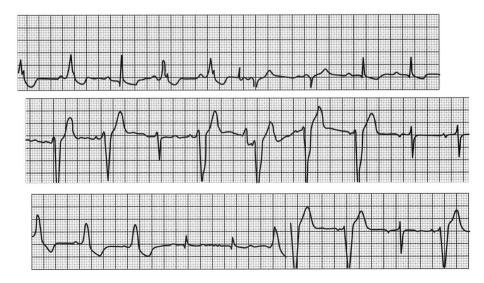

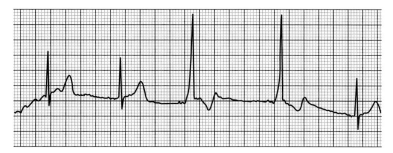

Figure 11–18.
Normal sinus rhythm interrupted by two WPW beats.

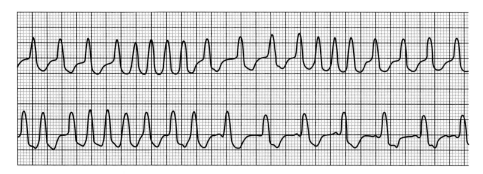

Figure 11–19.
Atrial fibrillation with WPW. Note the short runs of beats with a rate approximating 300 as well as the wide, deformed QRS complexes.

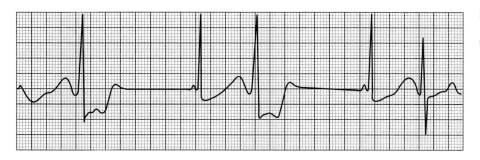

Figure 11–20.
LGL preexcitation with ventricular ectopic beats.

Note that in Figs. 11–15, 11–16, 11–17, 11–18, and 11–20, the preexcitation is intermittent. I find that this observation often comes as a surprise to physicians in training, but in fact, intermittent preexcitation is very common. *Moral:* Whenever you see mixtures of wide and narrow QRS complexes, look carefully at the P-R of the assorted beats to see if the wide complexes represent preexcitation!

Twelve

Fascicular Beats and Fascicular Tachycardia

For years, electrocardiographers were puzzled by the problem of the "narrow" ventricular premature contraction (VPC). Look at the ectopic beat in Figure 12–1. It looks like a VPC in every respect except that it's too narrow to qualify. This ectopic beat is about 0.10 to 0.11 second wide, whereas a real VPC should always be at least 0.12 second wide. Note the extreme left axis of the same ectopic beat: it's about −60 degrees.

The first thing everybody noticed about these narrow VPCs was that all had an extreme left or right axis. Another feature quickly became apparent; it's illustrated in Figures 12–2 and 12–3. In each of these tracings, the ectopic beat has an extreme right axis—about +120 to +130 degrees. If you look at V1 in each tracing, you'll notice one or more ectopic beats with an incomplete right bundle-branch block pattern. One explanation for these odd beats was that they were junctional beats that followed a different course through the ventricles because of their off-center origin.

Electrophysiologic studies, however, have demonstrated that, at least in many cases, these beats arise in a branch of the left bundle branch. Remember that the functional elements of the left bundle are called *fascicles*. Ectopic beats can originate in these fascicles. Cells high in the fascicles of the bundle-branch system may take on the characteristics of pacemaker cells and start generating beats. Because these beats are traveling down the specialized conducting cells of the bundle branches at 4 m/second, they move faster than ventricular ectopic beats moving "backward" through the subendocardium. That's why they're narrow.

A beat that arises in the posterior fascicle will naturally have an extreme left axis because that's where the posterior fascicle conducts. Anterior fascicular beats will have an extreme right axis for the same reason: because the fascicular impulse moves swiftly down the left ventricular network and invades the right bundle network before the retrograde impulse can travel backward up across the common bundle and into the right bundle branch. At that point, the right bundle branch, of course, will be refractory because of the retrograde stimulation (Fig. 12–4).

For a long time, this was nothing more than a curiosity, interesting only to investigators. Then observers began to notice tachycardias like the ones shown in Figures 12–5 and 12–6. These are wide-beat tachycardias with all the electrocardiogram (ECG) characteristics of paroxysmal ventricular tachycardia.

However, the ventricular complexes show a right bundle-branch block configuration with an extreme left axis. This tachycardia is clinically different from any other ventricular tachycardia. It usually appears in relatively young, otherwise healthy individuals, and it never causes catastrophic symptoms—that is, the patient doesn't collapse or go into shock. The usual complaints will be palpitation or breathlessness and apprehension.

This is the only wide-beat tachycardia you can treat with verapamil. It's perfectly safe in this specific form of tachycardia, and it usually stops the arrhythmia. In any other form of ventricular tachycardia, verapamil will probably cause ventricular flutter or fibrillation. Use of verapamil in any other type of ventricular tachycardia is malpractice. With this specific ECG configuration, it's perfectly safe and usually effective.

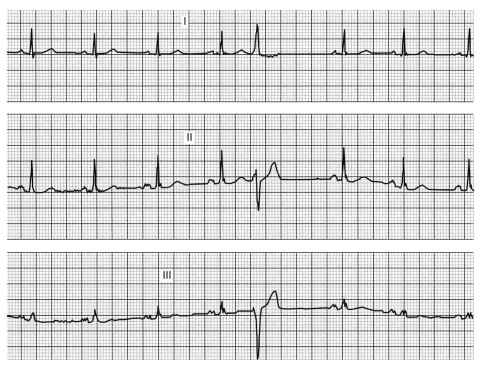

Figure 12–1.
Note the slightly narrow VPC with an extreme left axis. For years, these beats were a puzzle.

Figure 12–2.
Note the "narrow" ectopic beats (*arrowheads*). They are not preceded by P waves, and they have a completely different QRST shape from the sinus beats, but they're not as wide as ordinary VPCs. They have an extreme right axis and an incomplete right bundle-branch block configuration in V1.

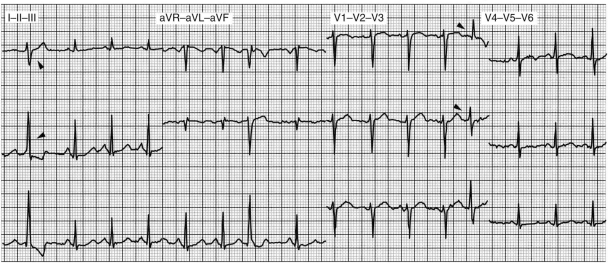

Rhythm [II] 10 mm/mV

This peculiar tachycardia is probably *fascicular*—that is, it arises in the posterior fascicle of the left bundle branch, producing the typical right bundle–left axis configuration. It's caused by accelerated automatic discharge of an ectopic focus rather than by a reentry circuit, the way most paroxysmal tachycardias are, hence the difference in prognosis and treatment.

Curious fact: When you administer verapamil for this type of tachycardia, the rate will slow progressively (e.g., 180–160–140–120–90–sinus). This is completely different from the all-or-nothing response of the common reentrant tachycardias and reflects the difference in the cause of the arrhythmia.

A combination of extreme right axis with right bundle-branch block almost certainly means an anterior fascicular tachycardia, but to date very few cases have been reported. Figure 12–7 is an example.

Figure 12–3.
Same phenomenon.
Ectopic beats about 0.09
second wide, extreme
right axis, incomplete right
bundle-branch block
pattern in V1.

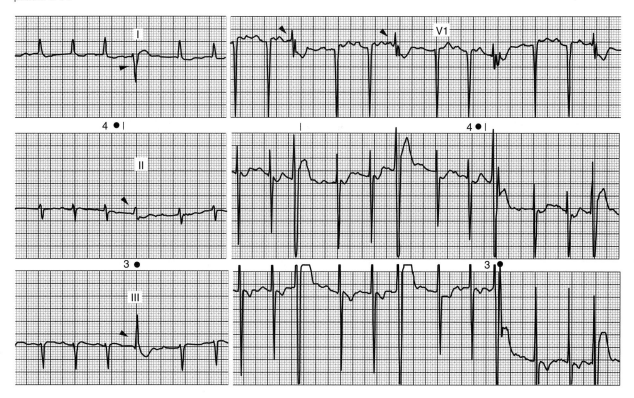

Figure 12–4.
Mechanism of fascicular
ectopic beats. **A,** Beat
arises in the posterior (left)
fascicle of the left bundle
at point A. It is conducted
leftward along the
posterior fascicle, causing
an extreme left axis. **B,**
There is slow retrograde
conduction into the right
bundle. **C,** As a result,
some variety of right
bundle-branch delay will be
present.

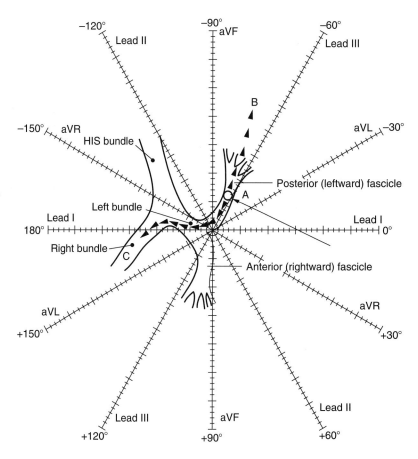

Note that when this kind of tachycardia arises in a patient with a compromised left ventricle, of course, it can be life-threatening simply because of the rapid, inefficient beating rather than because of the possibility of progression to a fatal arrhythmia.

More recent electrophysiologic studies have proved that these tachycardias are indeed fascicular. When the right bundle–left axis pattern is present, they originate in the posterior

Figure 12–5.
Wide-beat tachycardia with extreme left axis and V1 configuration mimicking right bundle-branch block.

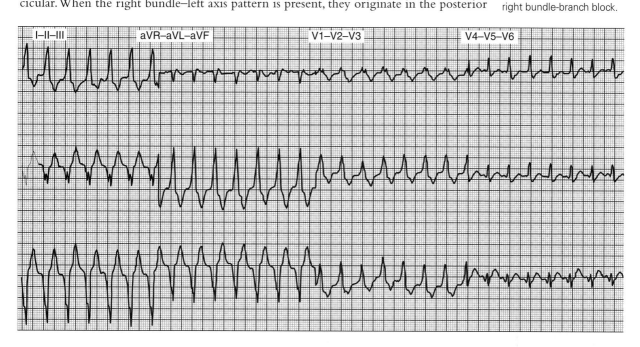

Figure 12–6.
Another wide-beat tachycardia with extreme left axis and a right bundle-branch block pattern in V1. In both these cases, the patient's blood pressure remained normal, and there was no serious hemodynamic compromise. Both responded to verapamil.

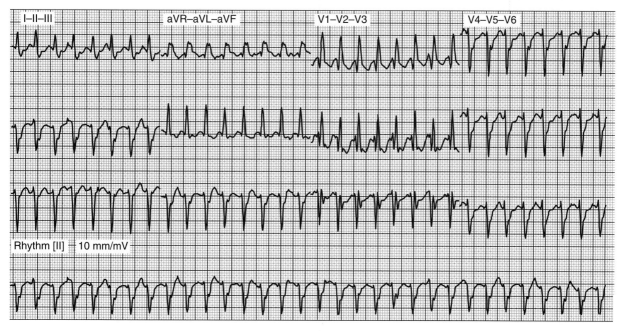

fascicle of the branch, exactly as one would have predicted from the ECG configuration. Another related type of ventricular tachycardia presents with a left bundle-branch pattern commonly with extreme inferior (rightward) axis deviation. This has been shown to originate in the outflow tract of the right ventricle.

Both types of tachycardia are lumped under the title of *idiopathic ventricular tachycardia* because they both appear in otherwise normal hearts. In response to treatment, however, the two types of tachycardia are radically different. As noted earlier, the right bundle–left axis variety responds to verapamil, and it does so in a way that is unique: instead of an abrupt ending of the tachycardia, there is stepwise reduction in rate until the tachycardia disappears. The left bundle-branch variety, however, responds to any of the usual drugs in the usual all-or-nothing manner. Class I agents like lidocaine, quinidine, or procainamide; beta blockers; sotalol; and amiodarone are all moderately effective, and when treatment is successful, the tachycardia stops at once.

These and other data suggest that the two varieties of idiopathic ventricular tachycardia have a different mechanism. The right bundle–left axis variety is probably the result of enhanced automatic firing from a single focus, whereas the left bundle–right axis variety is probably the result of a small reentry circuit or "triggered" after depolarizations.

Prognosis and Treatment

Prognosis in these tachycardias is excellent. They *never* progress to ventricular fibrillation, they *never* compromise circulation seriously, and they have no association with cardiac sudden death. In a rare case, they may be recurrent or persistent, and as a result, symptoms may be troublesome or even disabling.

Treatment in these cases is simple and specific—ablation! A skilled EP physician can locate the focus in the bundle-branch system and ablate it. Results are excellent. (Don't even consider anything else.)

Figure 12–7.
Wide-beat tachycardia with right bundle-branch block pattern and extreme right axis. This is probably a fascicular tachycardia arising in the anterior fascicle of the left bundle, but data on this configuration are still sparse.

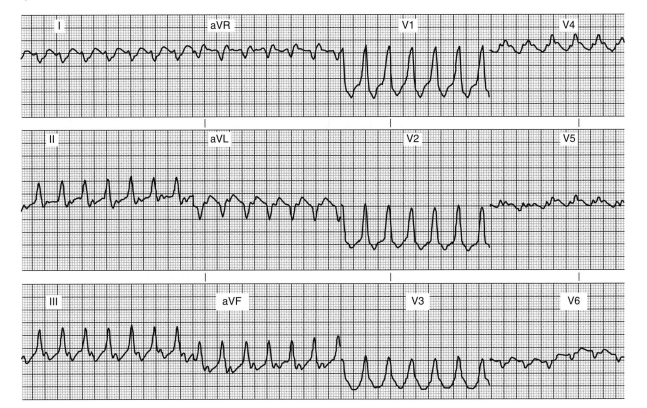

Thirteen

Concealed Conduction, Exit Block, Bundle-Branch Wenckebach, and Supernormal Conduction

Concealed conduction and exit block are two conditions you can't actually see on the surface electrocardiogram (ECG); these are diagnoses you have to make in the great Sherlock Holmes manner by finding the only possible explanation for what's happening. They are definite entities, not flights of theoretical fancy; both abnormalities have been certified by electrophysiologic study, and they're both important clinically.

Bundle-branch Wenckebach and supernormal conduction are both easy to recognize in the ECG, but they're very rare and often escape detection because physicians don't know they exist.

ECG Recognition of Concealed Conduction

Remember that conduction through the AV node is "silent"; that is, it doesn't produce any deflection on the surface ECG. Normally, you measure conduction through the atrioventricular (AV) node by measuring the P-R interval, but sometimes the AV node is only partially penetrated. This can happen from above or below; that is, either sinus beats or ventricular ectopic beats can penetrate some distance into the AV node without going all the way through. How can you tell this has happened? Usually, it's simple. The AV nodal tissues are unusually refractory when the next impulse comes along. This tells you they must have been partly penetrated and discharged.

The simplest example of concealed conduction into the AV node is what happens after a ventricular premature contraction (VPC). Often, the VPC will penetrate the AV node without penetrating all the way through to the atria. The next sinus beat will find the tissues fatigued, and the first P-R after a VPC may be prolonged. Figure 13–1 is an excellent example.

There are VPCs appearing every other beat, and the P-R of the sinus impulses is prolonged (0.29 second). When the VPCs were eradicated with lidocaine, the P-R interval became normal. Obviously, the VPCs were sending an impulse up into the AV node that

Figure 13–1.
Concealed conduction into the AV node from VPCs. The concealed conduction made the AV node refractory and produced the prolonged P-R. When the VPCs were eliminated, the P-R went back to normal.

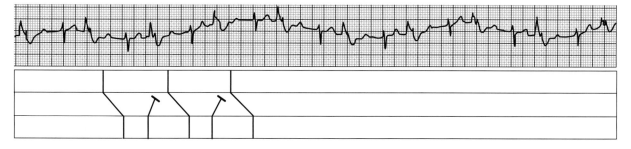

penetrated far enough into the nodal tissues to make them refractory when the next sinus impulse came along.

Figure 13–2 illustrates concealed conduction in the presence of a dissociated junctional rhythm. In the first part of the tracing, there is a junctional rhythm with dissociated P waves that come farther and farther after the QRS with each beat. After the third QRS, there is an abrupt pause in the junctional rhythm, and then it resumes.

The ladder diagram shows what happened. The sinus impulse came *so long after the junctional beat* that it found the upper nodal tissues out of their refractory state and was able to penetrate the AV node far enough to reach the site of the junctional pacemaker and discharge it. That's why there's a pause in the junctional rhythm. This is *concealed conduction* with "reset" of a junctional pacemaker. None of the sinus impulses reaches the ventricles because they arrive at the AV node when the cells below the site of the junctional pacemaker are still refractory.

Figures 13–3 and 13–4 provide another example of the same phenomenon. In Figure 13–3, there is a dissociated junctional rhythm: after the second QRS, the P wave comes late enough to find the AV nodal tissues ready to conduct, and the sinus impulse "captures" the ventricles for one beat.

In Figure 13–4, the same thing happens, except this time, the sinus impulse doesn't get all the way to the ventricles. It does penetrate as far as the junctional pacemaker and resets it, causing the obvious pause. Thus, you see concealed conduction into the AV node. You

Figure 13–2.
Concealed conduction in the presence of a dissociated junctional rhythm. When the sinus impulse comes a sufficiently long time after the junctional beat, it finds the upper AV nodal tissue out of its refractory period. The sinus impulse penetrates to the site of the ectopic junctional pacemaker and resets it; hence, the pause. The lower AV nodal tissues are refractory, so there's no conduction to the ventricles—just the pause in the junctional rhythm.

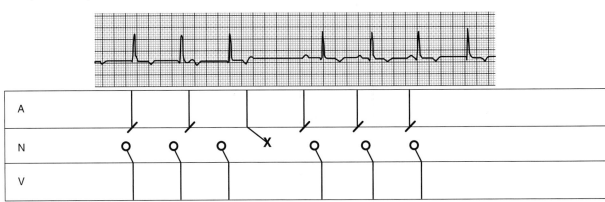

Figure 13–3.
A dissociated junctional rhythm with one capture beat by the sinus node (the third beat on the strip).

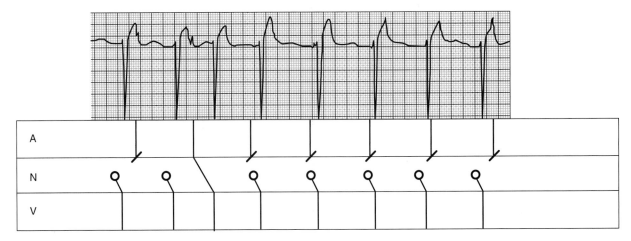

know it happened because there's a pause in the junctional rhythm, and the pause takes place every time the P wave comes a critical distance *after* the junctional beat, so that the nodal tissues have recovered enough to permit penetration to the site of the ectopic pacemaker.

These last two examples of concealed conduction are important because they tell you that *the AV block in each case is not complete*. How do you know? Simple. The sinus node can penetrate to the site of the junctional pacemaker and reset it. The junctional pacemaker can obviously reach the ventricles, because it does so most of the time. Therefore, there is a potential functioning track from atria to ventricles. It's only a matter of timing.

Concealed conduction can also take place in the bundle-branch system, but this is usually not significant in clinical terms. On the other hand, concealed conduction in the AV node, as in the examples given earlier, can be very significant indeed for the clinician trying to evaluate AV block.

Exit Block

You're familiar with block in the AV node and in the bundle-branch system. Now picture a kind of block in the tissue around the various pacemakers of the heart.

Start with the sinus node. The sinus node consists of two kinds of cells: the cells that form the activating impulse and those that conduct it out to the atria (Fig. 13–5). The activating impulse can encounter block in those conducting cells, just the way it can encounter block lower down, in the AV system. The difference is that this time you can't see the impulse in the activating cells; you can see it only when it reaches the atria and starts to form a P wave. This kind of block is called *exit block* because it keeps the impulse from making its exit into the conducting tissues. You can tell there's block because suddenly a P wave doesn't appear.

Figure 13–4.
Concealed penetration of the AV node by the sinus impulse. At X, the sinus impulse penetrates to the site of the junctional pacemaker but doesn't penetrate the lower AV node to reach the ventricles. The evidence of the concealed conduction is the pause in the junctional rhythm.

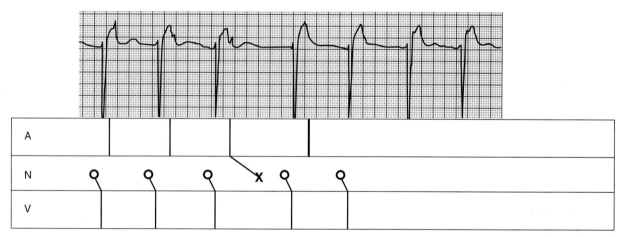

Figure 13–5.
Diagram of pacemaker and conducting cells of the sinus node.

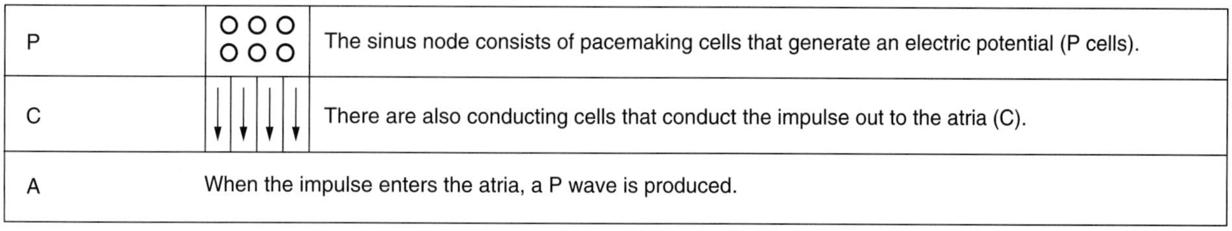

P	○ ○ ○ ○ ○ ○	The sinus node consists of pacemaking cells that generate an electric potential (P cells).
C	↓ ↓ ↓ ↓ ↓	There are also conducting cells that conduct the impulse out to the atria (C).
A		When the impulse enters the atria, a P wave is produced.

Failure of conduction in the "C" cells of the sinus node produces "exit block," preventing the sinus impulse from reaching the atria. This can take several forms.

In the classic type of sinoatrial exit block, there's a sudden pause equal to exactly twice the basic rate because the pacing cells of the sinus node go on firing normally. The problem is that one impulse doesn't reach the atria to form a P wave. The next impulse comes in right on time, so the pause equals a double interval, just like the pause in Mobitz-II block (Fig. 13–6).

Figure 13–7 illustrates typical exit block around the ectopic atrial pacemaker during paroxysmal atrial tachycardia (PAT) with block. Note that the pause is an exact double interval of the basic atrial rate. (This was the first case of its kind recorded; I was fortunate enough to run across it in our laboratory back in the early 1960s.)

Figure 13–8 illustrates the Wenckebach type of exit block around the sinus node. This is a 3:2 ratio of conduction. Two pacing impulses reach the atria and produce P waves, but the third one is blocked. Therefore, you see two P waves with pause. You know there's a Wenckebach type of exit block *because the pause is less than twice the basic rate*. Remember, that's typical of type I block.

Figure 13–6.
Sinoatrial exit block with pauses that are precise multiples of the basic rate.

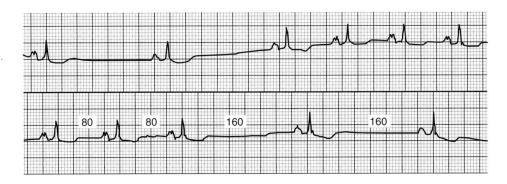

Figure 13–7.
Exit block around the ectopic atrial pacemaker during PAT with block.

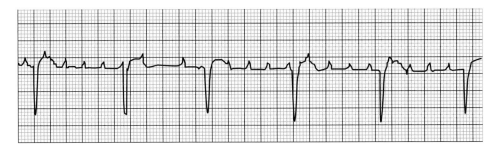

Figure 13–8.
Sinoatrial exit block, Wenckebach type, with 3:2 conduction to the atria.

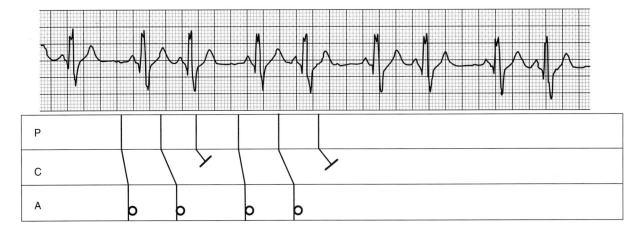

Accelerated idioventricular rhythms are common. So is exit block around the cells that cause the rhythm, down in the ventricular subendocardium. The block will most commonly be Wenckebach, or type I. You'll remember that another characteristic of type I AV nodal block is that as the P-R interval grows longer, the R-R interval, paradoxically, grows shorter. Of course that's because although the P-R grows longer, the *amount of increase* is progressively smaller with each beat. P-R values might run 0.16 to 0.24 to 0.26 to 0.27 in a typical Wenckebach cycle. The same thing happens when there's type I block in the tissues around an ectopic ventricular focus—you'll see a shortening R-R interval, typical of type I block (Figs. 13–9 and 13–10).

When you see a pause, it may be less than double the R-R interval of the beats ahead of the pause, exactly like the pause after a blocked P wave in AV nodal Wenckebach (see Fig. 13–10, top strip). In the bottom strip of Figure 13–10, the progressive shortening of R-R in the four-beat runs of ventricular beats leaves no question that there's an exit Wenckebach block around the ectopic focus. (The pause here is longer than you'd expect with a typical AV nodal Wenckebach, but the time required for an ectopic focus to "recharge" and start firing again doesn't always fit a precise pattern.)

Bundle-Branch Wenckebach and Supernormal Conduction

Figure 13–11 illustrates two rare phenomena that can be confusing if you don't understand them. Here and there through the strip, you see an obvious bundle-branch block. (It's lead I,

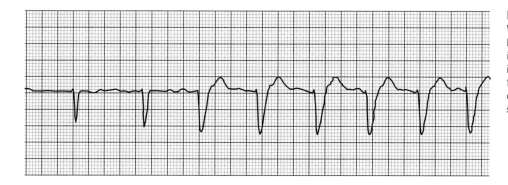

Figure 13–9.
Wenckebach type of exit block around an idioventricular focus interrupting atrial fibrillation. Note characteristic progressive shortening of R-R.

Figure 13–10.
Variable periods of Wenckebach exit block around an idioventricular focus.

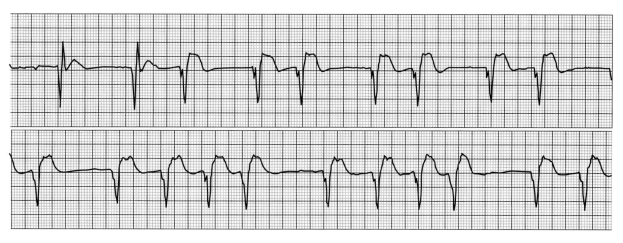

Figure 13–11.

Combination of rate-dependent left bundle-branch block, Wenckebach periods within the left bundle branch and supernormal conduction in the left bundle branch.

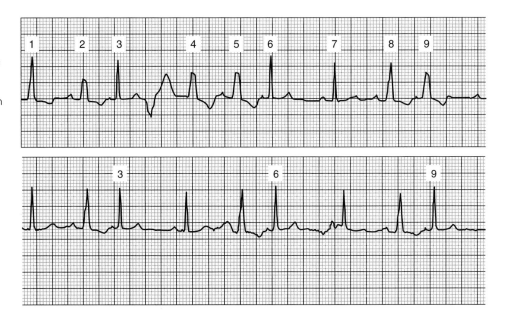

so it has to be left bundle-branch block.) In the first beat on the left (1), you see intraventricular conduction delay but not a full-blown bundle-branch block. Beat 2 is left bundle-branch block, and beat 3 is a normal QRS! The interval between the left bundle-branch block beat and the normal beat is short. The normal beat in fact comes early because it's a premature atrial contraction (PAC). Next you have a VPC followed by two left bundle-branch block beats (4 and 5) and another PAC *with a normal QRS* (6). After this second PAC, there's a pause and the next beat is normal (7).

Now you can begin drawing conclusions. First, beat 7 tells you that rate-dependent bundle-branch block is present because the normal QRS appears after a pause. Next look at beats 8 and 9. Beat 8 is wider than 7, but it's not a full-blown bundle-branch block. In beat 9, you see complete bundle-branch block. In other words, *there's a progression from incomplete to complete left bundle-branch block*. Look at the last six beats on the bottom strip, and you see the same thing. There's progressive widening of the QRS until there's complete left bundle-branch block in the last three beats. These are Wenckebach periods within the left bundle. The impulse is conducted with progressive slowing, with more widening of the QRS until it isn't conducted at all. At that point, complete bundle-branch block appears. So far, so good; everything is reasonable. Now you see all the rules broken. Look at beats 3 and 6 in the top strip and beats 3, 6, and 9 in the bottom strip. They're PACs. They come early—but the QRS is normal. The left bundle-branch block has disappeared! You can't explain the narrow QRS on the basis of rate; the bundle-branch block appears at a rate of 90 and up, but the R-R interval ahead of the narrow beat is equivalent to a rate of 150. You can't explain the narrow beat on an Ashman basis because the R-R relation is exactly opposite to what you would expect. You can't invoke bradycardia-dependent aberrancy to explain the left bundle-branch block because the narrow beats, like beat 7 in the top strip, also come after a long pause. The only explanation for these narrow beats is the *supernormal phase of conduction.* This is a rare bird, but here it is. Just after the T wave, there is sometimes a phase of supernormal conduction when you see conduction through tissues that are usually blocked—the left bundle in this case.

There's still no good electrophysiologic explanation, but the fact that it does occur is indisputable. Supernormal conduction probably occurs only in bundle-branch tissues. You will usually see it with rate-dependent bundle-branch block and bundle-branch Wenckebach periods, as in this example. In this setting, you may see an early beat with normal conduction that you can't explain on any of the usual bases of intraventricular conduction. You have to invoke supernormal conduction. Although this phenomenon is described in all serious works on arrhythmias, it isn't even mentioned in the current major textbooks of cardiology. Pity.

Note to all residents and fellows: You hereby have my permission to copy this tracing and spring it on the attending at morning report. Do it with a casual air, saying something like "Obvious, but interesting, don't you think?" (theory and practice of roundsmanship!).

Fourteen

Fatal Arrhythmias: Ventricular Fibrillation, Ventricular Flutter, Torsade, R-on-T Phenomenon, Standstill

Two arrhythmias can be instantly fatal: ventricular fibrillation and ventricular standstill. They're so simple to recognize that they hardly need any discussion.

Ventricular Fibrillation

When the ventricles fibrillate, the electrocardiogram (ECG) records a disorganized set of deflections. These may be large or small, fine or coarse. Of course, there aren't any P waves. These deflections are an accurate picture of what's going on in the heart muscle. When you look at a fibrillating heart or hold it in your hand, it's obvious that the muscle is quivering like a dying sea creature. There's absolutely no pumping activity of any kind (Figs. 14–1 and 14–2).

Ventricular Flutter

This is in fact a form of ventricular fibrillation that can be deceptive on the ECG. There are large, rapid, regular ventricular complexes that might make you think you are looking at ventricular tachycardia. The difference is that these complexes have no organized shape. You can't tell the QRS from the T because all you see is a simple wave; a physicist would call it a "sine wave." Ventricular flutter is the same as ventricular fibrillation in its effect on the heartbeat. The heart is twitching feebly but regularly. No blood is being pumped, and the victim dies almost at once unless the rhythm is changed (Figs. 14–3 and 14–4).

Torsade

We used to call this "polymorphic ventricular tachycardia," but then a French cardiologist coined the elegant name *torsade de pointes* because the changing of axis in successive beats made him think of a ballerina twisting on her toes—"sur les pointes." Glamorous foreign names have an unfair advantage, so that's the term we use now.

It's an important and dangerous arrhythmia. In torsade, the shape of the QRS complexes changes rapidly and progressively from upright to isoelectric to negative and back to upright again. In fact, the axis of the complexes really does "twist" around 180 degrees (Figs. 14–5 and 14–6).

It might be easy to mistake these for ventricular fibrillation, but you'll notice the progressive change in the QRS shape with reasonably well-defined QRS and T complexes. Torsade is usually brief, but if it's sustained, it can be fatal. Torsade is often seen when the Q-T interval is prolonged; usually that's the result of drugs like quinidine. Rarely it's the result of a congenital abnormality of cardiac activation that produces lifelong prolongation of the Q-T interval. (If the prolonged Q-T is associated with congenital deafness, it's called *Jervell and Lange-Nielsen syndrome*. If there's only Q-T prolongation, it's *called Romano-Ward syndrome*.)

Figure 14–1.
"Fine" ventricular fibrillation. The electric activity produces only minimal twitching in the baseline.

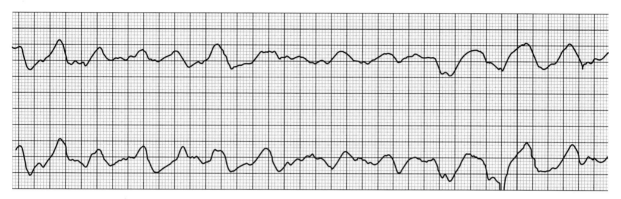

Figure 14–2.
"Coarse" ventricular fibrillation. There is some evidence that coarse ventricular fibrillation, with large deflections like the ones illustrated here, is more likely to respond to cardioversion.

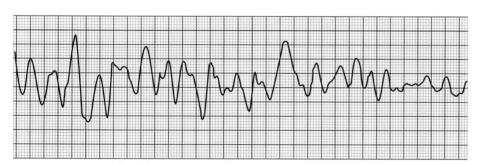

Figure 14–3.
Ventricular flutter. Note the large, regular deflections with no distinction between QRS and T. This arrhythmia is equivalent to ventricular fibrillation; no blood is being pumped, and death is almost instantaneous.

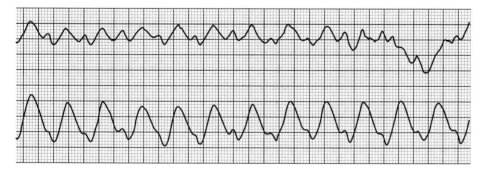

Figure 14–4.
On the left-hand side of this strip, there is well-defined ventricular tachycardia. On the right-hand side, this degenerates into ventricular flutter, with large, formless, regular waves.

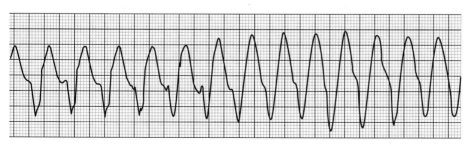

Figure 14–5.
Torsade. The ventricular complexes are first upright, then isoelectric, then negative, and finally upright again as the axis of the ectopic beat "twists" around 180 degrees.

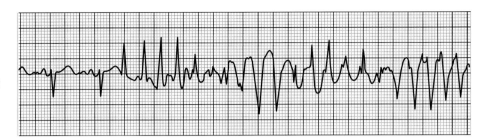

Figure 14–6.
Torsade. There are short bursts of torsade in both strips, with typical dramatic shift in axis of the ectopic beats. Note occasional abrupt prolongation of the Q-T in some beats just before a burst of torsade.

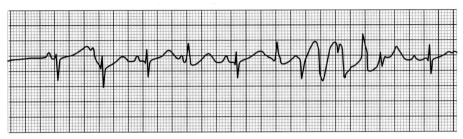

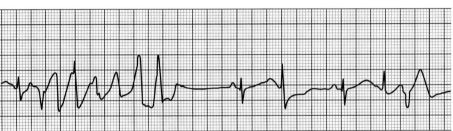

Treatment of torsade is completely different from treatment of ventricular flutter or fibrillation, and it's not covered in any of the usual texts or courses on cardiac resuscitation. Here it is:

1. **Intravenous magnesium (2 g) is given by bolus, and a drip of 2 mg/minute is started at the same time.**

2. **If torsade persists or recurs, accelerate the ventricular rate by atrial pacing. Drugs like atropine or isoproterenol would also work, but pacing's more reliable. *Warning:* Isoproterenol should never be administered when there's any question of myocardial ischemia—it's likely to lead to infarction or fatal arrhythmias. Atropine and pacing are simpler, safer ways of speeding the heart rate.**

Between these two measures, torsade can be controlled 100% of the time.

Prevention: If the prolonged Q-T is caused by drugs, stop them. If it's congenital, treat with beta blockers.

If beta-blockers fail, resection of the stellate ganglion often succeeds. The congenital form of torsade seems to represent an imbalance of left and right sympathetic innervation, so that resection of several left sympathetic ganglia has given very good results.

Finally, the perfection of implantable defibrillators has been a giant stride in the control of these arrhythmias. Defibrillators can be implanted with substantially no risk and with performance that is close to 100% in recognition and control of torsade. Torsade associated with congenital prolonged Q-T intervals may be the ideal indication for implantable defibrillators.

R-on-T Phenomenon

For many years, everybody knew that sometimes an electric shock would put the heart into ventricular fibrillation, and sometimes it wouldn't. Why the difference? Bernard Lown and his associates answered the puzzle. There's one small fraction of time during the heart cycle when the heart is vulnerable; a shock delivered during that time will produce ventricular fibrillation. During the rest of the heart cycle, the heart is relatively safe. This is the principle of elective cardioversion: the machine delivers the shock *outside* of the vulnerable zone. This vulnerable zone is about 0.01 second long and lies just ahead of the peak of the T wave (Fig. 14–7).

When a ventricular premature contraction (VPC) hits the vulnerable zone of the T wave, it can act as an electric shock and cause ventricular fibrillation (Fig. 14–8). This is commonly described as the *R-on-T phenomenon*. We now know a good deal more about this phenomenon than we used to. The R-on-T phenomenon is important in only three specific settings:

1. **In the presence of acute myocardial ischemia such as an infarct**
2. **In the presence of a low serum potassium level**
3. **In the presence of a prolonged Q-T interval**

In any other setting, a VPC hitting the vulnerable zone isn't any more important than any other VPC.

Standstill

There's really nothing to recognize on the ECG. Anybody can tell that a flat line is flat. The manipulations going on during a cardiac arrest can produce many twitches in the baseline that might look like ventricular fibrillation. It's important to have everyone take their hands off the patient for a few seconds to see if standstill is in fact present. After all, the treatment for standstill is quite different from the treatment for ventricular fibrillation, so the distinction can

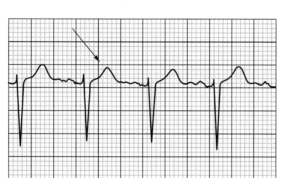

Figure 14–7.
The vulnerable zone of the heart cycle is a tiny segment of time just before the peak of the T wave (*arrow*). It is about 0.01 second in duration.

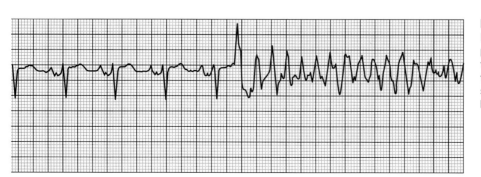

Figure 14–8.
Example of the R-on-T phenomenon triggering torsade. Note the VPC in the T wave of the last sinus beat before torsade begins.

be critical. Figure 14–9 illustrates a typical, very slow idioventricular rhythm degenerating into standstill.

The treatment of ventricular fibrillation and ventricular standstill is so widespread in the various advanced cardiac life support (ACLS) courses that there's no need to go into it here. (The surprising and somewhat shocking fact is that none of these courses teaches how to treat torsade.)

Measurement of the Q-T Interval

The Q-T interval is important in fatal arrhythmias, specifically in torsade. It's time to learn how to measure it and to recognize abnormal prolongation.

The Q-T interval varies with the rate: the faster the rate, the shorter the Q-T interval, and vice versa. The Bazet formula was an attempt to establish a normal value corrected for rate. The expression *Q-Tc* means "Q-T interval corrected for rate." Bazet[1] attempted to correct for rate by the formula Q-T/square root of R–R. This gives an upper normal level of 0.39 second for men and 0.44 second for women. The Bazet formula is relatively crude; Q-T intervals are best derived from the tables of Ashman and Hull,[2] and Lepeschkin[3] (Table 14–1).

Figure 14–9.
Two idioventricular beats ending in standstill.

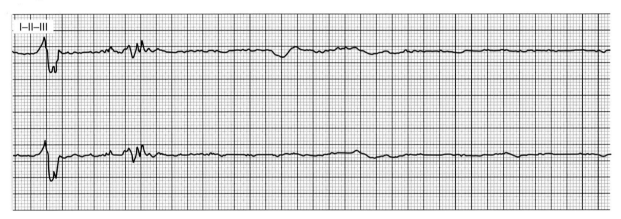

Table 14-1 Normal Variations of the Q-T Interval

Heart Rate	Lower Limit	Upper Limit	
		Men & Children	**Women**
40	0.42	0.49	0.50
43	0.39	0.48	0.49
46	0.38	0.47	0.48
48	0.37	0.46	0.47
50	0.36	0.45	0.46
52	0.35	0.45	0.46
55	0.34	0.44	0.45
57	0.34	0.43	0.44
60	0.33	0.42	0.43
63	0.32	0.41	0.42
67	0.31	0.40	0.41
71	0.31	0.38	0.41
75	0.30	0.38	0.39
80	0.29	0.37	0.38
86	0.28	0.36	0.37
93	0.28	0.35	0.36
100	0.27	0.34	0.35
109	0.26	0.33	0.33
120	0.25	0.31	0.32
133	0.24	0.29	0.30
150	0.23	0.28	0.28
170	0.22	0.26	0.26

The Lethal T Wave

Prolonged Q-T syndromes

Measurement of the Q-T interval often brings the cardiologist face to face with sudden cardiac death.

There are two syndromes associated with prolonged Q-T and sudden death:

1. **Jervell and Lange-Nielsen syndrome—congenital deafness, prolonged Q-T, and sudden death**

2. **Romano-Ward syndrome—same thing, without the deafness**

The danger in the prolonged Q-T syndromes is that the Q-T interval is so prolonged that a VPC is likely to fall on the vulnerable zone of the T wave and cause torsade (Fig. 14–10; see also p. 145).

The literature on the subject is vast, and there isn't room in a book like this for a detailed review, but a few general comments are in order:

1. **Always be aware of the Q-T interval as corrected in the Lepeschkin tables and don't trust ECG computer readings.**

2. **If a prolonged Q-T appears, always rule out toxic or metabolic causes (i.e., drugs, ischemic insult, electrolyte abnormality [depressed Ca$^+$] , and so forth; see Chapter 23 for effects of electrolytes and drugs).**

3. **If a prolonged Q-T is present without obvious cause, elicit a very careful family history of syncope or sudden death. (This is a chromosome-linked disorder, LQTS 1, 2, 3, and so on.)**

4. **Be aware that the Q-T interval can change dramatically in seconds in these congenital syndromes (Fig. 14–11). Q-T change and torsade can characteristically be invoked by fright, which is almost certainly the mechanism when people are supposed to have been "scared to death" or in the well-documented cases when primitives die because a witch doctor points the death bone). Q-T alternans is another marker for this lethal syndrome.**

5. **Learn to look for T wave "bumps"—little deflections on the descending limb of the T wave that seem to be characteristic of these syndromes (Fig. 14–12).**

Late Note: The Short Q-T Syndrome

Just to bedevil the cardiologist's life, several recent studies have documented another potentially lethal chromosome-linked abnormality of repolarization: the short Q-T syndrome. Although the numbers are small so far, there is no question that there is a heritable disorder that combines a short Q-T syndrome and sudden death[4] (Fig. 14–13).

The moral here is simple: if a corrected Q-T interval is short, rule out the one simple cause (i.e., hypercalcemia) and then confront the fact that a potentially lethal syndrome is at hand.

Corrected QTc in most reported case has been in the range of 252 ± 13 milliseconds.

The only definitive treatment for these syndromes is implantation of a defibrillator. Beta blockers are also helpful and will usually cut down the number of shocks.

(*Special note:* In these days of Internet access, a search of the literature is much easier than when we had to plow through the *Cumulative Index*. On the subject of sudden cardiac death

Figure 14–10.
Prolonged Q-T with VPCs striking on the vulnerable zone of the T wave. This zone (as first defined by Dr. Bernard Lown), lies in the 0.10 millisecond just before the peak of the T.

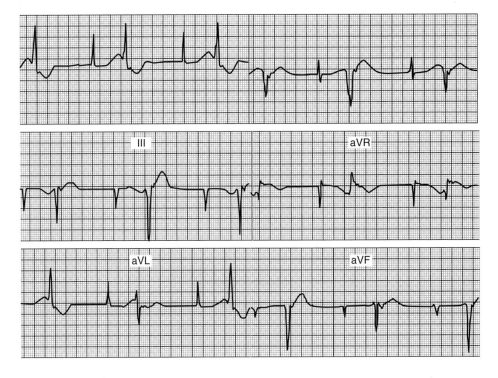

in general and prolonged Q-T syndromes in particular, the student is encouraged to call up the work of Dr. Arthur Moss of Rochester, New York, and Dr. Peter Schwartz of Milan, Italy, the two leading world authorities on the subject.)

The Lethal STT Complex: Brugada's Syndrome

Brugada's syndrome is another potentially deadly genetic pattern that can only be detected by the surface electrocardiogram—*repeat, only by the surface electrocardiogram*. It was first described in 1992 by the three Brugada brothers in Spain.

Brugada's syndrome presents as a peculiar elevation of the ST segments in the right precordial leads in the setting of right bundle-branch block. The really unusual aspect of this pattern is that the ST elevation is confined to leads V1, V2, and V3. It doesn't appear anywhere else, and there's no reciprocal change (Fig. 14–14).

The syndrome presents as abrupt, "drop-attack" syncope or sudden death because the patient suffers ventricular torsade or fibrillation. It is inherited as an autosomal dominant characteristic and has been detected all across the world in Spain, Italy, Southeast Asia, and the United States (including several cases here at the University of Arizona). The cause is a decrease in function of a subunit of the cardiac sodium channel.

The only treatment is implantation of a defibrillator, *but* there are major problems with diagnosis of Brugada's syndrome:

> 1. **The STT deformity is often intermittent; you're lucky if you catch it.**
> 2. **The right bundle-branch block itself is often intermittent.**

Victims of this syndrome may present with perfectly normal ECGs. In other words, this syndrome can be insidious.

What to do?

If a patient presents with a history of drop-attack syncope, and such obvious causes as aortic stenosis, heart block, prolonged Q-T syndrome, or hypertrophic subaortic stenosis have been ruled out, then proceed to the following:

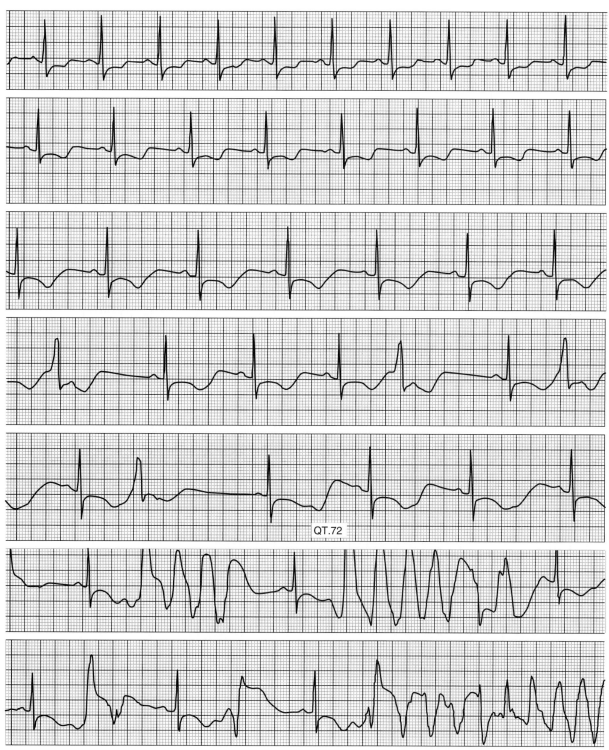

QT.72

Figure 14–12.
Minuscule "T bumps" (*arrows*) deforming the downslope of the T in leads V3 and V5. It's interesting that these bumps tend to disappear with beta-blocker therapy.

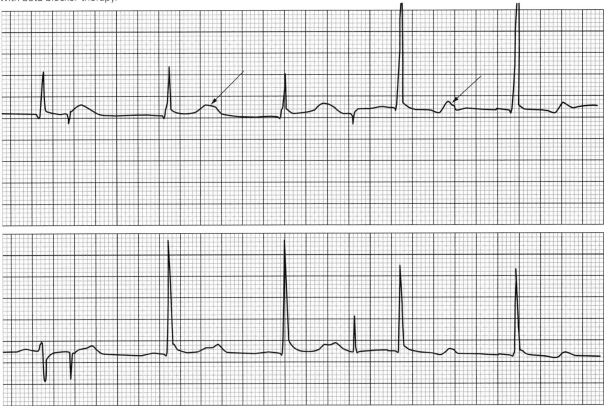

Figure 14–13.
Short Q-T. Q-T interval here is 238 milliseconds at a rate of 106—short by any standards.

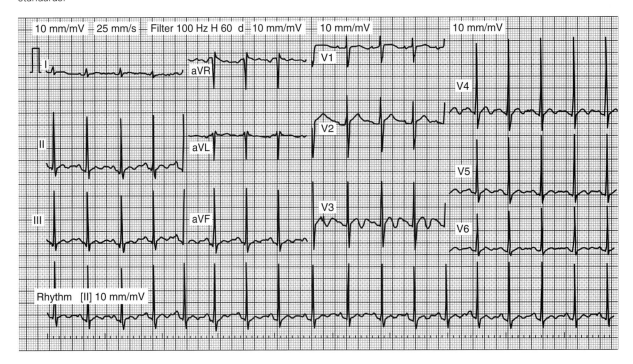

1. Take a very careful family history; remember the inheritance pattern.

2. Try to evoke the Brugada pattern with drugs. While monitoring the patient, administer a therapeutic dose of procainamide intravenously and watch for the emergence of the Brugada STT pattern. Other drugs, such as isoproterenol and disopyramide, have been used, but in the United States, procainamide is probably best and safest. In Europe, ajmaline has been the most specific drug for provocation of the pattern, but even with ajmaline, there are reports of false-negative results. A negative drug response does not rule out the syndrome, although a positive response is absolutely diagnostic.

3. Electrophysiologic study to provoke ventricular fibrillation is moot. Some workers insist that production of ventricular torsade or fibrillation by electrophysiologic stimulation is useful, whereas others insist it may be misleading. At this point, it is not clear whether invasive electrophysiologic study is helpful in the diagnosis of Brugada's syndrome.

4. Because this is an electrocardiographic diagnosis, record the ECG at great length! Use a loop recorder and make sure the electrodes are placed to record from the right precordium. With modern long-term recorders, it's possible to record for very long periods, and repeated recording is probably the best answer to this potentially fatal puzzle.

5. If there is reason to suspect the syndrome, and all tests are negative, genomic study by a leading authority (e.g., Dr. Arthur Moss at Rochester) is well worth pursuing.

Figure 14–14.
Typical Brugada's syndrome with elevation of ST segments in the right precordial leads. There's no reciprocal ST depression in opposed leads, which is what you'd expect if this were an acute anterior myocardial infarction.

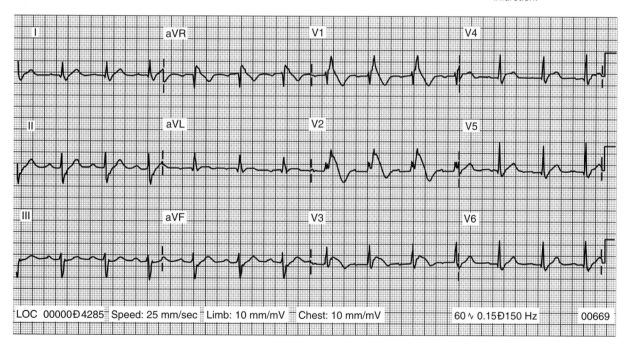

References

1. Bazet. Am. J Physiology, 1936;116:551.

2. Ashman, Hull, Lepeschkin. Ann Int. Med 1939;12: 1682.

3. Lepeschkin. Modern Electrocardiography. Baltimore: Williams and Wilkins, 1961.

4. Brugada R, Hong K, Dumaine R, et al. Sudden death associated with short QT linked to mutations in HERG. Circulation 2004;109:30–35.

Fifteen

The Sick Sinus Syndrome

The cells of the sinoatrial node are subject to all the slings and arrows of infection, ischemia, and degeneration. Disease of the sinoatrial tissues often produces an abnormally slow sinus rate. In extreme cases, the sinoatrial node may "die," with total replacement of active cells by scar tissue.

When depression of sinus node function causes symptoms, the *sick sinus syndrome* is said to be present. Thus, to diagnose the sick sinus syndrome, it isn't enough to read an electro-cardiogram (ECG). You have to be a clinician; you have to take a history.

The diagnosis of sick sinus syndrome can be established only when abnormally slow discharge of the sinus node produces symptoms. If there are no symptoms, there is no syndrome, no matter how alarming the bradycardia may appear on the ECG.

At least 90% to 95% of the time, the symptoms of subnormal sinus node function are *cerebral*. Inadequate perfusion of cerebral tissues may produce vertigo, "presyncope," or frank syncope. Less commonly, an inappropriately slow sinus rate may exacerbate or perpetuate congestive heart failure with symptoms ranging from generalized fatigue to incapacitating dyspnea. Very rarely, a sinus rate too slow to sustain circulation may cause ischemic pain—a kind of bradycardia-dependent angina. (I've seen only one case like this in the past 30+ years.)

ECG Diagnosis

Subnormal sinus node function can take one of three forms.

Inappropriate Sinus Bradycardia

This takes some careful defining. Normally, the sinus rate varies on demand within wide limits. Rates of 30 or 40 are common during sleep, whereas vigorous activity may produce rates of 150 or higher. *Inappropriate sinus bradycardia* means that the sinus rate is persistently too low to support the circulation at any given level of activity. In other words, the sinus rate can be assessed only in terms of the immediate needs of the body. A rate of 40 or 50 might be adequate during sleep, but it won't support the circulation when the patient is climbing stairs.

Figure 15–1 illustrates severe, sustained bradycardia. The rate remained in the range of 40 even when the patient walked or performed other exercise that would normally increase the heart rate. With this persistently low rate, the patient became dizzy and sometimes started to faint.

Sinus Pauses

The sinus node may suddenly pause so that there's no activity for several seconds or even longer. Sinus pauses are common; everybody has them. They are significant only if they produce symptoms.

(Cardiology, like the rest of medicine, is haunted by myths. The legend of the 3-second pause ranks right up there with the tooth fairy for pure mendacity. An author of a text once

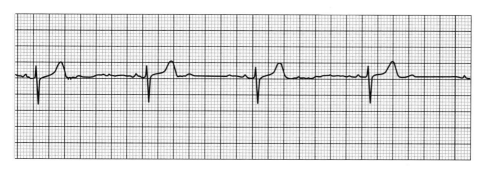

Figure 15–1.
Severe symptomatic sinus bradycardia recorded during light exercise (walking).

made a casual comment that 3-second pauses might be dangerous and might justify implantation of a pacemaker. This was no more than an offhand opinion, without supporting data. Large-scale studies subsequently proved that 3-second pauses are common and harmless and should be disregarded unless they produce symptoms, but the genie was out of the bottle. Uninformed or unscrupulous physicians to this day persist in inserting unnecessary pacemakers on the basis of an occasional 3-second pause even though the patient has no symptoms whatsoever.)

Sinus pauses can take one of two forms:

1. **The first is true sinoatrial exit block. This is relatively rare. Suddenly there's no P wave and, of course, no QRS. The next beat comes in exactly on time. The pause is exactly double the basic rate—in other words, it's equal to two R-R intervals (Fig. 15–2). This precise double interval means that the pace-making cells of the sinus node actually went on firing at regular intervals, but suddenly one impulse wasn't conducted out to the atria. Go back to Figure 13-5 and recall that there are pace-making cells and conducting cells in the sinoatrial node. With this kind of block, the pacing cells are normal, but the conducting cells occasionally fail.**

2. **Random sinus pauses are much more common. Suddenly there's no P wave and hence no heartbeat for a long time. The pause has no relation to the basic sinus rhythm (Fig. 15–3). Sometimes these pauses can come out of the blue, interrupting a normal sinus rhythm, and they can be very prolonged indeed.**

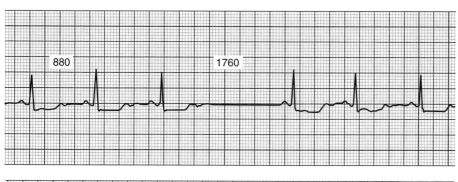

880   1760

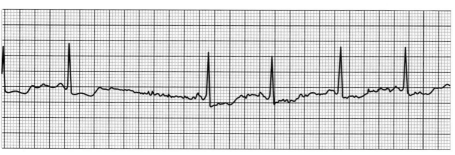

Figure 15–2.
Sinoatrial block. The pauses are an exact multiple of the basic sinus rate. This means that the pacing cells of the sinus node have gone on building up their charge and discharging normally, but an occasional impulse isn't conducted out to the atria.

Figure 15–3.
Random sinus pauses with no relation to the basic sinus rate.

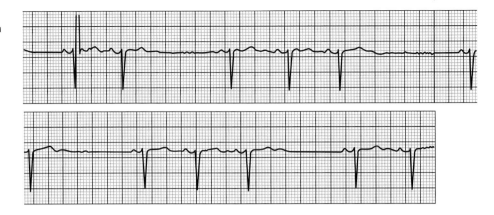

If sinus pauses produce symptoms, and if they are recurrent and not drug induced, a pacemaker will probably be needed.

Fortunately, the automatic demand pacemakers in the junction and the ventricles are usually ready to pick up the rhythm if the sinus node fails. In Figure 15–4, you see a sinus rate of about 40 with two junctional escape beats between successive sinus beats. When you see junctional or idioventricular escape beating, always check the sinus rate to see if an abnormally slow sinus rate is the reason for the "escape" of the ectopic focus.

In Figure 15–5, there is evidence of atrioventricular (AV) nodal block together with long sinus pauses and junctional escape beating. AV nodal block commonly accompanies sick sinus behavior and may be a reflection of the same pathologic process. All the hallmarks of the sick sinus are present in this tracing: Now you have to ask the patient about symptoms!

Figure 15–4.
Junctional escape beating. The slow sinus rate (40) permits the junction to escape and set the rhythm for several beats at a time. Note the occasional pairing, or bigeminal, rhythm when a junctional beat is followed by a sinus beat. This is escape-capture bigeminy, typical of sick sinus patterns.

Bradycardia-Tachycardia Syndrome

Sometimes periods of slow sinus rhythm are interrupted by bursts of abnormal rapid rhythms in the atria—flutter, fibrillation, or atrial tachycardia. It's common to have a patient present with one of these tachyarrhythmias and then convert to an abnormally slow sinus rate or to one interrupted by frequent long pauses (Figs. 15–6 and 15–7).

Figure 15–5.
AV nodal block associated with severe sinus bradycardia and occasional escape junctional beats. The AV block is actually first-degree block, with a P-R interval of 0.38 second. The occasional apparent short P-R is caused by junctional escape beats that have no connection to the preceding P waves.

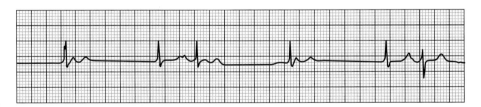

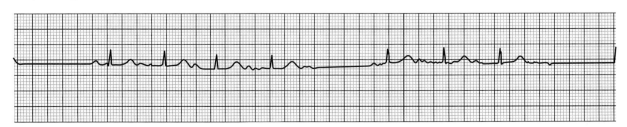

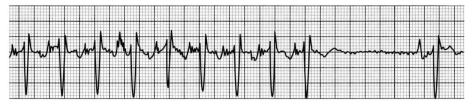

Figure 15–6.
Bradycardia-tachycardia syndrome. A run of paroxysmal atrial tachycardia (PAT) is followed by severe, symptomatic sinus bradycardia.

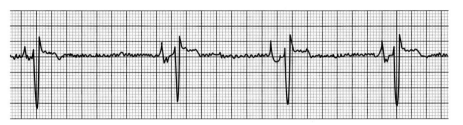

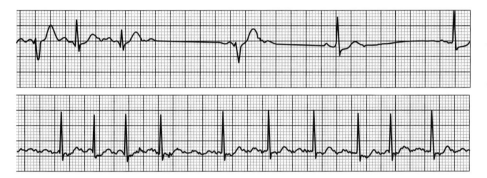

Figure 15–7.
Bradycardia-tachycardia syndrome with atrial flutter as the "tachy" component. Note the sustained bradycardia when the sinus rhythm resumes.

This is the bradycardia-tachycardia form of the sick sinus syndrome. What causes this combination of events? It is possible that the absence of sinus node impulses for long periods allows the abnormal rapid rhythm to "take over," although this cannot be the entire explanation.

Caution: To diagnose the bradycardia-tachycardia syndrome, you have to document significant periods of bradycardia between the episodes of tachyarrhythmia. Don't diagnose a "brady-tachy" syndrome just because you see paroxysms of flutter, fibrillation, or tachycardia. In most cases, you'll see periods of normal sinus function between episodes of tachyarrhythmia. Be sure you document symptomatic bradycardia before you diagnose the brady-tachy syndrome.

Figure 15–8 illustrates this point. Here you see paroxysms of atrial fibrillation with short periods of sinus rhythm. This is *not* a brady-tachy phenomenon because there's no "brady." There are three sinus beats in V1 and two in V2; these sinus beats appear at a rate of about 80 to 88, indicating normal sinus node function.

A variant of brady-tachy is pseudoblock with the sick sinus syndrome. In Figure 15–9, there's a severe sinus bradycardia, rate about 43. This slow rate permits a junctional pacemaker to escape, setting the rhythm of the heart until a sinus beat arrives between ectopic beats and captures the rhythm of the heart momentarily.

Important: Even though there are periods of complete AV dissociation, there's no AV block—just a dearth of P waves. This particular patient didn't need a pacemaker; he just needed relief from the toxic drugs that were suppressing his sinus node (clonidine and digitalis in this case).

Figure 15–8.
Not the brady-tachy syndrome. There are paroxysms of coarse atrial fibrillation with a perfectly normal sinus rhythm and rate between paroxysms. This patient can safely be treated with suppressive drugs like quinidine or procainamide. No pacemaker needed.

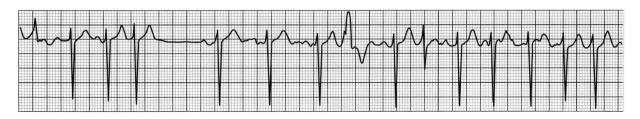

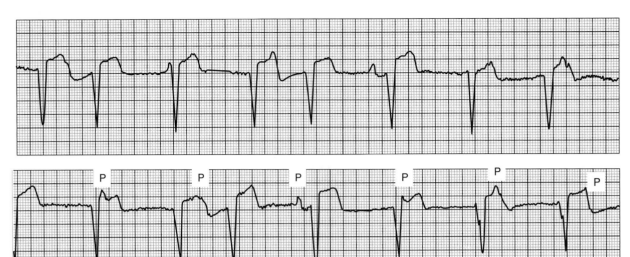

Figure 15–9.

Pseudoblock. Severe sinus bradycardia, rate 40, with escape of a junctional pacemaker. Note occasional sinus capture beats, such as the beat produced by the second P wave in the bottom strip. Two capture beats are also apparent in the top strip. These capture beats tell you that this is interference-dissociation caused by the slow sinus rate—it is *not* complete AV block.

Mystery of the Sick Sinus Syndrome

Normally the "demand" ectopic pacemakers in the junction and in the ventricles will set the rhythm if the sinus node fails. In the sick sinus syndrome, they often don't. That's why there are long pauses, and that's why symptoms appear. If the subsidiary pacemakers functioned normally, there would be no symptoms, hence no syndrome. In the sick sinus syndrome, there is really a failure of all pacing systems from the sinus node to the ventricles; nobody has even come close to explaining how or why this happens.

Caution: It's safe to say that more than 90% of all cases of subnormal sinus node function are caused by physicians. There's an alarmingly long list of drugs that can depress sinus node function:

1. **Digitalis**

2. **Quinidine**

3. **Procainamide**

4. **Calcium blockers**

5. **Beta blockers**

6. **Clonidine**

7. **Morphine and other opium derivatives**

8. **Psychotropic drugs**

9. **All the newer antiarrhythmic drugs, such as amiodarone, sotalol, and propafenone**

The sinus node may be temporarily depressed during myocardial infarction. Retching and vomiting can stimulate the vagus, with some spectacularly long pauses. Hyperkalemia typically slows the sinus node; so does hypothyroidism. In other words, be sure to rule out the effect of drugs or other metabolic abnormalities before you decide the sinus node itself is "sick." True sick sinus syndrome is rare. In our busy county hospital, where many of our patients are old and sick, I might see only one genuine sick sinus syndrome in a year.

The sick sinus syndrome isn't usually a threat to life. One large-scale British study was unable to find a single case of cardiac arrest caused by the sick sinus syndrome. There are anecdotes of rare cases of cardiac arrest caused by sinus node failure, but there is no authenticated list of such occurrences in the world medical literature. (Obviously, the sick sinus syndrome is a threat to life if it causes syncope while someone is driving a car!)

The only treatment of the sick sinus syndrome is permanent pacing. When the brady-tachy syndrome is present, it's also essential to treat the tachyarrhythmia with suppressive drugs.

Occasional happy outcome: When a patient has paroxysms of atrial fibrillation as part of a brady-tachy syndrome, the physician should pray that the atrial fibrillation becomes permanent. When that happens, the sinus node is irrelevant, and the treatment is the same as for any ordinary case of atrial fibrillation. No pacemaker is needed because there are plenty of fibrillary impulses bombarding the AV node. All the physician has to do is to control the rate.

The diagnosis of the sick sinus syndrome is made by recording an ECG during symptoms. This can be done by an ordinary ECG, by an event recorder, or by Holter recordings. The event recorder has been a boon; it can be worn for 2 weeks, can record up to 15 episodes, and has a 5-minute memory loop. In other words, it is now *always* possible to record an ECG during symptoms. An ECG recorded during symptoms is the gold standard—no other studies are necessary.

In past years, there were attempts to measure sinus node function by invasive means, but these were never very sensitive and are now totally obsolete. If some invasive electrophysiology enthusiast wants to study your sick sinus syndrome, bar the door and burn his catheter. Invasive electrophysiology studies have no place in the modern diagnosis of the sick sinus syndrome.

Sixteen

Digitalis-Toxic Arrhythmias

In recent years, the uses of digitalis have become precisely defined. Digitalis can slow the ventricular rate by depressing atrioventricular (AV) nodal conduction, it can suppress atrial and junctional ectopic activity, and it is a mild inotrope. Digitalis may also be the most overused drug in the world. It's often prescribed in a kind of knee-jerk clinical reflex for old sick people who don't really need it, and it often does more harm than good. Specifically, it causes arrhythmias, some of them dangerous; in the current jargon, it is powerfully proarrhythmic. Digitalis-toxic arrhythmias are much less common than they were a few years ago, but they still emerge with distressing frequency. They're dangerous!

Figure 16–1 explains the double-toxic effect of digitalis. First, it stimulates the vagus nerve. Second, it "turns on" ectopic firing anywhere in the heart. Remember, the vagus nerve is the "slowing" nerve in the heart. When the vagus nerve is overstimulated, it can depress the sinus node so that it fires very slowly and sometimes stops firing entirely. In other words, digitalis can produce a sick sinus syndrome (see Chapter 15).

Diagnosis of Digitalis Toxicity: The Four Commandments

Commandment One

If you see subnormal sinus node function in a patient taking digitalis, *always* assume that digitalis toxicity is the cause.

Overstimulation of the vagus nerve can also produce block in the AV node. This is a very common effect of digitalis toxicity. AV block caused by digitalis is always localized in the AV node, never in the bundle-branch system. The reason for this is simple: digitalis produces block in the AV node by stimulating the vagus nerve. The vagus nerve doesn't reach the bundle-branch system. It stops around the bottom of the AV node (Fig. 16–2).

Digitalis toxicity can produce any type of AV nodal block—first-degree, 2:1 or other "fixed ratio," type I (Wenckebach), and complete block.

You will *never* see Mobitz-II block as a result of digitalis toxicity because Mobitz-II block never occurs in the AV node. Because the vagus nerve does not send fibers to the bundle-branch system, digitalis toxicity has no effect on the bundle-branch tissues, where Mobitz-II block takes place.

Commandment Two

When you see AV nodal block in a patient taking digitalis, *always* assume that digitalis toxicity is the cause.

Digitalis-toxic AV nodal block is always temporary. The immediate antidote is atropine. Sometimes temporary pacemakers are necessary.

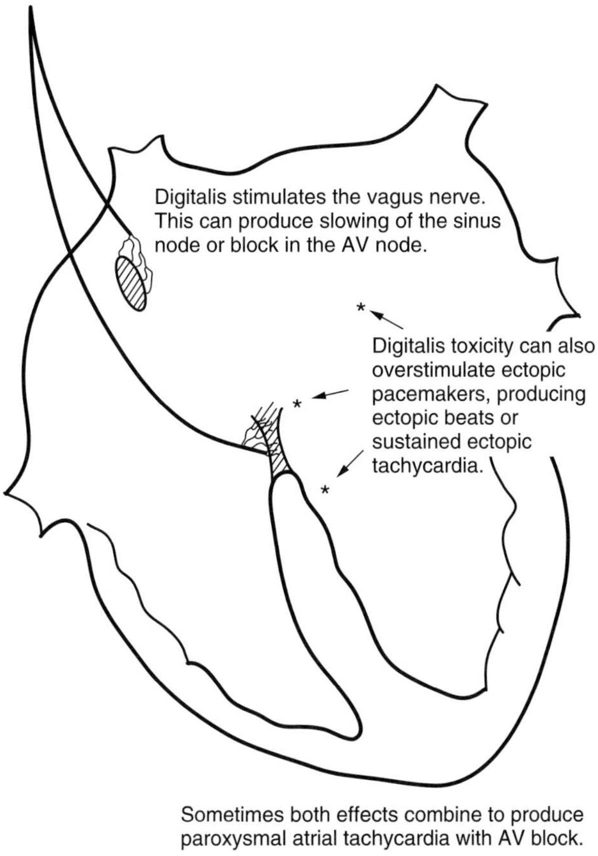

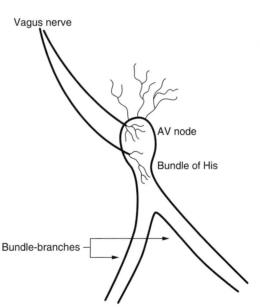

Figure 16–1.
The double-toxic effect of digitalis.

Digitalis stimulates the vagus nerve. This can produce slowing of the sinus node or block in the AV node.

*Digitalis toxicity can also overstimulate ectopic pacemakers, producing ectopic beats or sustained ectopic tachycardia.

Sometimes both effects combine to produce paroxysmal atrial tachycardia with AV block.

Vagus nerve

AV node

Bundle of His

Bundle-branches

Figure 16–2.
Vagus nerve anatomy. The fibers of the vagus nerve reach the AV node and may penetrate the bundle of His. Vagal fibers do not reach the bundle-branch system. Block produced by vagal stimulation will therefore always be localized in the AV node.

The other effect of digitalis toxicity is a kind of stimulation of ectopic foci anywhere in the heart—atria, junction, or ventricles. Ectopic firing as single beats or as sustained tachycardia will be the result.

The VPC is the most common single arrhythmia caused by digitalis toxicity. When frequent VPCs appear in a digitalized patient, especially if they start forming couplets or triplets, it's a good bet that digitalis is the cause. It's also a good time to stop the digitalis to see if the beats go away.

Commandment Three

Any ectopic beats that appear in a digitalized patient should be assumed to be the result of digitalis effect. This is especially important if the ectopic beats are ventricular.

Commandment Four

This is a golden rule. You'll save lives if you learn it and observe it: Certain types of paroxysmal tachycardia in a digitalized patient should always be regarded as digitalis toxic until you prove otherwise. On the other hand, some types are never the result of digitalis toxicity.

For instance, AV nodal reentrant tachycardia will never be the result of digitalis toxicity, nor will AV nodal reciprocating tachycardia (bypass tract) or true ectopic atrial tachycardia of childhood.

On the other hand, whenever you see accelerated junctional rhythms, ventricular tachycardia, or paroxysmal atrial tachycardia with AV block in a digitalized patient, the diagnosis is digitalis toxicity until you prove otherwise.

> 1. **Rapid junctional rhythms are the most common type of digitalis-toxic sustained tachycardias. These rhythms may appear in several forms. Figure 16–3A illustrates a true paroxysmal junctional tachycardia with a rate of 148. Figure 16–3B illustrates an accelerated junctional rhythm with a rate of 90. Both rhythms were the result of digitalis toxicity. Thus, digitalis toxicity may produce either an accelerated junctional rhythm in the high-normal range or a true paroxysmal junctional tachycardia.**
>
> 2. **Ventricular tachycardia is of course the most dangerous type of digitalis-toxic paroxysmal tachycardia. It looks exactly like any other kind of ventricular tachycardia; you make the diagnosis by taking a history.**

Digitalis Levels

AV nodal block or paroxysmal tachycardia caused by digitalis can be diagnosed only by discovering that the patient is taking digitalis and making the assumptions listed earlier. Digitalis levels in the blood are useful only to tell you that the patient has in fact been taking the drug.

Serum levels of digitalis (digoxin) do not correlate with toxicity or with therapeutic effect. The patient can be toxic at low levels (0.9 ng/mL) or subtherapeutic at high levels (2.8–3.0 ng/mL). You make the diagnosis of digitalis toxicity from the history and the electrocardiogram (ECG) findings.

One more time: In everything described so far, you make a clinical assumption. If AV nodal block or certain types of paroxysmal tachycardia appear in a patient taking digitalis, you assume that digitalis is the cause until it's proved otherwise. Why is all this so important? The digitalis-toxic tachyarrhythmias are very dangerous. As an overall risk, it's conservative to say that giving more digitalis will produce a 36% mortality rate.

Paroxysmal Atrial Tachycardia with Block

Now we come to a dangerous digitalis-toxic arrhythmia that you can recognize from the ECG. It's a combination of the two elements in Figure 16–1, that is, acceleration of an atrial ectopic focus together with AV nodal block.

Look at Figure 16–4. You see P waves coming rapidly and regularly with a rate of 214. Every other P wave is blocked. There is 2:1 AV nodal block. (You know the block is in the AV node because the QRS is narrow.) These are the two elements in this critical diagnosis: paroxysmal atrial tachycardia (PAT) with block. Remember, to make the diagnosis you note

A

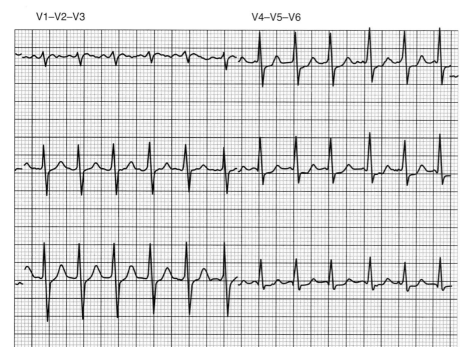

V1–V2–V3   V4–V5–V6

B

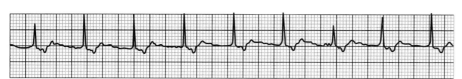

Figure 16–3.
A, Paroxysmal junctional tachycardia, rate 150. **B,** Accelerated idiojunctional rhythm, rate 90. Both are examples of digitalis-toxic junctional rhythms.

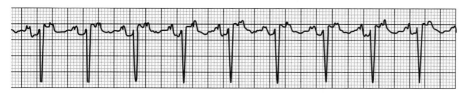

Figure 16–4.
Paroxysmal atrial tachycardia with 2:1 AV block.

first that P waves are appearing rapidly and regularly. Therefore, there is a PAT. Now you make another simple observation: not all the P waves are reaching the ventricles. Therefore, there is some degree of AV block. That's all you need to know. The block may be first or second degree, of any of the usual nodal types. The type of block isn't important.

Remember the two simple elements in the diagnosis of PAT with block:

1. **You see rapid, regular P waves in the tachycardia range.**

2. **Some of the P waves are blocked.**

PAT with block is caused by a combination of digitalis toxicity and a low serum potassium about 90% of the time. The treatment is intravenous potassium, administered rapidly. More digitalis at this point is likely to be fatal.

Figure 16–5.
PAT with block. In the first five beats, the P-R prolongs progressively until one P wave is blocked. The sixth beat is a junctional escape beat, and then a three-beat Wenckebach cycle follows. Wenckebach periods are present through the rest of the tracing. Note the irregular ventricular response as the degree of block changes.

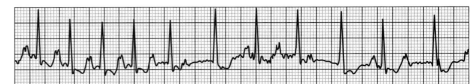

Figure 16–6.
PAT with variable block. On the right-hand side of the strip, you'd have a hard time making a diagnosis. On the left side, you can see P waves very clearly; the atrial rate is 210. There's obviously atrial tachycardia. Not all the P waves reach the ventricles, so there is AV block. That's all you need for the diagnosis of PAT with block. If you march the rest of the P waves out you can see that there are P waves hidden in the QRS complexes on the right-hand side of the strip with a variable degree of AV block. The exact type of block isn't important; what *is* important is that there is atrial tachycardia with some kind of AV block.

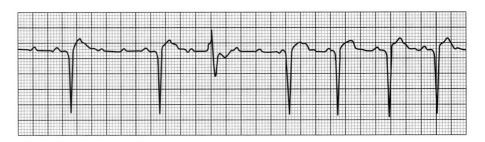

Figures 16–5 through 16–9 illustrate variations of PAT with block. Notice that the ventricular rate can be fast or slow, regular or irregular, depending on the atrial rate and the degree of block. It could be very easy to confuse this with atrial fibrillation.

One of the silliest medical myths is that an "irregular irregularity" of the heart means atrial fibrillation. By now the student should be able to list a half dozen other arrhythmias that can cause "irregular irregularity" of the heartbeat. PAT with block is one of them.

If you decided that the rapid irregular rhythm in Figure 16–4 was caused by atrial fibrillation and gave more digoxin, the patient would probably die. Any intelligent jury would call it malpractice. You'd have no defense.

Special distinction: The thoughtful student will note that there are similarities between atrial flutter and PAT with block. In each, there's a rapid abnormal regular atrial rhythm. In each, there's some kind of failure of conduction to the ventricles. Thus, it might be easy to confuse them.

However, there are several important differences. The diagnosis of flutter is made by detecting typical flutter waves in the ECG. The atrial waves of PAT are typical separate

Figure 16–7.
PAT with block. The degree of block is variable, ranging from 3:1 to 6:1 in various parts of the strip. The two essentials for the diagnosis are obvious: (1) there are P waves appearing rapidly and regularly in the paroxysmal tachycardia range, and (2) they don't all reach the ventricles. That's all you need to see to diagnose this very dangerous arrhythmia.

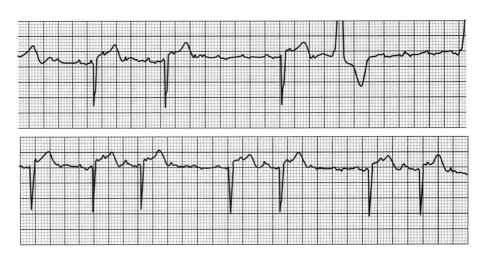

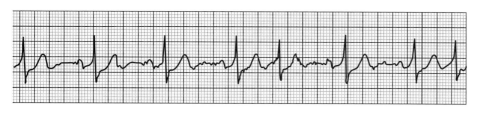

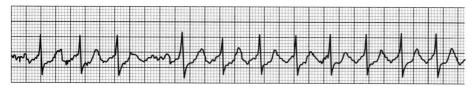

Figure 16–8.
This illustrates a number of types of AV block with PAT. In the *top strip,* there are periods of 2:1 block that shift into Wenckebach cycles with a 3:2 response. The *bottom strip* begins with a 4:3 Wenckebach period and shifts to first-degree block with a P-R of 0.30 second. It's hard to see the P waves buried in the T waves during 2:1 block, but the changing shape of the T waves during Wenckebach periods makes it clear that there's a P wave hidden in them. This gives you the clue to the atrial rate—about 128.

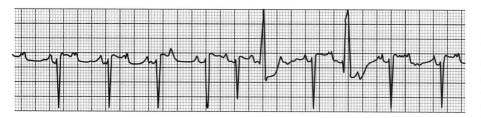

Figure 16–9.
PAT with 2:1 block interrupted by VPCs. *Warning:* Except for the VPCs, this is a slow regular rhythm with a rate of 80. It would be impossible to distinguish this from a normal sinus rhythm at the bedside! Rely on the ECG, and always be suspicious when patients are taking digitalis.

P waves with an isoelectric period between them. The atrial flutter rate can be very fast. If you see an atrial rate of 300 in the adult, it has to be flutter. PAT never goes that fast; in fact, PAT very rarely goes over 250. Flutter is almost never a digitalis-toxic arrhythmia. PAT with block almost always is. Digitalis is an excellent treatment for flutter; it's lethal with PAT with block.

Study Figure 16–10 carefully because you will certainly have to make the distinction between these two arrhythmias. The wrong answer can be fatal.

Digitalis Toxicity and Atrial Fibrillation: A Very Special Case

Practically every case of atrial fibrillation is treated with digitalis, and it's safe to say that most cases of digitalis toxicity appear in exactly this setting. It's extremely important, therefore, to be able to recognize digitalis toxicity in the presence of atrial fibrillation. If you remember what digitalis does, it's not difficult.

Digitalis-Induced AV Block in the Presence of Atrial Fibrillation

In incomplete block, there will be no P waves to measure from, so you simply go by the rate. Figure 16–11 is an example of atrial fibrillation with a very slow ventricular rate. The rhythm is irregular, so you know that the fibrillating impulses are still driving the ventricles, but they're coming through the AV node so slowly that common sense tells you there's a high degree of block. Stop the digitalis!

The diagnosis of complete AV block in the presence of atrial fibrillation is simple (Fig. 16–12). The ventricular rhythm is regular, and the rate is 45 or less. The regular ventricular rhythm tells you that there's complete AV dissociation—in other words, an "idio" pacemaker is driving the heart, and none of the fibrillating impulses are coming through the

Figure 16–10.
Typical flutter waves. At the right-hand end, carotid sinus pressure has been applied to block conduction through the AV node; the flutter waves are seen without QRS complexes. Note how the end of one wave is the beginning of the next. There is no flat, or isoelectric, period between waves. Compare these typical flutter waves with the P waves in Figs. 16–3 through 16–8. Even though the atrial rate is in the same range as the flutter rate, there is no mistaking the well-defined P waves with a flat, or isoelectric, period between them.

AV node. The slow rate tells you that the block is complete. (Another one of those beautiful, high-fidelity golden oldies from my intern days!)

Interference-Dissociation and AV Block

Remember the phenomenon of interference-dissociation back in Chapter 7. You'll often see the same thing when the atria are fibrillating and there's incomplete block in the AV node. Conduction from the atria slows just enough to let an ectopic focus in the AV junction or in the ventricles "escape" and set the rhythm of the heart. In Figure 16–13, you see atrial fibrillation. The first beat, marked f, is conducted from the fibrillating atria; so are the other beats marked f later in the tracing. Most of the time, you see a regular rhythm with wide QRS complexes (V). This is an idioventricular rhythm. It tells you that there's some degree of block in the AV node, but the occasional conducted beats tell you that the block is not complete.

When the pulse turns regular in a fibrillating patient, look out! It doesn't necessarily mean that you've restored a sinus rhythm. If the pulse is slow and regular, there's probably

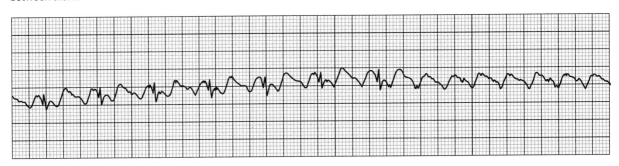

Figure 16–11.
Atrial fibrillation with high degree of AV nodal block and frequent VPCs. Concealed retrograde conduction from the VPCs into the AV node can make block more severe, as it did in this patient.

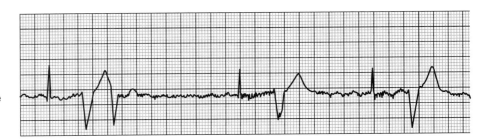

Figure 16–12.
Atrial fibrillation with complete AV nodal block and VPCs forming a bigeminal rhythm.

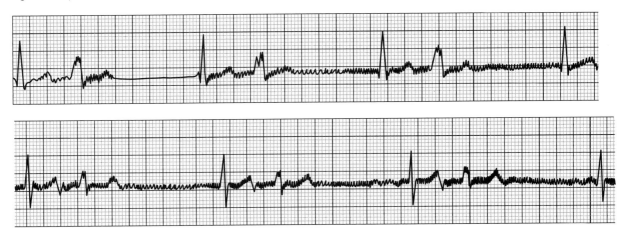

complete AV block. If it's regular in the normal range, there may be an idiorhythm with partial AV block. In either case, the patient is digitalis toxic.

Ectopic Beats

Ventricular ectopic beats are the most common single manifestation of digitalis toxicity in the ECG. Figure 16–14 is typical. When ventricular premature contractions (VPCs) begin appearing frequently or in couplets, assume digitalis toxicity.

Paroxysmal Tachycardia

When the rhythm turns regular and the rate is rapid, paroxysmal tachycardia is interrupting the atrial fibrillation. You recognize junctional and ventricular tachycardia just the way you do in any other setting (Figs. 16–15 and 16–16).

Diagnostic Algorithm for Digitalis Toxicity in the Presence of Atrial Fibrillation

Here's an "algorithm," or systematic approach to detecting digitalis toxic rhythms in the fibrillating patient:

Figure 16–13.
Atrial fibrillation interrupted by long runs of an idioventricular rhythm (V), rate 60. A few beats are conducted from the fibrillating atria (f). There is a high degree of block, not complete.

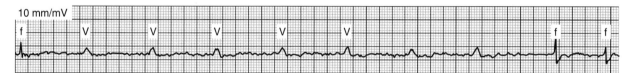

Figure 16–14.
Atrial fibrillation interrupted by many multifocal VPCs, ending in ventricular fibrillation. This is a graphic illustration of the possible fatal outcome of digitalis toxicity.

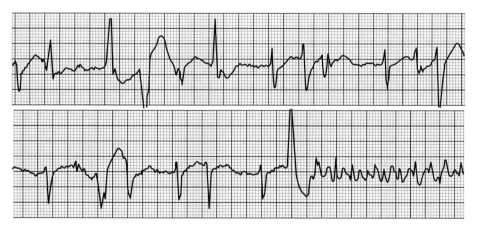

Figure 16–15.
Digitalis-toxic ventricular tachycardia interrupting chronic atrial fibrillation.

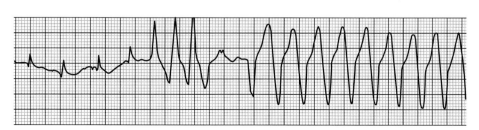

Figure 16–16.
Digitalis-toxic long runs of junctional tachycardia interrupting chronic atrial fibrillation. Note the regularity of the complexes and occasional periods of aberrant conduction. The tachycardia appears in runs of varying length, so the pulse has periods of irregularity. Bedside distinction from atrial fibrillation would be very difficult.

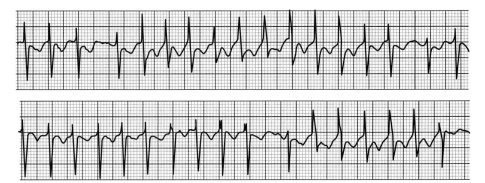

A. Rhythm irregular, rate slow. Incomplete AV block

B. Rhythm regular, rate slow to normal, three possibilities:

   1. Normal sinus rhythm has been restored.

   2. Atrial fibrillation persists with complete AV dissociation. Check an ECG at this point!

     a. If rate is 45 or less: complete AV block.

     b. If rate is in the normal range, an idiorhythm is present with partial AV block.

C. Rhythm regular, rate rapid (140 or more): paroxysmal tachycardia is present.

Unless a normal sinus rhythm has been restored, all the other possibilities listed above mean digitalis toxicity!

Tips on Treatment

There's no specific drug therapy for digitalis-toxic supraventricular tachycardia. Make sure electrolytes, especially potassium and magnesium, are in the high-normal range, and support the patient until the digitalis wears off. If the tachycardia threatens life, treat with specific antibodies, such as FAB fragments. Remember, you can do this only once in the patient's lifetime, so be sure it's needed! I've never had to use it.

The specific therapy for digitalis-toxic ventricular tachycardia is *intravenous diphenylhydantoin*. The effect is specific, immediate, and gratifying. This is the only arrhythmia that responds to diphenylhydantoin. One good protocol is 100 mg slow push every 5 minutes until the arrhythmia ends *or* toxic central nervous system symptoms appear *or* 1 gram has been given. Then go to maintenance.

Potassium for PAT with block should be given relatively rapidly—10 mEq/hour, or even more if the patient is severely distressed.

Seventeen

Myocardial Infarction

It's sound practice to start with pathophysiology. Myocardial infarction (MI), of course, is always caused by abrupt occlusion of a coronary artery. In most cases, this is the result of thrombus formation in a diseased vessel. Rarely, an atheroma can be "levered out" by subintimal bleeding so that it blocks the artery totally even without a thrombus. Even more rarely, a thrombus can form in an apparently normal artery. Spasm in an anatomically normal artery can cause total occlusion with infarct formation, and with distressing frequency, the combination of spasm and accelerated atheroma formation in cocaine addicts can kill young people in their 20s and 30s. For whatever reason, the artery is occluded, and within seconds, electrophysiologic changes take place in the insulted myocardial cells.

You may remember crushing a frog's gastrocnemius in the physiology laboratory and recording an "injury current." That's exactly the same kind of current that's generated in acutely ischemic myocardial cells (Fig. 17–1). If you were to place an electrode on the epicardium directly over the injured area, you'd record an S–T deviation: the S–T segment would be elevated (Fig. 17–2). The injury current registers during the S–T segment because the balancing currents introduced by the electrocardiogram (ECG) offset the injury current during the rest of the heart cycle.

Now comes an extremely important principle in ECG diagnosis of MI: if you were to go around to the other wall of the heart, exactly 180 degrees from the site of the occlusion, you'd record depression of the S–T segment (Fig. 17–3). This illustrates the phenomenon of image cancellation. In plain language, whatever you record on one side of the electric field of the heart can be recorded upside down on the opposite side. It's like a mirror image, except that it's not right to left—it's upside-down. Changes seen on the side of the heart opposite the site of the infarct are called the *reciprocal* pattern. Changes recorded directly over the infarct site are called the *infarct* pattern.

Stay with the lead "facing" the infarct for the time being. Suppose it's an inferior infarct and you're looking at aVF. If you stood at the junction of the thigh with the trunk and looked straight up, you'd be looking at the inferior or diaphragmatic surface of the heart, and that's exactly what aVF records (Fig. 17–4). The S–T elevation may be a millimeter or less, or it may be very high indeed—5 to 10 mm or more (Fig. 17–5).

In Figure 17–6, there's a further progressive change. You'll note that the S–T segment has an upward concavity. This curve is called the *Pardee cove-plane curve* after the man who described it. Our interns describe this as the "tombstone" curve, and it's not a bad term, all things considered.

Distortion of depolarization may be the next change. As the cells undergo the changes of ischemia, there is dispersion and slow conduction of the depolarizing impulse. This will of course distort the depolarizing impulse with change in the QRS. The most common and most specific form of QRS distortion is the initial negative deflection or Q wave. In Figure 17–7, the central shaded area represents the zone of early necrosis where the Q wave probably originates. When you see a combination of a pathologic Q wave with S–T elevation and beginning T wave inversion, you have an absolutely specific ECG diagnosis of MI. A "pathologic" Q wave is one that is 0.04 second wide. Many older studies emphasized the depth of the Q wave compared with the R in the same lead, but careful pathologic

Figure 17–1.
A thrombus occludes a diseased coronary artery. The changes of ischemia begin within seconds.

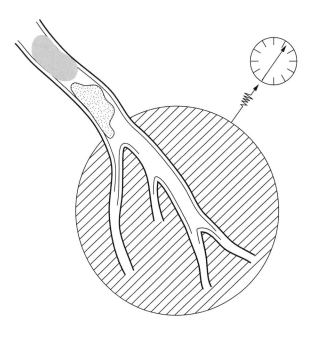

Figure 17–2.
The acutely ischemic tissue produces an injury current—a small, steady potential that registers during the S-T segment. In the lead that "faces" the infarct, the S-T segment will be elevated.

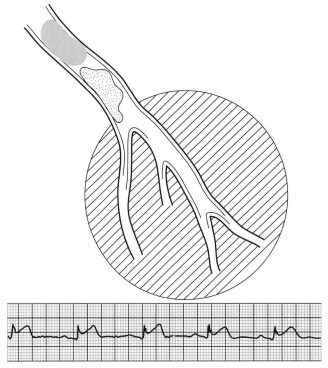

Figure 17–3.
Reciprocal or upside-down electrical pattern on the part of the electric field of the heart opposite the infarct.

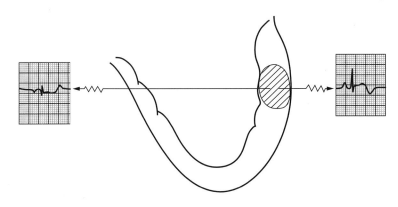

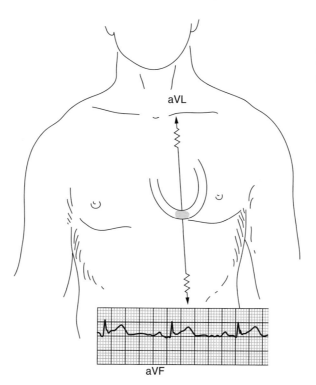

Figure 17–4.
Infarct pattern with elevated S-T segment in the inferior leads—II, III, and aVF.

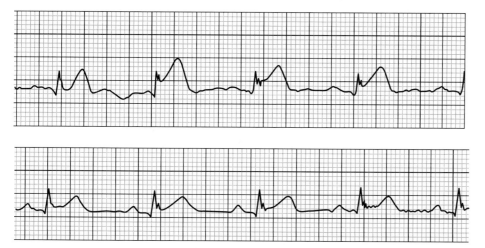

Figure 17–5.
Varieties of S-T elevation with MI.

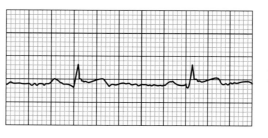

Figure 17–6.
Further progression of S-T change with upward coving of the S-T segment and beginning inversion of the T wave.

correlation has proved that it is the *width* of the Q that is important. Look at Figure 17–8. The Q in the bottom strip is much deeper than the one in the top strip, but both are wide—at least 0.04 second wide—and that's what makes them pathologic Q waves.

Sooner or later, all the injured tissue either dies or recovers. Either way, the injury current disappears, and the S-T segment returns to the baseline. As this happens, the T waves progressively change shape in a direction opposite to the S-T deviation. This "opposite deviation" is what distinguishes the S-T-T pattern of infarction from that of hypertrophy.

Figure 17–7.
The pathologic Q wave (q) presumably arises from distortion of electric forces in the necrotic core of the infarct.

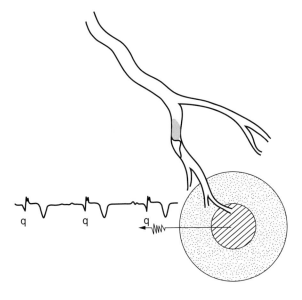

Figure 17–8.
Varieties of pathologic Q waves. The important point is that they're both 0.04 second wide. Note beginning inversion of T waves.

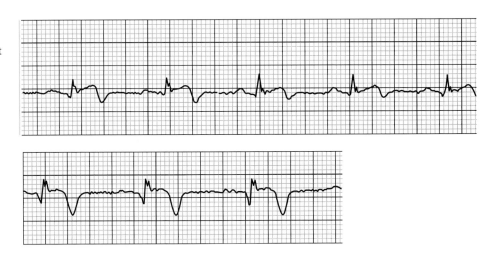

Figure 17–9 represents the "stable" stage of evolution of an MI. The S-T segment was elevated, but now it's back to baseline, and the T wave is inverted. This whole process may take minutes, hours, or days. The whole evolution may be complete in 24 hours, or it may take as long as 2 weeks. This last fact is important to note. Studies by Gorlin and others have shown that the evolution of the ECG in an ordinary, uncomplicated MI may take as long as 2 weeks. Don't become anxious and start thinking of catheters just because there's still some S-T deviation after a week or so. This is well within the range of normal.

You're now ready to apply the principle of reciprocal deviation or "upside-down image" to the diagnosis of MI. Just to make sure you're clear about what the reciprocal pattern is, try drawing the full-blown ECG of MI, complete with Q wave, elevated S-T segment, and inverted T wave (Fig. 17–10). Now turn the paper back to front and upside down and look at it against the light. Where part A is, you see the pattern inscribed in part B, and vice versa. In part B, you recognize that instead of a Q wave, you see an R; instead of an elevated S-T segment, you see one that's depressed; instead of an inverted T wave, you see one that's upright. This is the reciprocal pattern of infarction, and it's just as important as the "direct" infarct pattern in diagnosis. From here on, we're going to use the terms *infarct pattern* and *reciprocal pattern;* be sure you understand what they mean.

Now look at Figure 17–11. There is very striking S-T elevation in aVF, leaving no doubt that there's acute ischemia in the inferior wall. Note the reciprocal pattern in aVL, exactly opposite the deviation in aVF. You diagnose an inferior MI, therefore, when you see infarct

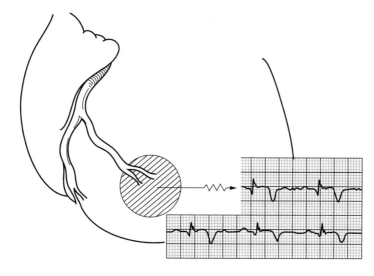

Figure 17–9.
Stable stage of evolution of an infarct pattern with Q, S-T segment almost back to baseline, and inverted T waves.

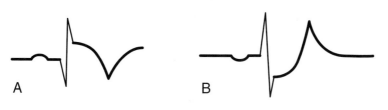

A   B

Figure 17–10.
A simple way to visualize reciprocal patterns. The ECG recorded from one side of the electric field of the heart (**A**) will be seen in an upside-down mirror image on the other (**B**).

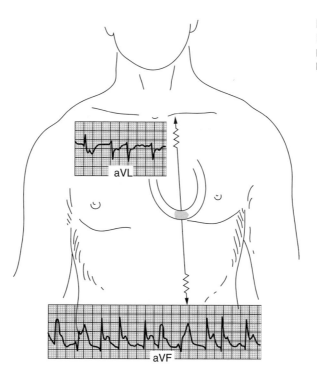

Figure 17–11.
Inferior infarction. Infarct pattern in aVF; reciprocal pattern in aVL.

changes in the "left leg" leads—II, III, and aVF. You confirm the diagnosis when you see reciprocal changes in the leads that are 180 degrees opposite—I and aVL.

When you see reciprocal changes like these, the diagnosis of acute MI is established with 100% confidence. (It's unfortunate that the investigators in the various studies of thrombolysis in MI didn't include anybody with a primary interest in electrocardiography. They produced criteria for thrombolysis like "2 mm S-T elevation in adjacent leads" but totally overlooked the most specific S-T-T deformity for infarction—the reciprocal deviation described here. Most experienced electrocardiographers will agree that the finding of reciprocal S-T-T changes together with significant symptoms is much more specific than simple S-T elevation.)

A Critical Point about Q Waves

A pathologic Q wave is one that's 0.04 second wide. Q waves this wide are always abnormal and practically always indicate necrotic change in the myocardium, new or old. Go back to Chapter 5 and look at Figure 5-1 to refresh your memory about normal, physiologic septal Q waves. Remember that activation of the septum normally produces a narrow Q. The rules are simple:

> 1. **A Q wave that's 0.02 second wide is normal, or "septal."**
>
> 2. **A Q wave that's 0.04 second wide is pathologic.**
>
> 3. **A Q wave that's 0.03 second wide is borderline, possibly pathologic.**

Keep a hand lens handy because you're going to be measuring hundredths of a second.

With These Basic Elements, You're Ready to Detect an Infarct and Localize It Anatomically

Here are the basic rules.

Anterior Infarcts

The infarct pattern is present in the precordial leads. There are usually no reciprocal changes because you can't record from the opposite, or posterior, aspect of the left ventricle (Fig. 17–12). Anterior infarcts can be usefully divided into anteroseptal (V1 and V2, possibly V3) and anterolateral (V5 and V6). (See examples later in the chapter.)

Figure 17–12.
Anterior MI. Q waves, elevated S-T segments, and inverted T waves in V1 to V4.

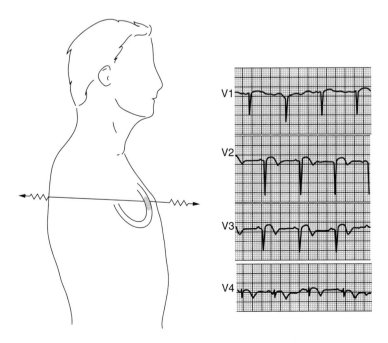

> **1. Inferior infarcts:** infarct pattern in II, III, and aVF; reciprocal pattern in I, aVL (see Fig. 17–11)
>
> **2. Lateral infarcts:** infarct changes in I, aVL, sometimes in V5, V6; reciprocal pattern in II, III, aVF (Fig. 17–13)

Posterior Infarcts

These can be diagnosed only by finding the reciprocal pattern in the precordial leads because the posterior wall of the heart can't be recorded directly by the ECG (Fig. 17–14). Note the tall R in V1—it's really an upside-down Q. The depressed S-T segments are the reciprocal recording of elevated S-T segments on the other side of the electric field of the heart. Often, inferior infarcts will include the posterior wall; when there are infarct changes in II, III, and aVF with reciprocal changes in V1, V2, or V3, there is an inferior-posterior combination (Fig. 17–15). This is an important combination of findings to recognize because it usually means there's a great deal more jeopardized myocardium than in a simple inferior MI. Later in the chapter, you'll have a chance to study a series of examples of infarction, illustrating a number of variations from the basic infarct patterns described earlier.

At this point, a little recent medical history must be cleared up. With all this talk about "reciprocal changes," some of you may be thinking back to studies published 10 or more years ago suggesting that these upside-down S-T relations were really the result of remote, coincidental ischemic events in a different coronary artery. Some investigators looked at coronary angiograms recorded at the time of infarction, and of course, they found disease in other coronary arteries as well. That's not surprising; it's safe to say that in about half of all infarcts, there is multiple vessel disease. These investigators concluded that reciprocal changes were the result of two coincidental ischemic processes evolving at exactly the same time, with identical but opposite S-T changes hour by hour and even minute by minute. If you think about that very long, you're confronting a staggering coincidence. Subsequent investigations have established

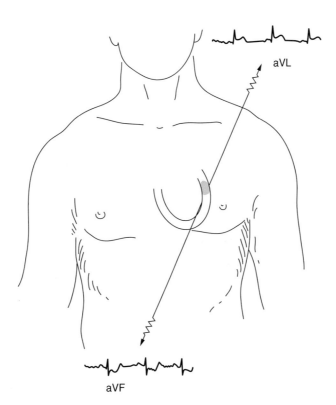

Figure 17–13.
"High" lateral MI. Infarct pattern in aVL, reciprocal pattern in aVF.

Figure 17–14.
Posterior-wall MI. You can't
record directly over the
posterior wall, so you have
to rely on the reciprocal
pattern in the right
precordial leads, V1 to V3.
Remember that the farther
the reciprocal ST
depression of a posterior
infarct extends out across
the precordium, the worse
the prognosis—thus, ST
depression all the way to
V6 would imply a very
large posterior infarct.

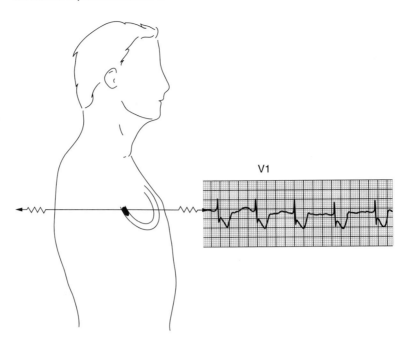

Figure 17–15.
Infarction of inferior and
posterior myocardium. This
is a common combination.

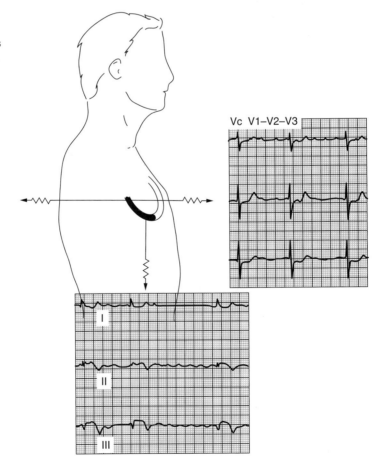

the "reciprocal" basis for S-T deviation and cleared the air of the "remote-coincidental" phenomenon; but there may still be echoes around to worry the student. Forget it.

Special note on right ventricular infarction. Infarction of the right ventricle will always occur in association with the ECG pattern of inferior MI. In addition, right precordial leads can be diagnostic. These are recorded from positions over the right precordium that are analogous to the left-sided leads. Thus, V4-R is recorded in the right midclavicular line, and so on. The ECG diagnosis of right ventricular infarction in these leads is simple: any S-T elevation of 1 mm or more in the right precordial leads is both sensitive and specific for right ventricular infarction. The typical "cove-plane" or tombstone configuration will appear, just as in the left-sided leads.

Some Commandments about the ECG and the Diagnosis of Myocardial Infarction

1. **Don't over-read! The ECG may help you diagnose an infarct, but it won't tell you how large it is or how dangerous it is, or whether it's subendocardial or transmural. A patient can go into cardiogenic shock with one inverted T wave, whereas another patient with S-T elevation all across the precordium may hardly be aware that anything has happened. You can't prognosticate from the ECG!**

2. **You've been looking at typical examples of infarction. Remember that you may see only fragments or parts of these patterns—one deviated S-T segment, one deformed T wave, one pathologic Q. If the symptoms are typical or even suspicious, any acute change in the ECG should be regarded as supporting evidence in the diagnosis of MI.**

3. **Don't forget the distinction between normal septal Q waves and pathologic Q waves.**

4. ***One more time:* The evolution of an MI may be complete in a few hours, or it may take 2 weeks. Don't overreact if the ECG evolves slowly; unless there are symptoms or other signs of further ischemic insult, there's no reason to intervene. (In this day of the overanxious catheter, that's a very important bit of advice.)**

5. **When are wide Q waves normal? In two places: V1 and sometimes V2 and in lead III.**

The right precordial leads "look down" into the negatively charged cavity of the heart, and many normally record a QS—much the same as the potential recorded in aVR. On the other hand, if V1 has a small R wave, and if the leads to the left, such as V2, V3, or V4, *then* record a Q; that Q is 100% diagnostic of infarction.

Since the earliest days of electrocardiography, it has been known that Q waves and inverted T waves are found in lead III in about 15% of normal individuals. It wasn't until Goldberger invented the unipolar limb leads that we understood why that happened. The aVL and aVF leads actually record the electric potential at the left shoulder and the left thigh. Lead III is based on the difference between those two points. When the left leg—aVF—is positive compared with the left arm—aVL—there's an upstroke in III. When aVF is negative compared with aVL, lead III records a downstroke. "Negative" also can mean simply "less positive."

Suppose you have a 2-mm R in aVF and an 8-mm R in aVL. The aVF lead is less positive than aVL, so there's a downstroke, or Q, in III. This is a "false" Q based on the fact that aVL is recording a higher potential than aVF. This problem doesn't arise in I and II because the indifferent electrode is aVR, which is all negative. For practical purposes, ignore lead III and look at aVF. That's the actual left leg potential, and that's all you need to see.

Q Wave Equivalents

A Q wave is a deformity of the initial forces of depolarization that emerges as a negative deflection in the surface ECG. Will this deformity always appear as a negative deflection? Of course not. It can appear as a positive deflection, depending on the lead being recorded, such as the tall R in V1 and V2 in posterior infarction. In fact, MI can distort any part of the QRS and can do it in many different ways.

When you think of the varieties of location and type of pathology associated with MI, it's obvious that a whole spectrum of changes can be produced in the QRS. The middle and terminal forces of the QRS can be distorted just as easily as the initial forces. The surface ECG can show gain or loss of potential, difference in speed of inscription, and change of direction. Many investigators have recorded these changes, and they can be lumped under the heading of *Q wave equivalents*. If you're not prepared to recognize them, you'll miss critical diagnostic information. The notion that infarction will distort only the initial forces of the QRS and that it will always produce a negative deflection has been described as "electrocardiographic naïveté," yet many studies comparing Q wave and non–Q wave infarcts have been based on this crude distinction.

Types of Q Wave Equivalent Deformities

1. **The tall R in the right precordium with posterior infarction is the best known and most widely accepted Q wave equivalent (Fig. 17–16).**

2. **A drastic shift in frontal plane axis is another common change with infarction. Typically, an inferior infarct produces a loss of inferiorly directed forces so that the R in aVF becomes smaller and the R in aVL becomes taller, with a leftward and superior shift of axis toward the remaining viable myocardium (Fig. 17–17).**

3. **Striking localized loss of R in the precordial leads is widely recognized as a Q wave equivalent (Fig. 17–18).**

4. **Notching or slurring of various elements of the QRS is common (Figs. 17–19 and 17–20).**

5. **Sudden, otherwise unaccountable shift of axis—to the right in this case. This can be produced by a lateral wall infarction as a simple result of loss of leftward-conducting myocardium (Fig. 17–21).**

Myth 1: Death of a Myth

You may have heard that Q wave infarcts are transmural and that non–Q wave infarcts are subendocardial. There was never any basis for this notion; it was based on a mistake by Prinzmetal, which he later acknowledged, but every text for a generation repeated it as gospel. In fact, every careful pathologic study has shown that about half of all Q wave infarcts are in fact subendocardial and about half of all non–Q wave infarcts are transmural. The Q wave tells you there's an infarct, but it doesn't tell you anything about the pathology. I had the pleasure of helping to lay this myth to rest in one of the first editions of the *Journal of the American College of Cardiology* back in 1983.[1]

Myth 2: Another Myth Debunked

Many cardiologists were so wedded to the idea that the pathologic Q must mean *something* specific that they produced another bit of nonsense that dominated medical literature for 5 or 6 years. It was alleged that non–Q wave infarcts were somehow "incomplete" or "unstable," grounds for aggressive intervention. Some of my colleagues and I were able to demol-

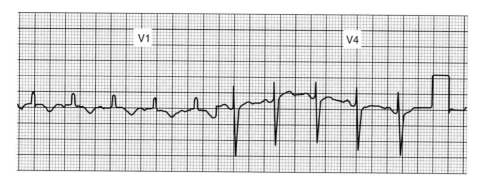

Figure 17–16.
Q wave equivalent. The tall R in V1 is in fact an upside-down Q.

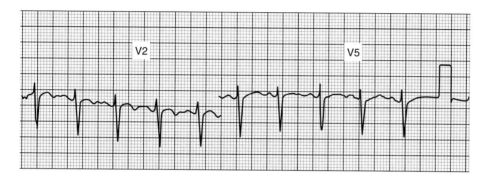

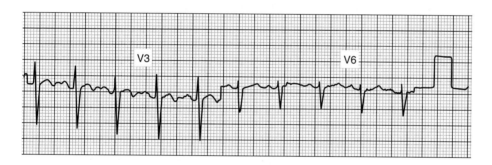

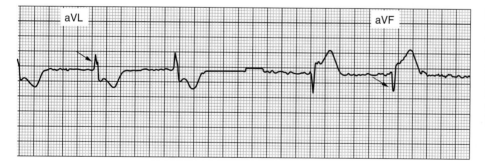

Figure 17–17.
Q wave equivalent. A new tall R appears in aVL and a new deep S in aVF, reflecting loss of inferior forces in an inferior wall MI. The axis has shifted superiorly, away from the infarcted area.

ish this chimera as well. We found that no valid study had ever supported this claim. We found further that the studies alleging the unstable character of the non–Q wave infarct to be so flawed in protocol that any intelligent fourth-year medical student could discredit them.[2]

What does the pathologic Q wave tell you? It tells you that there is necrotic myocardium, usually from infarction. Period. Q wave infarcts on average tend to be larger than the non–Q wave variety, but the two categories overlap to such an extent that you can't draw any practical clinical conclusions from the distinction.

Special final note: When is aVL significant and when isn't it? As you know, aVR normally records a totally negative complex because it's recording a "cavity" potential. Sometimes aVL

Figure 17–18.
Q wave equivalent. Abrupt loss of precordial R voltage in the presence of an anterior infarct.

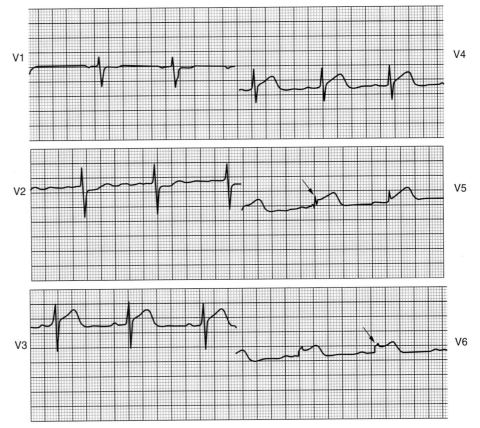

Figure 17–19.
Q wave equivalent. Loss of R in aVF in 1 day during the course of an inferior MI, reflecting loss of viable inferior myocardium.

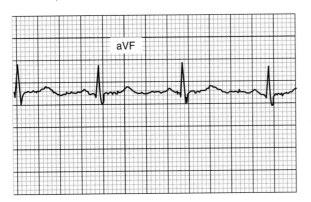

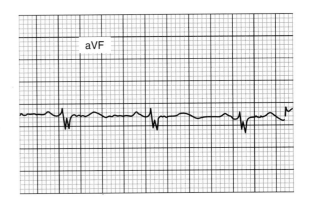

records the same kind of potential because of a "vertical" heart (Fig. 17–22). When aVL looks like aVR, you can ignore the negative deflections. On the other hand, when aVL is recording from left of the septum, you'll see the usual septal Q followed by an R or a plain tall R. A pathologic Q wave appearing in that setting of course is a very specific marker of infarction.

The last part of the chapter, from Figures 17–23 to 17–41, presents a variety of ECGs recorded in the course of documented MIs. These tracings illustrate a number of the possible variations and combinations of the simple elements presented so far. Take time to review them carefully.

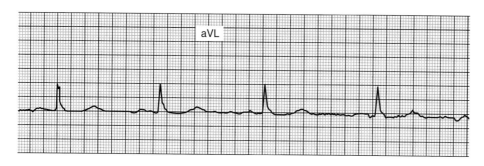

Figure 17–20.
Q wave equivalent. The previous day, aVF had consisted of a tall R and aVL of a small r followed by a deep S. Twenty-four hours after inferior infarction, aVF is a tiny, slurred complex (arrow) and aVL has changed to a simple tall R.

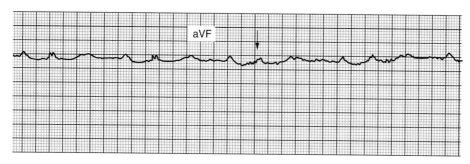

Figure 17–21.
Q wave equivalent. The ECG had been normal 2 weeks previously. Now the axis has shifted dramatically to the right, and there's a striking loss of R in V5 and V6 together with a tall R in V1. All these QRS changes are as significant as the presence of a simple pathologic Q: they mean infarction.

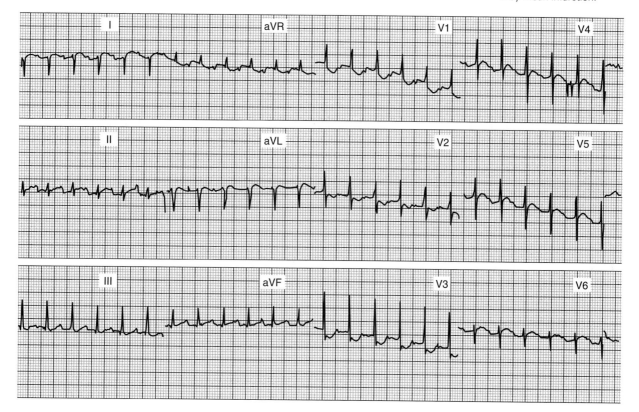

Figure 17–22.
"Cavity" potential in aVL. The aVL looks exactly like aVR, which means that the aVL electrode is recording from the negatively charged interior aspect of the left ventricle. The configuration of the QRS in aVL, therefore, has no practical significance in this setting.

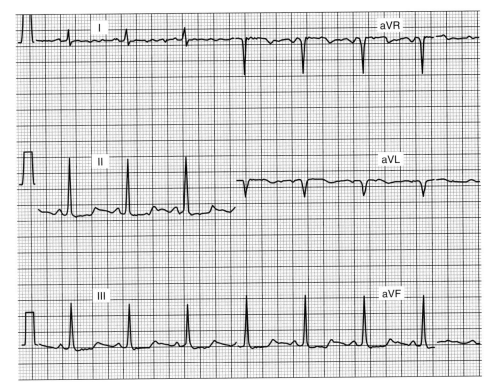

Figure 17–23.
Note Q waves in V2 to V4. The whole QRS complex consists of a simple downward deflection, or Q wave. This is sometimes referred to as a "QS" complex. There is S-T elevation in V2 to V5 and beginning T wave inversion in V2 to V5 together with an inverted T in aVL. Diagnosis: anterior MI with lateral wall involvement (aVL).

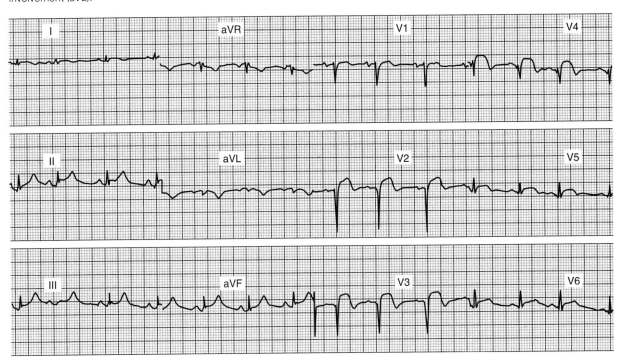

Figure 17–24.
Q waves in II, III, aVF, and V6. Elevated S-T segments in the same leads as well as in V5. S-T depression, aVL. This is a typical pattern of inferior MI with the infarct pattern in II, III, and aVF and the reciprocal pattern in aVL. It is very common for the infarct pattern to appear in V5 and V6 in inferior infarcts because the artery supplying the inferior myocardium almost always supplies the lower lateral wall of the left ventricle. It's important to realize that the changes in II, III, and aVF and V5 and V6 are all part of the same process, *not* part of two separate infarcts.

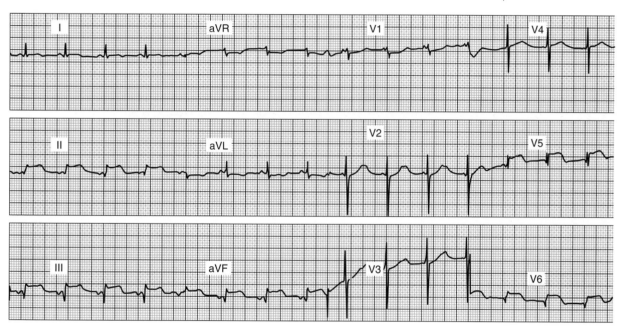

Figure 17–25.
Typical reciprocal S-T
deviation with elevation in
II, III, and aVF and
depression in I and aVL.
Seeing these leads alone,
you can predict inferior
infarction with 100%
accuracy.

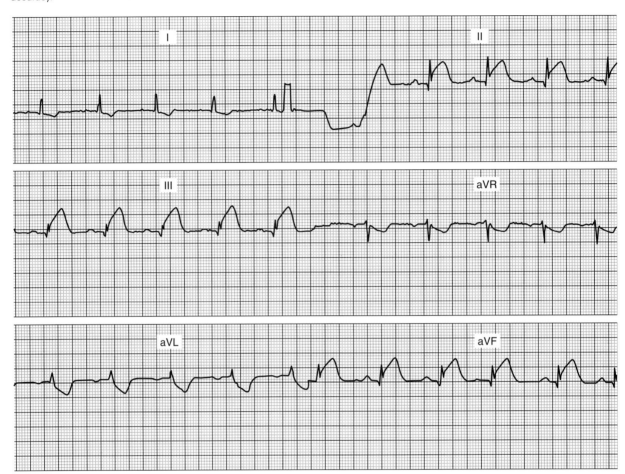

Figure 17–26.
V leads for tracing shown in Fig. 17–25. There are tall R waves in the right precordium with deeply depressed S-T segments, indicating infarction of the posterior wall with equal accuracy. (Turn these leads upside-down in your mind's eye, and you see what you'd record if you applied an electrode directly to the posterior wall over the infarcted area.)

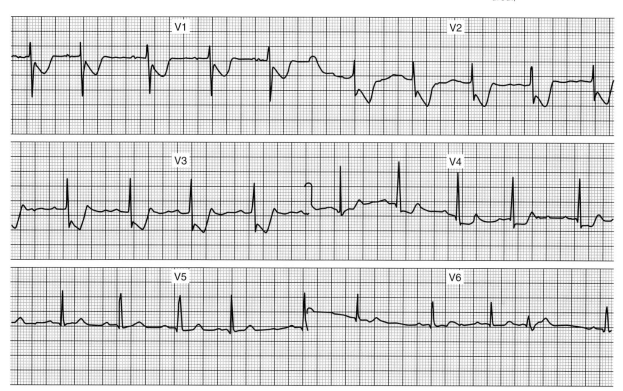

Figure 17–27.

Q waves, I, aVL, V2 to V5. Elevated S-T, aVL, V2 to V5. Evidence of anterior and lateral MI. Important point about Q waves: there's a small r in V1. This r disappears in V2 to V5, and true Q waves appear. Sometimes there's a QS complex in V1 or V2 simply because of the electric "position" of the heart, but when you see an rS complex in the right precordial leads, such as in V1, and then the r disappears and Q waves appear in the leads to the left of that point, it's 100% evidence that these are pathologic Q waves and that you're dealing with an anterior MI.

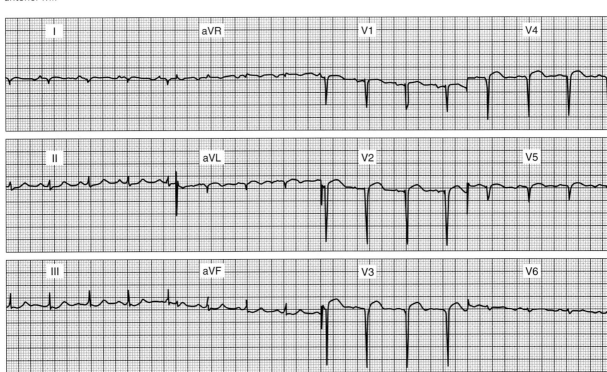

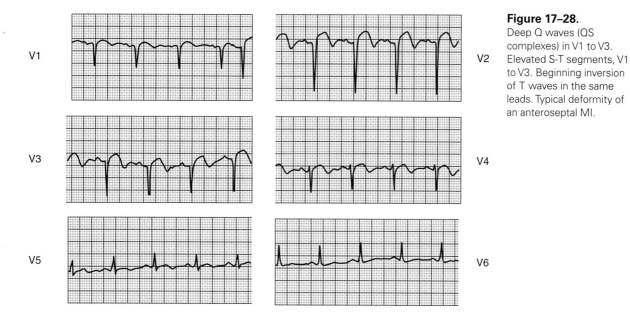

Figure 17–28.
Deep Q waves (QS complexes) in V1 to V3. Elevated S-T segments, V1 to V3. Beginning inversion of T waves in the same leads. Typical deformity of an anteroseptal MI.

Figure 17–29.
Q waves and elevated S-T segments in leads I and aVL. Reciprocal pattern in II, III, and aVF. This is a true "high lateral" infarct, in sharp contrast to the "low lateral" deformity in V5 and V6 often seen as part of inferior infarction.

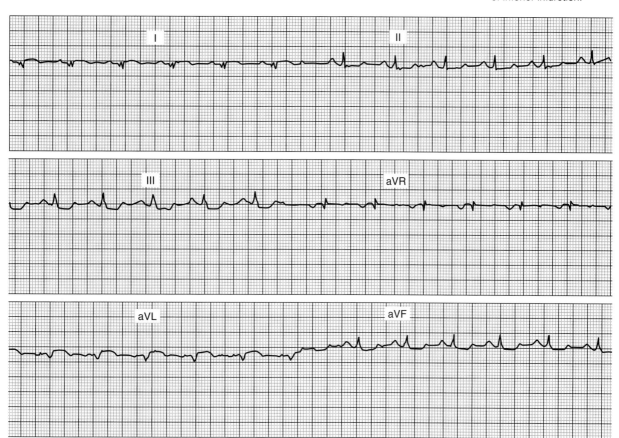

Figure 17–30.

"Hyperacute" S-T-T
changes. (How can
something be more acute
than acute? Bad
semantics, but a useful
term.) Dramatic S-T
elevation in V2 and V3,
with tall, upright T waves.
This is a reliable indicator
of acute anterior MI.

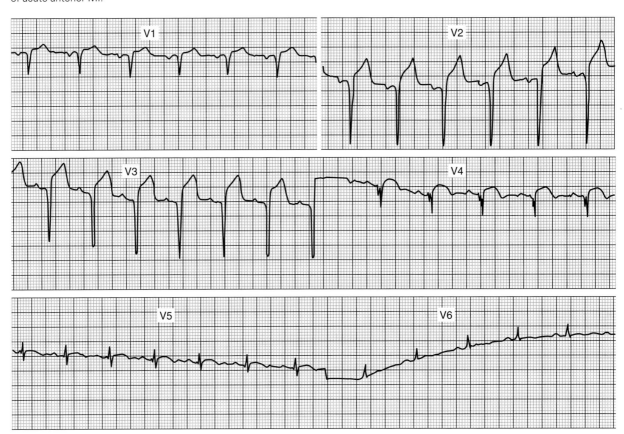

Figure 17–31.

Now put together some of the things you've learned. There's a regular ventricular rhythm, rate 41. The QRS complexes are narrow. The P waves have no relation to the QRS complexes. Diagnosis: (1) complete AV dissociation with junctional rhythm, (2) ventricular rate less than 45, and (3) no capture by an adequate number of P waves to test the system. Conclusion: complete heart block in the AV node (narrow QRS). Depressed S-T in leads I and aVL; elevated S-T in II, III, and aVF; Q in III and aVF. Inferior MI. (AV nodal block is common with inferior MIs because the artery that supplies the inferior surface also supplies the AV node about 85% of the time.)

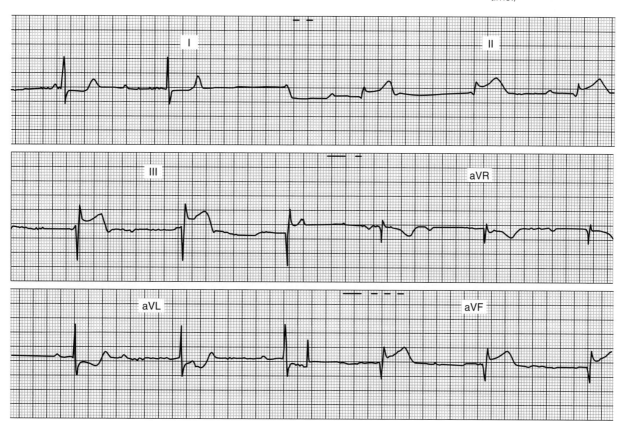

Figure 17–32.
Tiny r in V1. QS in V2 and
V3. Inverted T in V1 to V4.
Anteroseptal MI, almost
always an LAD lesion. LAD,
left anterior descending.

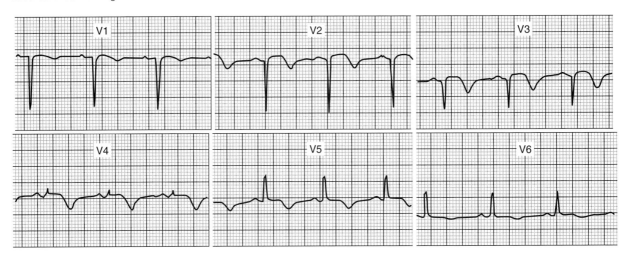

Figure 17–33.
Here's an infarct pattern
developing before your
eyes in about 23 seconds.
This is lead V4, recorded
during chest pain. Note the
change in shape of the T
wave from upright to
inverted and back to
upright across the top
strip. Across the bottom
strip, you can see the
typical injury current
emerging with tombstone
S-T elevation progressing
to T wave inversion within
five heartbeats. It can
happen fast!

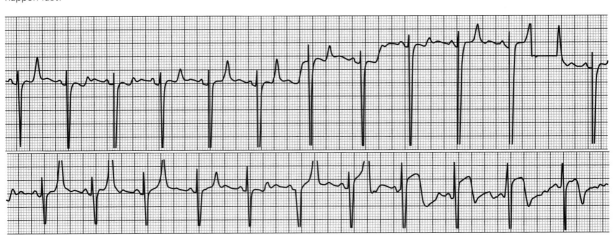

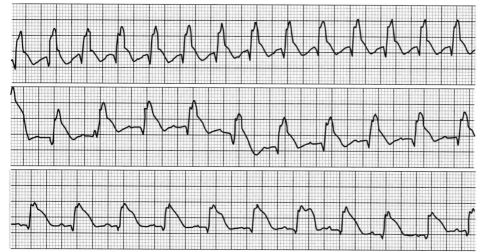

Figure 17–34.
Another example of extreme S-T elevation in the early stage of an infarct. The top strip suggests bundle-branch block, but as you can see in the bottom two strips, there's simply extreme S-T elevation, so high that the S-T segment takes off from the top of the R wave.

Figure 17–35.
Hyperacute S-T elevation in V2 to V4; reciprocal S-T depression in leads II, III, and aVF.

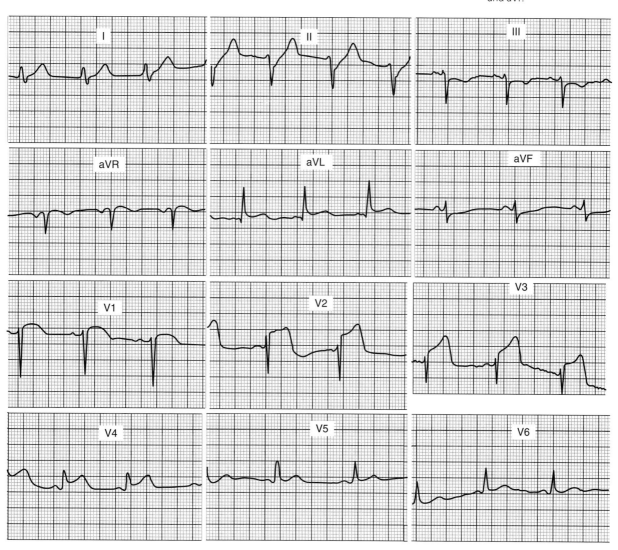

Figure 17–36.
High lateral MI with infarct
changes confined to leads
I and aVL. Interesting
configuration of aVR with
tall R; this is a reciprocal
manifestation of the
Q aVL.

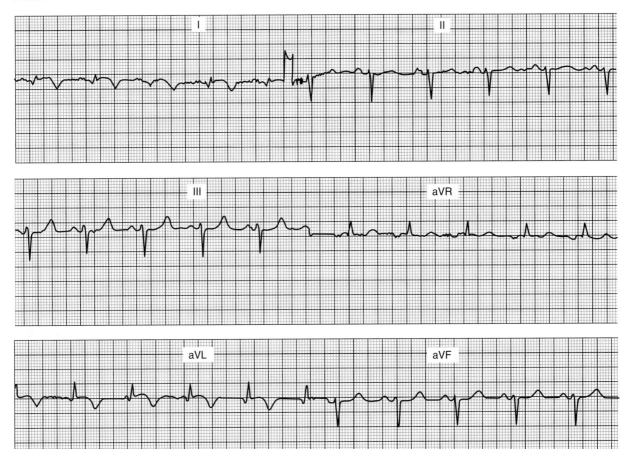

Figure 17–37.
Precordial leads with a variation of the hyperacute pattern. Q waves are present from V1 through V5. Note interesting beginning of reciprocal S-T-T change in V6.

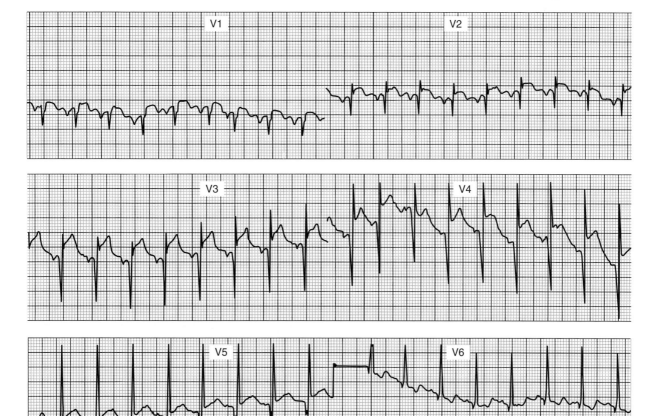

Figure 17–38.
This is an extreme example of hyperacute S-T-T deformity. Note also absence of P waves with an accelerated junctional rhythm interrupted by VPCs. (Oddly, this patient subsequently had an uneventful course; the initial appearance of the ECG can be really deceptive in terms of the subsequent course.)

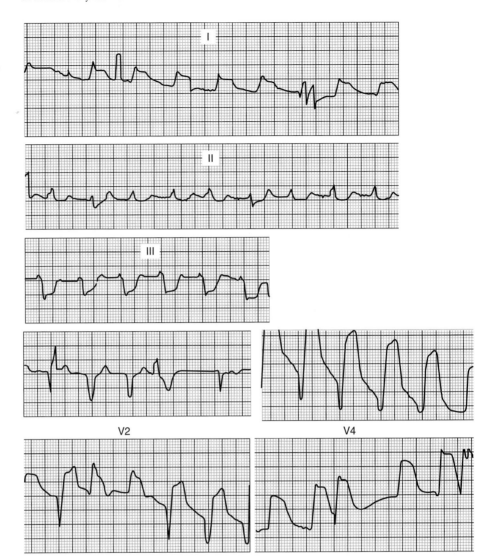

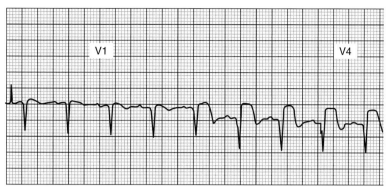

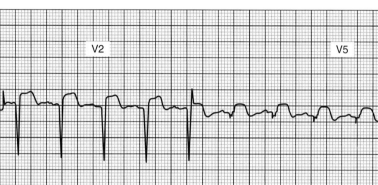

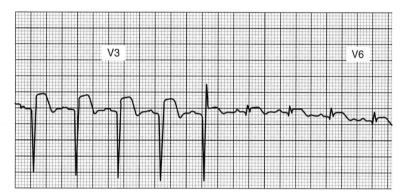

Figure 17–39.
Q waves and Q wave equivalents everywhere— QS complexes from V1 through V5 plus aVL (Q wave equivalent low voltages in frontal place leads). This is one time you can do some prognosticating: really widespread Q waves connote a large area of infarction.

Figure 17–40.
Minimal but dangerous! S-T depression in the precordial leads of the resting ECG raises four possibilities: digitalis effect, low serum K, hypertrophy, or ischemia. When you've ruled out the first three, *always* assume that precordial S-T depression means ischemia. This is a point not sufficiently emphasized by many authors, but it's absolutely reliable.

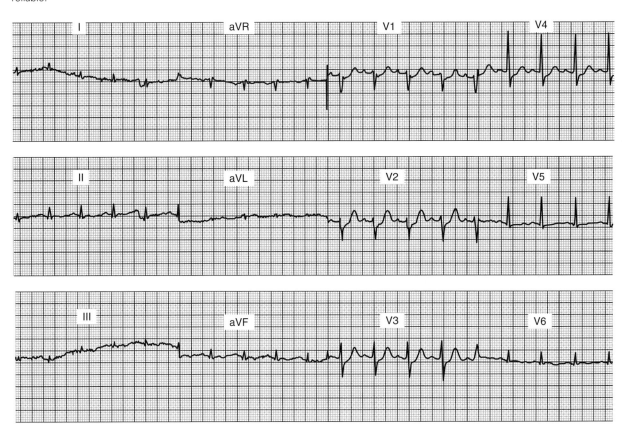

Figure 17–41.
Here's the same phenomenon of precordial S-T depression, much more pronounced than in Fig. 17–40. It is further reinforced by reciprocal S-T in V6. It's important to remember that you can see reciprocal S-T deviation in opposite precordial leads, such as V1 and V6. This is sometimes a really important marker for infarction.

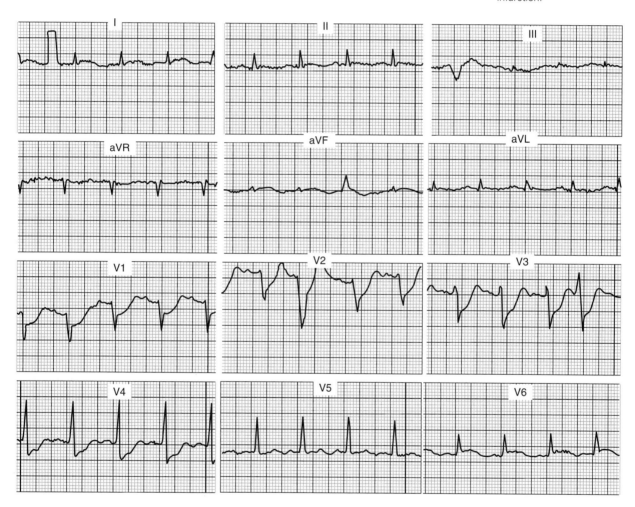

References

1. Phibbs B: "Transmural" vs. "subendocardial" myocardial infarction: an electrocardiographic myth. J Am Coll Cardiol 1983;1:561–564.
2. Phibbs B, Marcus F, Marriott HJC, et al: Q wave versus non–Q wave myocardial infarction: a meaningless distinction. J Am Coll Cardiol 1999;33:2:576–582.

Eighteen

Diagnosing Myocardial Infarction in the Presence of Bundle-Branch Block

Myocardial Infarction in the Presence of Right Bundle-Branch Block

This is easy. Most infarcts take place in the left ventricle. Because the left ventricle is activated normally when right bundle-branch block (RBBB) is present, you read the electrocardiogram (ECG) the way you always would—with two obvious differences. First, you ignore the terminal wide deflection that characterizes RBBB—the wide terminal R in V1 and the wide terminal S in I and V6. Those wide deflections are, of course, the result of the conduction defect and have nothing to do with infarction. Second, remember that it's normal to see inverted T waves over the blocked ventricle. In other words, expect to see inverted T waves in the lead with the wide terminal R—usually V1 and V2 and occasionally V3. Again, this T wave inversion is a result of the conduction defect and is a normal part of RBBB (Fig. 18–1).

Otherwise, you use exactly the same criteria for infarction you'd use if the RBBB weren't present. A Q wave is still a Q wave and has exactly the same significance with or without RBBB. You read the changes in the S-T-T complex exactly the way you always would. As you can see in Figures 18–2 and 18–3, there are obvious pathologic Q waves, and the characteristic "tombstone" S-T-T deformity is obvious even in leads over the blocked ventricle.

Important Note about T Waves and RBBB

Although it's normal to see inverted T waves over the blocked ventricle, you should not see inverted T waves when you start recording over the left ventricular area—that is, when you're recording from V4, V5, or V6. When you lose the wide terminal R wave, you've left the electric field of the blocked ventricle. T waves to the left of this point should be upright. If the T waves are inverted over the normally activated ventricle, it's abnormal (Fig. 18–4).

Myocardial Infarction in the Presence of Left Bundle-Branch Block

This is much more difficult and sometimes impossible to diagnose. Much of the time, all you can say is that left bundle-branch block (LBBB) is indeed present, and that's the end of it (Fig. 18–5). However, there are sometimes clues that are very precise:

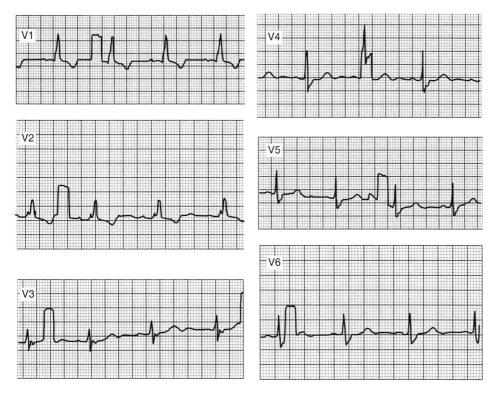

Figure 18–1.
Normal T wave configuration in RBBB. Note that the T waves are inverted only in the precordial leads with the wide R'—in other words, over the blocked ventricle.

Figure 18–2.
Anterior myocardial infarction in the presence of RBBB. Note pathologic Q waves in leads II, III, and aVF as well as in V1 to V6. The characteristic tombstone S-T elevation with reciprocal T wave inversion is present across the precordium. In other words, all the ECG elements of myocardial infarction are obvious despite the RBBB.

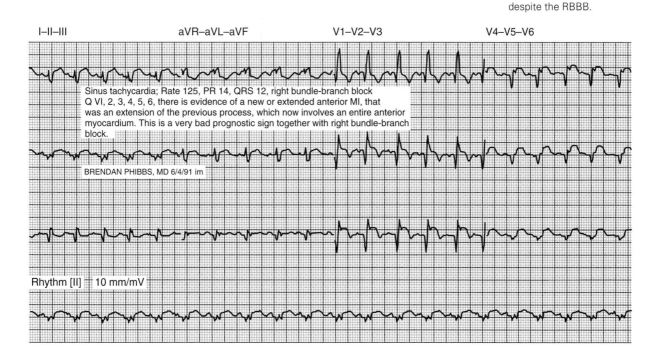

Sinus tachycardia; Rate 125, PR 14, QRS 12, right bundle-branch block Q VI, 2, 3, 4, 5, 6, there is evidence of a new or extended anterior MI, that was an extension of the previous process, which now involves an entire anterior myocardium. This is a very bad prognostic sign together with right bundle-branch block.

BRENDAN PHIBBS, MD 6/4/91 im

Figure 18–3.
Striking changes of anterior myocardial infarction in the presence of RBBB and atrial fibrillation, with Q waves in V2 to V5 and unmistakable tombstone S-T-T pattern in the same leads.

Figure 18–4.
Abnormal S-T-T configuration in the *left* precordial leads in the presence of RBBB. The T wave deformity in V1 and V2 can be attributed to the conduction defect, but from V3 to V6, the electrodes are clearly recording from the unblocked, or left, ventricular aspect of the field, and the T waves should be upright. If they're not, the ECG is abnormal (*arrowheads*) and is consistent with myocardial pathology on some basis.

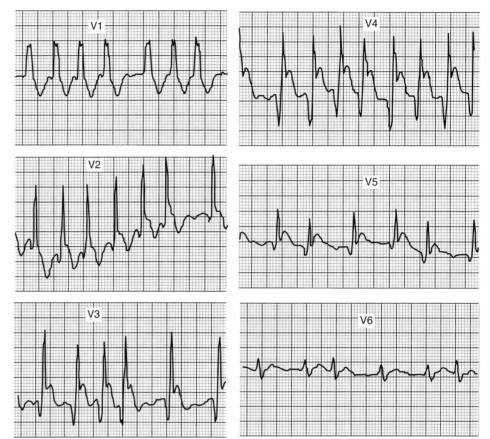

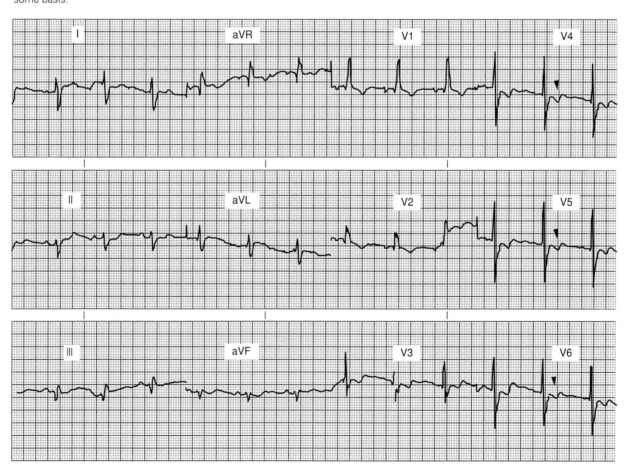

1. **Any pathologic Q wave is still a significant Q even in the presence of LBBB (Figs. 18–6 and 18–7). LBBB per se never produces a pathologic Q; when you see one, it's always the result of pathology and never the result of the conduction defect.**

2. **There's a specific kind of S-T-T deformity that characterizes LBBB. The S-T-T forces are directed away from the QRS forces, so that in the lead with the wide R wave, there's a depressed S-T segment and a diphasic or inverted T (Fig. 18–8). However, you may see patterns of S-T-T deformity that don't fit the LBBB configuration. Sometimes you'll see a typical tombstone S-T-T in the presence of LBBB, and then you can diagnose an acute ischemic process despite the presence of LBBB (Fig. 18–9). In other words, there's a kind of S-T elevation or depression you expect to find as a result of the LBBB. When you encounter S-T elevation or depression that doesn't fit the pattern of LBBB, you can diagnose ischemia. Therefore, in the leads with a wide R wave like I, aVL, and V6, you should see S-T depression as a result of the bundle-branch block. When you see elevation in these leads, it's never the result of the conduction defect; it indicates ischemia. Conversely, in leads with wide S waves like V1, V2, and V3, LBBB should produce S-T elevation. When you see S-T depression in these leads, it's a very reliable marker of acute ischemia.**

With all this in mind, take a look at Figure 18–10, and you'll recognize a typical infarct pattern in leads III and aVF, complete with pathologic Q waves and typical tombstone S-T-T. You can now diagnose myocardial infarction with perfect confidence despite the LBBB.

Figures 18–11 and 18–12 are striking examples of obvious myocardial infarction in the setting of RBBB and LBBB, respectively. As this book was going to press, a study of more than 21,000 cases of myocardial infarction confirmed these observations about diagnosing LBBB in the presence of myocardial infarction, especially with reference to S-T depression in leads V1 to V3 in the setting of LBBB; the conduction defect itself never produces S-T depression in those leads.

Figure 18–5.
Typical LBBB. The S-T-T deformity is obviously consistent with the conduction defect.

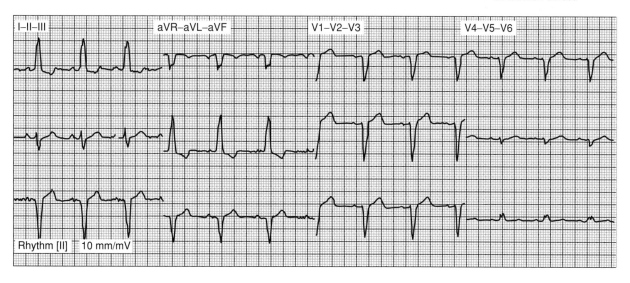

I–II–III   aVR–aVL–aVF   V1–V2–V3   V4–V5–V6

Rhythm [II]   10 mm/mV

Figure 18–6.
LBBB with pathologic Q waves in leads II, III, and aVF, and V5 and V6. These are in fact QS complexes. Note particularly that in V1 to V4, there are R waves. When these disappear with the change to a QS complex in V5 and V6, there is hard-core, 100% evidence of infarction or comparable pathology. The QS deformity cannot possibly be attributed to the conduction defect.

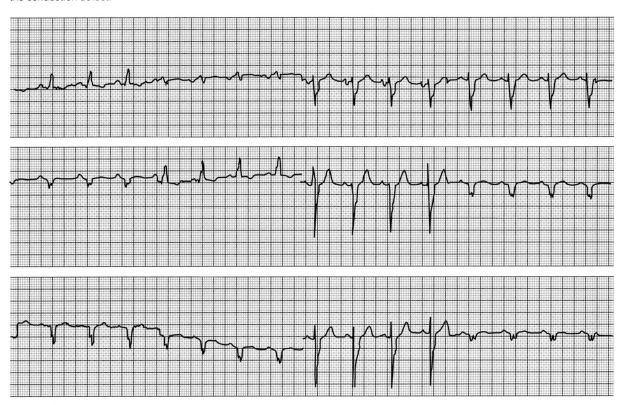

Figure 18–7.
A and **B**, Pathologic Q waves in leads I, aVL, and V6 in the setting of LBBB. This is 100% reliable as a marker of lateral wall myocardial infarction. Note also the typical tombstone deformity of S-T V6.

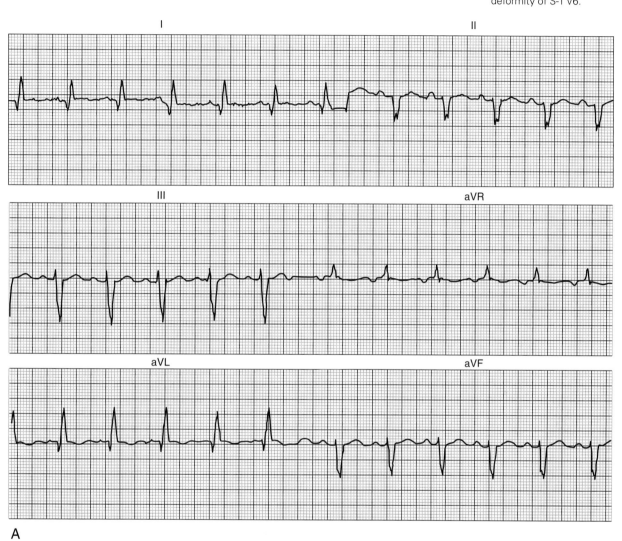

A

(continued)

Figure 18–7, cont'd.

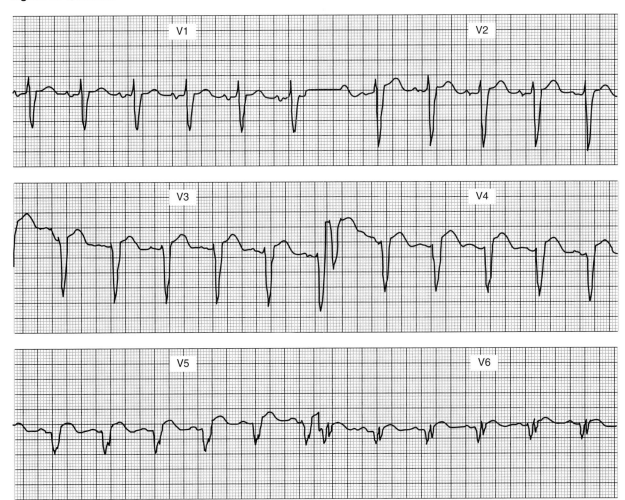

B

Figure 18–8.
LBBB with very striking
S-T-T deformity of the type
consistent with the
conduction defect. Note
again the depressed S-T
and inverted T hockey-
stick configuration in the
leads with the wide R, and
the opposite configuration
in the leads with the wide
S. Contrast this with the
tombstone S-T-T in the
preceding illustrations; the
difference is striking and
diagnostic.

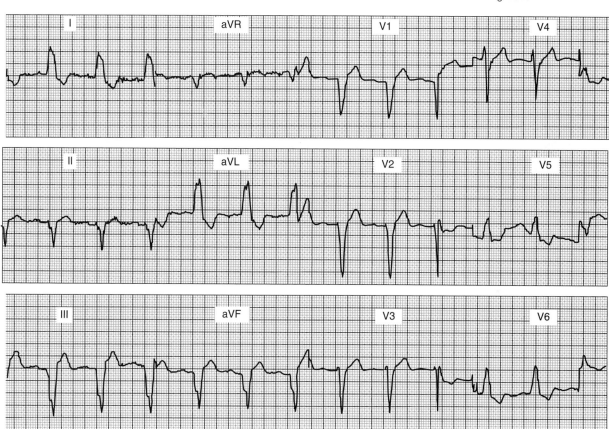

Figure 18–9.
Comparison of the S-T-T pattern of LBBB with the tombstone S-T-T superimposed on preexisting LBBB (*arrowheads*). When the typical S-T-T pattern of infarction appears in the presence of LBBB, it is possible to make a precise diagnosis despite the conduction defect.

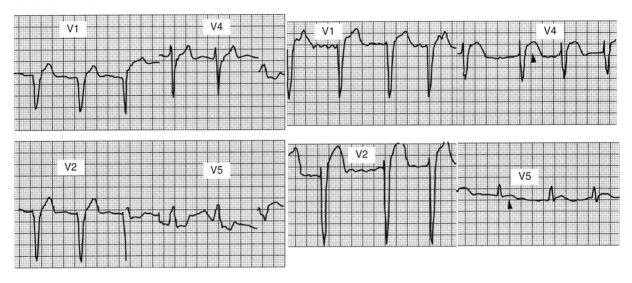

Figure 18–10.
Obvious pattern of inferior myocardial infarction in the setting of LBBB.

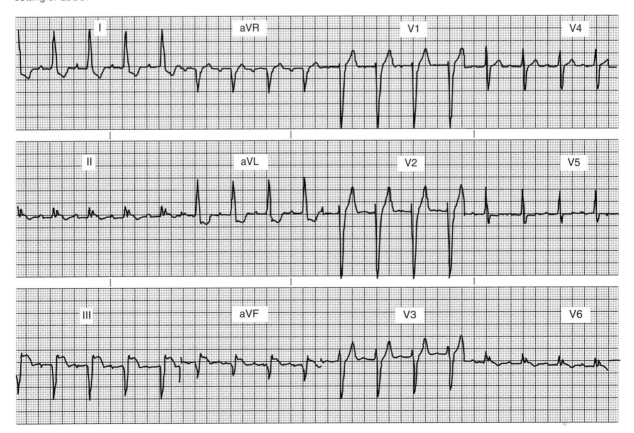

Figure 18–11.
Acute anterior ischemic
S-T changes in the setting
of RBBB. The S-T
elevation in V2 to V5 is
totally different from the
pattern you'd expect with
RBBB. Note also the
reciprocal S-T deviation in
II, III, aVF, and aVL.

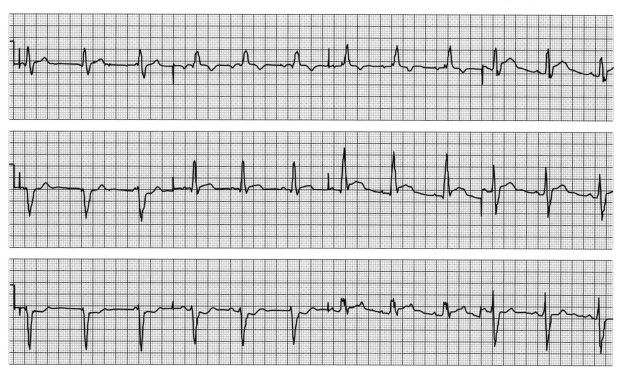

Figure 18–12.
Striking hyperacute S-T-T
deformity of anterior
myocardial infarction in the
presence of LBBB. Note
also reciprocal S-T
deviation with elevation in I
and aVL and depression in
II, III, and aVF.

I–II–III   aVR–aVL–aVF   V1–V2–V3   V4–V5–V6

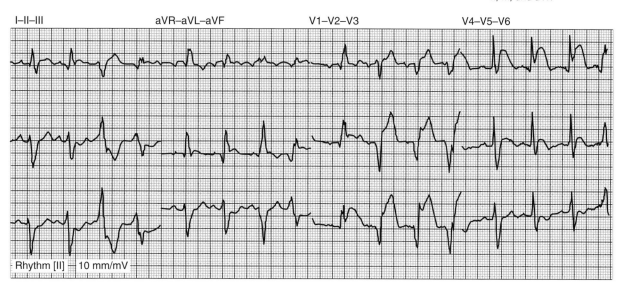

Rhythm [II]   10 mm/mV

Nineteen

Transient Myocardial Ischemia and Angina Pectoris

Angina pectoris is a *symptom;* to be more precise, it's a collection of symptoms. Transient myocardial ischemia, on the other hand, is a *pathologic state.* It means that there's a temporary lack of adequate blood flow to some area of heart muscle. Sometimes transient myocardial ischemia produces the kind of discomfort we call angina pectoris. Sometimes it doesn't.

What are the symptoms of transient myocardial ischemia? To quote Ernest Hemingway, they're various. In the first place, there may not be any symptoms at all. Transient myocardial ischemia may be totally "silent." TMI (as we may now call it) may depress left ventricular function acutely, causing any or all of the symptoms of left heart failure. TMI may cause arrhythmias and can lead to sudden death. In other words, TMI can produce a whole spectrum of different signs and symptoms; classic angina pectoris is only one (Table 19–1).

The electrocardiogram (ECG) is useful in transient myocardial ischemia in two ways:

> **1. It may demonstrate change during anginal symptoms, thus confirming the clinical diagnosis of angina pectoris.**
>
> **2. It may demonstrate change when there are no symptoms, or when the symptoms are atypical, thus providing objective evidence that coronary artery disease is in fact present.**

Transient myocardial ischemia is exactly what the name implies: transient. So are the ECG changes that accompany it.

The common ECG change during TMI is S-T deviation—elevation or depression (Fig. 19–1A–C). There may also be deformity of the T waves; they may change from upright to inverted, or vice versa (Fig. 19–2). (The reader may recognize this as the first part of Fig. 17–33, recording the S-T-T changes in the seconds immediately before an MI.)

There are no specific S-T-T changes that characterize TMI; any acute change can be significant. The point to remember is that TMI sometimes produces change in the S-T-T complex and even in the configuration of the QRS. The absence of acute change doesn't rule out angina, but the presence of ECG change during pain is the strongest possible evidence of an acute ischemic process.

So far so good, but now the reader comes up against an odd gap in modern cardiologic knowledge: What are the specificity and sensitivity of acute S-T-T change in detecting TMI? Nobody can really answer this question because nobody's ever done an adequate study of the subject. When a patient lying in a hospital bed suffers pain that may be anginal, the nearest nurse will always administer nitroglycerin long before there's time to record a 12-lead ECG. That's as it should be—you'd have to be pretty cold-blooded to stand around watching a patient suffer while you waited for the ECG machine to be connected just to let

Table 19–1. Symptoms of Transient Myocardial Ischemia

1. Angina pectoris
2. Transient depression of left ventricular function with typical symptoms of congestive heart failure
3. Arrhythmias
4. Nonspecific symptoms, e.g., apprehension, paresthesias
5. Sudden death
6. No symptoms ("silent" ischemia)

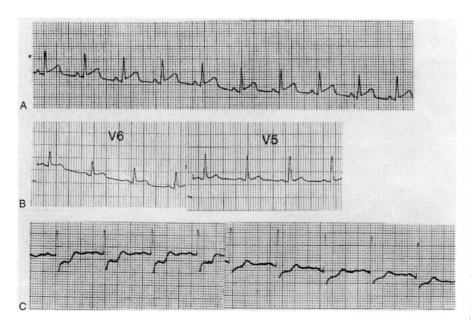

Figure 19–1.
Examples of S-T deviation during transient myocardial ischemia, in these cases manifested by anginal pain. The S-T elevation is obvious in **A**. The minor S-T elevation in **B** is equally significant because it represented a change, during symptoms, from the baseline S-T previously recorded. On the left side of **C**, there is typical horizontal S-T depression of 4 mm, diagnostic of ischemia. The upsloping S-T depression on the left side is less significant, but when changes of this magnitude accompany symptoms, the diagnosis of transient myocardial ischemia is established, for all practical purposes.

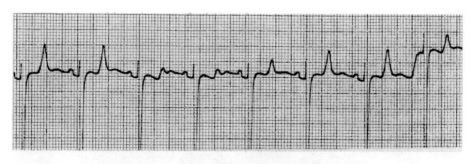

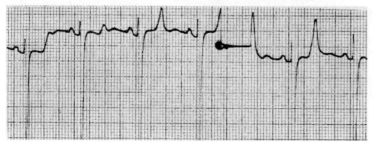

Figure 19–2.
Very dramatic changes in both S-T and T wave morphology taking place within a few seconds during anginal pain. These strips are continuous.

you carry out some research! This small practical point has precluded any definitive study of S-T-T change during spontaneous angina. Everybody assumes that acute ECG change during pain is highly specific for TMI, but how sensitive is it? How often does the ECG remain normal during genuine spontaneous angina? Nobody knows.

In contrast to the ignorance that surrounds the question of S-T change during spontaneous angina, there is voluminous information about the kind and degree of S-T change during deliberate stress, for example, during stress testing. Certain reliable, well-correlated rules have emerged:

1. **Any S-T elevation caused by physical stress is significant. It practically always connotes ischemia.**

2. **S-T depression is usefully divided into two types: *junction depression* and *horizontal or downsloping depression*.**

3. **Junction depression means that only the junction of the S-T with the QRS is depressed; the rest of the segments slope *upward* to the T wave (Fig. 19–3). Junction S-T depression during exercise is significant only if the depression is very severe, that is, if it equals 4 mm or more. It's also necessary to take into account the *rate of rise* of the S-T segment. If it's still depressed 2 mm or more, 0.08 second from the QRS, it's significant. In either case, this type of marked junction depression usually connotes ischemia (Fig. 19–4).**

4. **Horizontal or downsloping depression means that the S-T segment is depressed with a horizontal or downsloping configuration for at least 0.08 second from the junction (Fig. 19–5). When this kind of depression is present, the following numbers apply:**

   a. **0.5 mm depression: possibly ischemia (odds about 50%)**
   b. **1 mm depression: probably ischemia (odds about 75%)**
   c. **1.5 mm to 2 mm depression: almost certainly ischemia (odds about 90%)**

These criteria have been assessed against angiographically demonstrated coronary artery disease in many thousands of cases, so there's no question that they're reasonably reliable in the right setting.

Figure 19–3.
Moderate junction depression of the S-T segment with upsloping configuration. This is often a normal variant during stress testing.

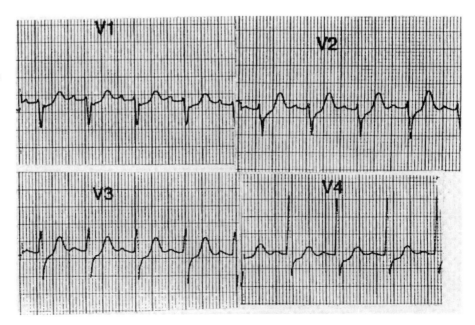

Figure 19–4.
Deep junction S-T depression. When the junction of the QRS with the S-T segment is depressed 4 mm or more, it has a high correlation with ischemia.

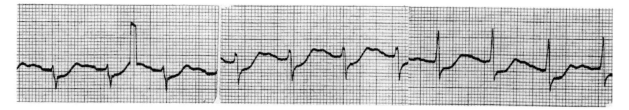

Figure 19–5.
A–C, Horizontal or downsloping depression of S-T segments. See text for correlation of degree of S-T depression with confidence of diagnosis of transient myocardial ischemia.

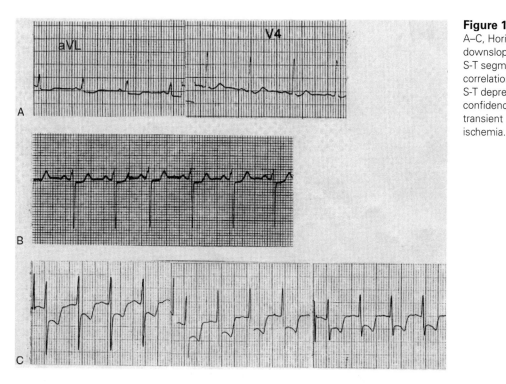

1. **How significant is silent myocardial ischemia?** The best available data suggest that silent ischemia has exactly the same significance as symptomatic ischemia. The important fact is that ischemia is present; whether it produces symptoms or not is incidental, an accident of autonomic innervation.

2. **How common is silent myocardial ischemia?** Two colleagues and I published what was probably the first study in the field, in 1968.[1] We studied a large number of patients with documented coronary artery disease and recorded their symptoms at the time of acute S-T change during exercise testing. Only 41% described painful discomfort, whereas 46% described other symptoms such as severe abrupt dyspnea, paresthesias, or apprehension, and 10.8% reported no symptoms of any kind. Thus, myocardial ischemia is either silent or is accompanied by symptoms other than pain in about half of all cases. A glance at Table 19–1 will aid in understanding this phenomenon: many of the symptoms of TMI are in fact manifestations of acute, transient left heart failure.

How often does myocardial ischemia occur without ECG change? Nobody knows. One clue lies in the fact that about 20% of treadmill tests are "false negative"; that is, coronary disease is present, but there's no ECG change with exercise. Every clinician knows that the ECG often remains normal during obvious anginal pain in patients with documented coronary artery disease. There's no question, therefore, that TMI may occur without electrocardiographic change, but there are simply no data to suggest how often this occurs.

Reference

1. Phibbs B, Holmes R, Lowe C. Transient myocardial ischemia, the significance of dyspnea. Am J Med Sci 1968;256:210–221.

Twenty

Pericarditis

Only a few specific disease entities can be diagnosed from the electrocardiogram (ECG) with a high degree of accuracy. Myocardial infarction, of course, is one. *Pericarditis* is another. Pericarditis produces an injury current on the epicardium only. The myocardium is not involved (Fig. 20–1). Because the myocardium is not involved, there are two important differences between the ECG of pericarditis and the ECG of myocardial infarction:

1. The S-T segments in one or more leads will be elevated. They will never be depressed. *Repeat: There is no reciprocal S-T depression in pericarditis; there is only S-T elevation.* You may see the S-T elevation in many leads or in only a few; most of the time, the S-T elevation will be widespread.

2. Since the myocardium is not involved, the QRS is not affected. There are no Q waves or other changes in the QRS complex. Changes are limited entirely to the S-T-T.

Study Figures 20–2 and 20–3. These are typical examples of ECG deformity in pericarditis. Note the widespread S-T elevation without reciprocal depression (except in aVR, where it doesn't count). As the pericarditis resolves, the S-T segments come back to baseline—usually within 72 hours. Sometimes that's all that happens. In other cases, the T waves will invert progressively, moving opposite to the direction of S-T deviation, exactly as in the evolution of an infarct (Fig. 20–4). The whole evolution may take 3 to 5 days—a shorter time, on average, than the evolution of an infarct.

Dr. David Spodick is one of the leading investigators in this field. He pointed out a distinctive sign that often clinches the diagnosis. In acute pericarditis, the P-R segment will often show a peculiar downward displacement—an actual downslope as the segment approaches the QRS (Fig. 20–5). This finding appears to be highly specific for acute pericarditis—the sensitivity of this particular sign has not yet been documented. In other words, when you see it, it's important evidence of pericarditis, but don't rule out pericarditis just because it's not there.

Pericardial Effusion with Tamponade

Figure 20–6 illustrates the curious phenomenon of electrical alternans. In the precordial leads, the ventricular complexes actually alternate polarity—up and down. In the other leads, they simply alternate size. Nobody knew what caused this until catheterization and echocardiography made it possible to see the heart's movements. With tamponade, the heart actually swings back and forth like a pendulum—hence the electrical alternation.

Figure 20–1.
The injury current of pericarditis. Only the pericardium and occasionally the epicardium are involved. The injury current will record only an upward deflection, never a reciprocal downward deflection (except for aVR, which you don't consider in this setting).

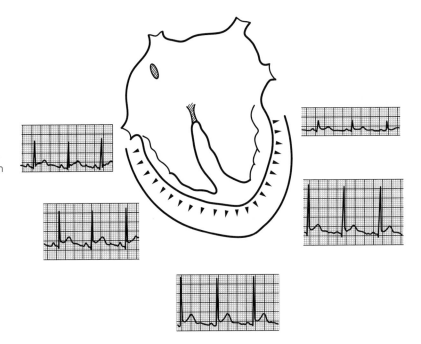

Figure 20–2.
Typical pattern of pericarditis with S-T elevation in I, III, aVF, and V3 to V6.

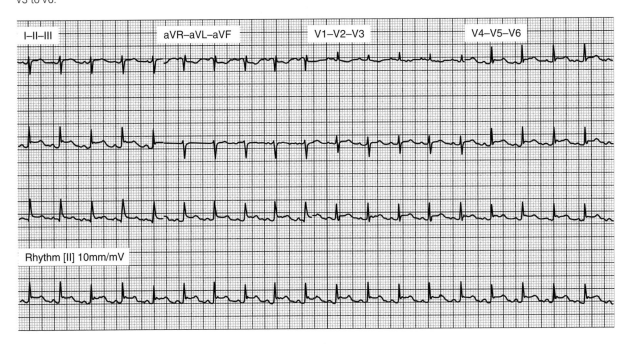

Figure 20–3.
Pericarditis. There is obvious S-T elevation in all leads except aVR, aVL, and V1. Note downward deflection of P-R segment.

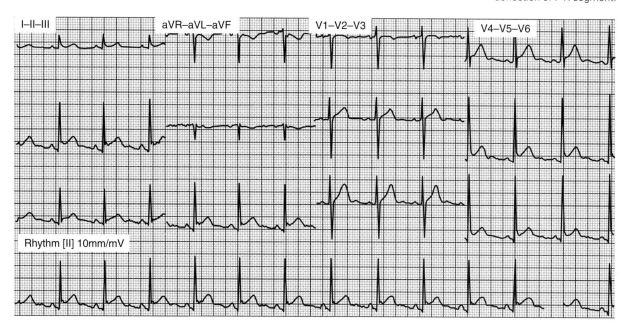

I–II–III aVR–aVL–aVF V1–V2–V3 V4–V5–V6

Rhythm [II] 10mm/mV

Figure 20–4.
End stage of evolution of pericarditis with T wave inversion in V1 to V4. If you saw only this tracing, it would be very hard to differentiate this from an anterior myocardial infarction.

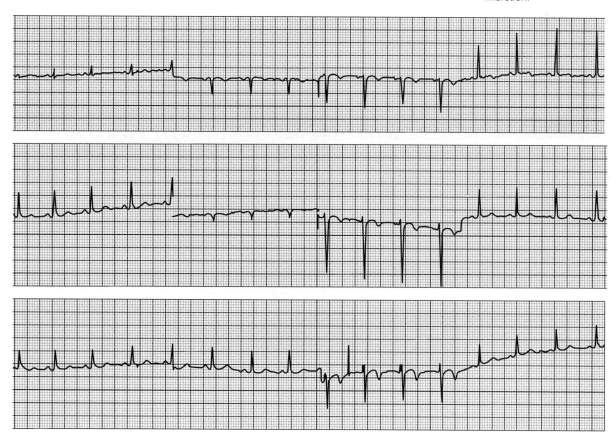

Figure 20–5.
Spodick's sign. Enlarged ECG to illustrate the downward deflection of the P-R segment (*arrows*).

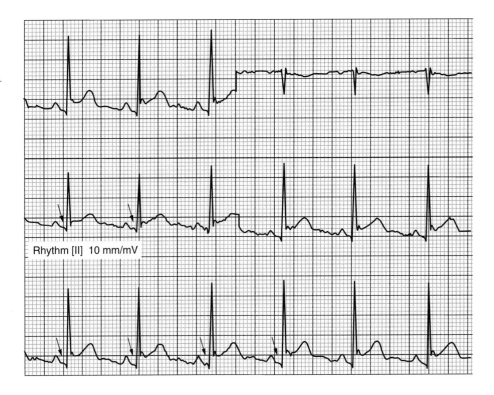

Rhythm [II] 10 mm/mV

Figure 20–6.
ECG during pericardial tamponade. Note striking change in direction of ventricular complexes in the precordial leads. (From Spodick, D. The Pericardium: A Comprehensive Textbook. New York: Dekker, 1997.)

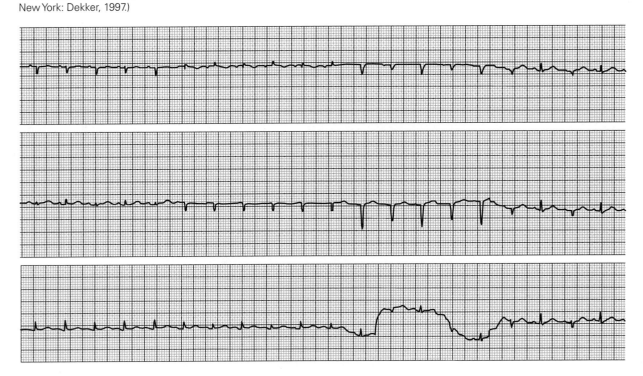

Twenty-one

Enlargement of the Chambers of the Heart: Hypertrophy and Dilatation

Measurement of mean frontal plane axis is important in the diagnosis of the various types of chamber enlargement. Presumably, anyone reading this book knows how to calculate axis. If there's any doubt, look at Appendix II.

"Normal" Axis: Effect of Age and Body Habitus

Many texts make the statement that a "normal" axis lies between 0 and 90 degrees. This is dangerously misleading. You have to correct for age and body habitus before you decide whether an axis is normal or not.

Infants are born with a rightward axis because of high pressure in the pulmonary circuit during fetal life. An axis to the right of 100 degrees is normal in infants. The axis moves leftward during life, so that an axis of 0 degrees or even slightly minus is common in adult life. Tall slender people tend to have a rightward axis because of the near-vertical position of the heart. Short stocky people commonly have a left axis because the heart tends to lie out to the left, sometimes almost horizontal. If you saw a 10-year-old with an axis of +10, you'd have to call it abnormal; the axis would be much too far to the left for a youngster of that age. If you saw an overweight 65-year-old with an axis of +90, it would be grossly abnormal. You'd look for something that would impose a load on the right heart, such as a pulmonary embolus. *Before you decide whether an axis is normal, always correct for age and body habitus.*

Chamber Enlargement

Enlargement of the chambers of the heart may be caused by dilatation, hypertrophy, or both. The ventricles *dilate* when there's an increased volume of blood at the end of diastolic filling; this may be the result of valvular regurgitation or a ventricular septal defect. The ventricles *hypertrophy* when they contract against an abnormally high pressure; aortic stenosis and hypertension are of course the most common causes. Dilatation may appear after hypertrophy when a failing heart can no longer balance inflow and outflow of blood. Many physicians do not realize that chronic ischemia can produce ventricular hypertrophy. In fact, ischemic cardiomyopathy may be the single most common cause of ventricular hypertrophy.

Atrial enlargement will always be the result of passive distention—e.g., dilatation.

For a time, there was an effort to distinguish between ventricular hypertrophy and dilatation—systolic and diastolic overload—on the basis of the electrocardiogram (ECG), but that effort has been totally discarded. You can't make the distinction. In fact, the ECG is only moderately successful in detecting chamber enlargement of any kind; false-positive and false-negative readings must be expected, and the wise electrocardiographer will never be too dogmatic.

Electrocardiogram Diagnosis of Atrial Enlargement

Start with the "rule of three," just as in bundle-branch block. If the P wave in the limb leads is 0.12 second wide or 3 mm tall, there's evidence of atrial enlargement. If the P wave is 0.12 second wide and *notched*, the left atrium is almost certainly enlarged. This is the classic *P-mitrale*, so named by the French because it appears most commonly with the large left atrium of mitral disease (Fig. 21–1A). The P-mitrale will most commonly be seen in II and III. If the P waves in II, III, and aVF are 3 mm tall and peaked (the "gothic" P because it's supposed to look like a cathedral), the right atrium is enlarged. This is commonly called *P-pulmonale* because it's most commonly seen with severe lung disease accompanied by pulmonary hypertension (see Fig. 21–1B). Some writers pick the number 2.5 in the diagnosis of atrial enlargement—thus, if the P wave is 0.10 second wide or 2.5 mm tall, they read hypertrophy. I prefer to be more specific even though possibly less sensitive—hence the criteria outlined above.

The P wave in V1 can also be helpful. Think of the right atrium as the anterior atrium and the left as the posterior. Look closely at P-V1 in most ECGs and you'll see a small upward deflection followed by a small negative deflection (Fig. 21–2). Because the right atrium is anterior, the wave activating it moves *toward* V1, producing the upward deflection. By the same token, because the left atrium is posterior, the wave activating it moves *away* from V1 and produces a negative deflection. If either the positive or negative components of the P wave enclose an area equal to a generous square millimeter, there's evidence of atrial abnormality—either enlargement or slow conduction through a diseased syncytium (Fig. 21–3A and B).

Figure 21–1.
A, Left atrial enlargement, as reflected in the limb leads. **B,** Right atrial enlargement, as reflected in the limb leads.

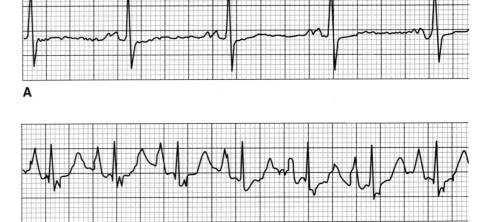

A

B

Figure 21–2.
Normal diphasic P in V1. Note that the P wave consists of a small upward deflection followed by a small negative deflection. These deflections represent right atrial and left atrial activation, respectively.

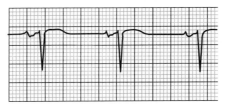

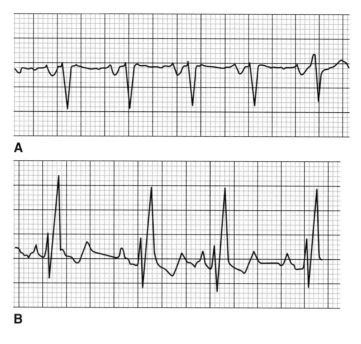

A

B

Figure 21–3.
A, Left atrial enlargement, reflected in the deep negative component of P in V1. In this strip, the enlarged left atrium is posterior. There is a large negative P wave in V1 because the wave activating the left atrium is moving *away from* V1. The negative P wave must enclose at least 1 mm^2 to be significant. **B,** Right atrial enlargement, reflected in a tall, wide, positive component of P in V1. The right atrium is anterior. The large P wave is positive in V1 because the wave activating the right atrium is moving *toward* V1. The positive P wave must also enclose at least 1 mm^2 to be significant.

Electrocardiogram Diagnosis of Left Ventricular Hypertrophy

The diagnosis of hypertrophy of ventricular musculature is based on a few simple concepts:

1. **The thicker the heart muscle, the taller the R wave it produces. Thus, an abnormally tall R is one of the important criteria of hypertrophy. Obviously, an abnormally tall R on one side of the electric field of the heart means that there'll be an abnormally deep S on the opposite side. Excessive voltage, positive or negative, is therefore the key criterion for hypertrophy (Fig. 21–4).**

2. **The mean electric axis will swing toward the thickest mass of myocardium. If the left ventricle is enlarged, the mean axis will swing leftward. (Correspondingly, of course, right ventricular hypertrophy [RVH] will move the axis to the right.)**

3. **A peculiar S-T-T configuration may appear in leads over the hypertrophied ventricle. The S-T segment is depressed and downsloping, and the T wave is inverted in a hockey-stick configuration with a low, slow descent and a rapid upstroke (Fig. 21–5).**

4. **Left atrial enlargement. Because the mitral valve is open all through diastole, increased left ventricular pressures will be transmitted back to the left atrium, with subsequent left atrial enlargement. In the absence of mitral disease, left atrial enlargement is a fairly reliable reflection of the pathophysiology that has produced left ventricular enlargement and failure.**

5. **Delayed onset of intrinsicoid deflection. The thicker the myocardium, the longer it takes for the activating wave to traverse it. When the myocardium is abnormally thickened, therefore, it takes longer than normal for the R wave to complete its rise from base to peak. This time interval has the clumsy title of *time of onset of intrinsicoid deflection*. The intrinsicoid deflection is defined as the time to the beginning of the rapid fall from the peak of the R. (A more logical term would be *R wave inscription time*, but medical jargonists will never settle for a simple term if they can come up with something more complicated.) Normal value is less than 0.05 second.**

Now you can put these elements together into a system for diagnosing left ventricular hypertrophy (LVH). The most authoritative correlation of these five variables was accomplished by Romhilt and Estes.[1] These investigators measured postmortem wall thickness and

Figure 21–4.
Increased voltage in LVH.

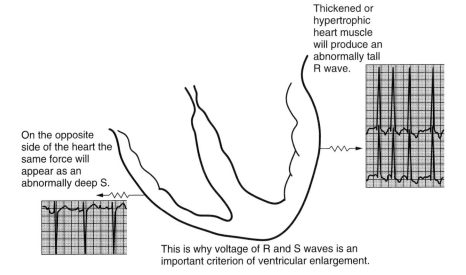

Thickened or hypertrophic heart muscle will produce an abnormally tall R wave.

On the opposite side of the heart the same force will appear as an abnormally deep S.

This is why voltage of R and S waves is an important criterion of ventricular enlargement.

Figure 21–5.
S-T-T "strain" pattern in LVH.

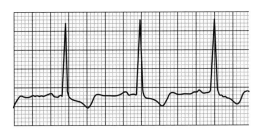

ventricular mass as their basis for comparison. They produced a point-score system reproduced in Table 21–1. Note that in this system, "increased voltage" means 30 mm in a precordial lead and 20 mm in a limb lead. This point-score system still gives the best correlation with LVH.

An older study by Sokolow and Lyons[2] was carried on before the days of catheterization or echocardiograms, and the authors did not use postmortem measurements as their basis of comparison. They simply compared patients with and without hypertension on the assumption that hypertensive patients were more likely to have LVH. On this tenuous basis, they concluded that if the sum of the S wave in V2 and the R in V5 equaled 35 mm, LVH was likely to be present. Other studies subsequently added voltage in aVL greater than 11 mm as a criterion of LVH. These voltage criteria are widely used today, and it's worthwhile examining their accuracy.

Cumming and Proudfit[3] tested these voltage criteria against postmortem findings and found that if the criterion of the sum of R V5 and S V2 was applied, there were 39% false-positive readings. In other words, the voltage criteria of Sokolow and Lyons indicated LVH

Table 21–1. Romhilt-Estes Point-Score System for Detection of Left Ventricular Hypertrophy

1. Voltage. Any of the following: R or S wave in limb leads, 20 mm; S V1–V2, 30 mm, R V5–V6, 30 mm. 3 points
2. S-T-T deformity of "strain" type: 2 points
3. Left atrial enlargement: 3 points
4. Left axis, 30 or greater: 2 points[*]
5. QRS duration 0.09 second or greater (<0.12 second): 1 point[†]
6. R wave inscription time in V5, V6, 0.05 second or more: 1 point
7. Left ventricular hypertrophy: 5 points
8. Probable left ventricular hypertrophy: 4 points

[*]"Left axis" should mean axis in the −20 to −30 range. Extreme left axis of −40 or higher means that there is a conduction defect in the left ventricle (anterior fascicular block), and such an axis cannot be used to establish presence of LVH.

[†]"QRS" duration of 0.09 second or greater applies only if the widening is less than 0.11–0.12, that is, if the widening is not caused by bundle-branch block.

From Romhilt DW, Estes EH. Point-score system for the ECG diagnosis of left ventricular hypertrophy. Am Heart J 1968;75:752.

when the heart was in fact normal about 40% of the time. Increased voltage in aVL was similarly inaccurate: false-positive readings equaled about 36%. If increased precordial voltage was combined with increased voltage in aVL, the accuracy was improved, although the design of this study precluded an exact percentage.

Reicheck and Devereux[4] carried out a precise study correlating ECG criteria for LVH with postmortem findings. Their conclusions are worth repeating:

1. In a clinical population with a moderate incidence of LVH, both Romhilt-Estes and Sokolow-Lyons voltage criteria are highly specific: when present, they indicate LVH with about 95% confidence.

2. Neither set of criteria is acceptably sensitive. The fact that these criteria are *not* fulfilled doesn't mean that LVH isn't present. With Romhilt-Estes criteria, sensitivity is only 50%, whereas with Sokolow-Lyons, it is 21%. In other words, a normal ECG doesn't rule out LVH. With the best current criteria, the ECG will miss the diagnosis about half the time.

3. In a population with a low prevalence of LVH (less than 10%), there will be more false-positive than true-positive readings. In other words, the ECG will give a false reading of LVH in this group more often than a true one. The moral here is that the physician reading ECGs for routine physical examinations or for life insurance applications should not diagnose LVH from the ECG alone. This is especially true when only voltage criteria are present.

Figure 21–6 illustrates many of the criteria for LVH.

Figure 21–6.
LVH with all the elements of the Romhilt-Estes system: voltage, axis, "strain" S-T-T pattern, left atrial enlargement, and delay of onset of intrinsicoid deflection.

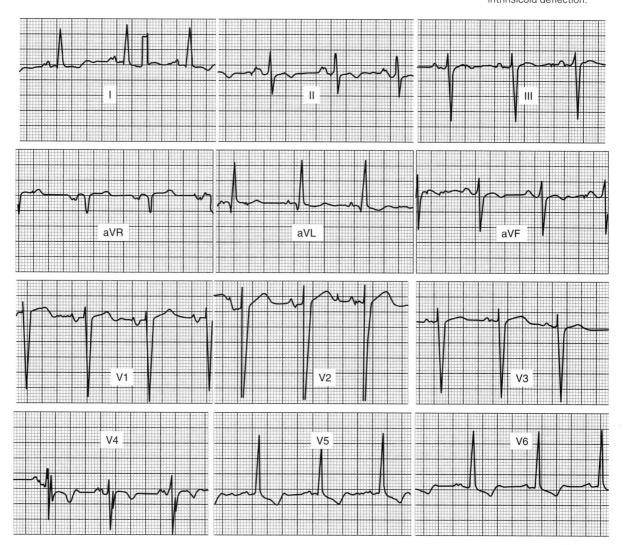

Electrocardiogram Diagnosis of Right Ventricular Hypertrophy

Here the ECG correlation is probably better than it is with LVH. The classification of Chou and Helm[5] is very useful.

1. **Type A RVH. This is a very simple diagnosis. V1 consists of a simple R wave and hence looks like the letter** *A*. **There's an extreme right axis (Fig. 21–7). This is the most severe type of RVH. The type A pattern means that the pressure in the right heart is extremely high—at least two thirds of systemic pressure. The pulmonary artery systolic pressure will be in the range of 85 mm Hg or higher. It's the kind of RVH you would expect with pulmonic stenosis or with severe congenital left-to-right shunts. Figure 21–8 is a typical example of type A RVH.**

2. **Type B RVH. This connotes a less severe type of RVH than type A. V1 consists of an initial tall R followed by an S. The R will be at least equal to the S. This terminal S in V1 is the important distinction between type A and type B. There will be a right axis in the frontal plane leads (Fig. 21–9). Type B RVH appears with moderate elevation of pulmonary artery and right heart pressures—a pulmonary artery pressure of 60/40, for example. It's the kind of pattern you often see with mitral stenosis. Figure 21–10 is a typical example of type B RVH.**

3. **Type C RVH. This is the most specific pattern in terms of correlation with disease. Careful correlative studies by Dr. Carl Schmock and his colleagues at the University of Colorado proved that this occurs exclusively with chronic obstructive lung disease, predominantly in the "pink puffer" subgroup, in which the principal pathology consists of hyperdistention of terminal bronchioles and alveoli. Leads I, II, and III are all negative—in other words, there's a dominant S in I, II, and III. The frontal axis is therefore in the quadrant between –90 and –180. The axis is in fact so far to the right that it's left. This is called** *axis illusion* **or** *pseudo left axis.* **The precordial leads consist exclusively of a small r with a deep S in every lead from V1 to V6 (Fig. 21–11). This pattern is amazingly specific. When you see it, diagnose the type of chronic obstructive lung disease associated with predominant emphysema with complete confidence (Fig. 21–12).**

Figure 21–7.
Anatomy and ECG of type A RVH. There is extreme elevation of right ventricular pressure, as in pulmonic stenosis or severe pulmonary hypertension. Right ventricular forces are larger than left ventricular forces throughout depolarization. If pulmonary hypertension is the cause, the pulmonary artery pressure will be at least two thirds of systemic.

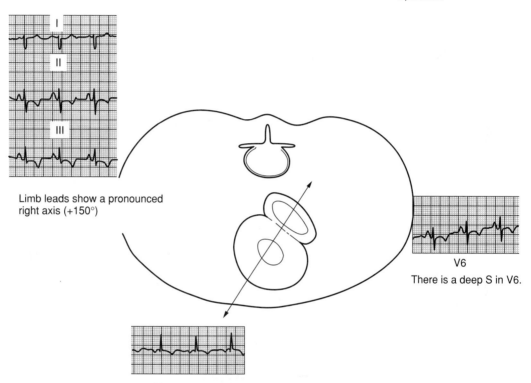

Limb leads show a pronounced right axis (+150°)

V6
There is a deep S in V6.

V1   V1 consists of a "pure" R wave not followed by an S. (There may or may not be a tiny "septal" q.)

Figure 21–8.
Typical ECG of type A RVH,
reflecting extremely high
pulmonary artery and right
ventricular pressures.

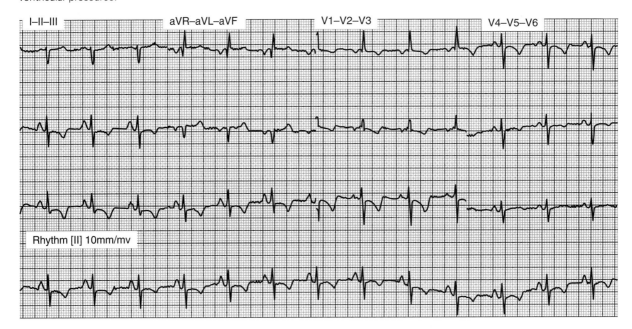

I–II–III   aVR–aVL–aVF   V1–V2–V3   V4–V5–V6

Rhythm [II] 10mm/mv

Figure 21–9.
Anatomy and ECG of type B RVH. This is the pattern seen with moderate RVH. Mitral stenosis with pulmonary artery pressure of 60/40 would be a typical example. Right ventricular forces dominate initially, but left ventricular activation finally pulls the forces of depolarization back and to the left.

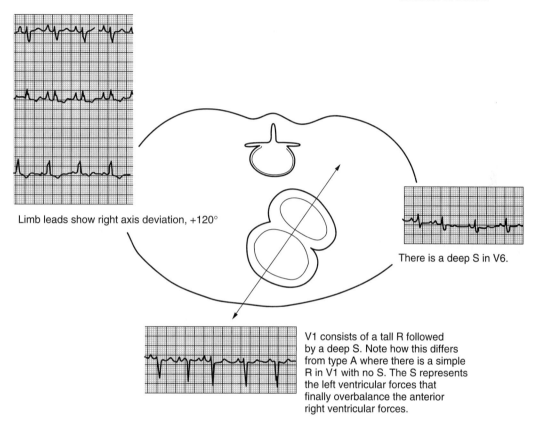

Limb leads show right axis deviation, +120°

There is a deep S in V6.

V1 consists of a tall R followed by a deep S. Note how this differs from type A where there is a simple R in V1 with no S. The S represents the left ventricular forces that finally overbalance the anterior right ventricular forces.

Figure 21–10.
Typical type B RVH
associated with moderate
elevation of pulmonary
artery and right ventricular
pressures.

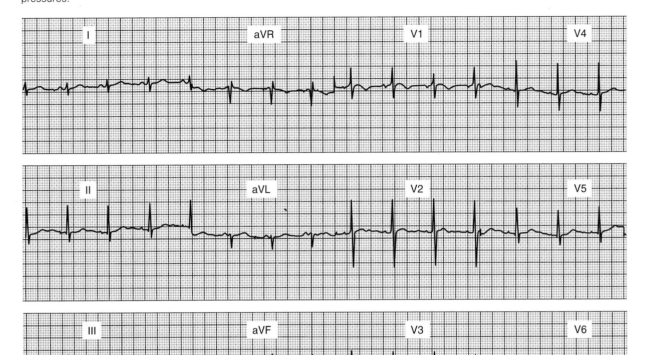

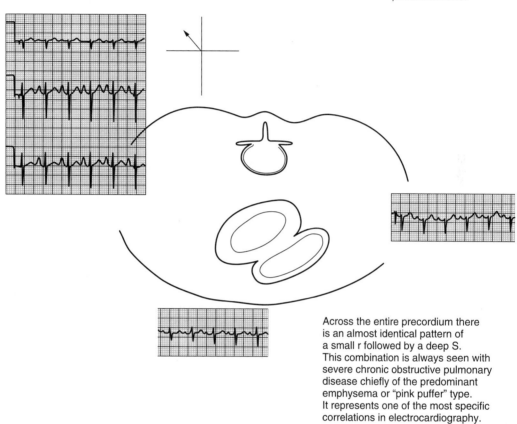

Figure 21–11.
Anatomy and ECG of type C RVH. This is a curious and highly specific pattern. The axis in the limb leads is "so far right that it's left." In other words, it's about +240 degrees, as shown in the diagram. This is sometimes called the S1-S2-S3 pattern in the limb leads; it has also been termed *axis illusion* and *pseudo left axis*.

Across the entire precordium there is an almost identical pattern of a small r followed by a deep S. This combination is always seen with severe chronic obstructive pulmonary disease chiefly of the predominant emphysema or "pink puffer" type. It represents one of the most specific correlations in electrocardiography.

Figure 21–12.
Typical type C RVH
associated with severe
chronic obstructive
pulmonary disease.

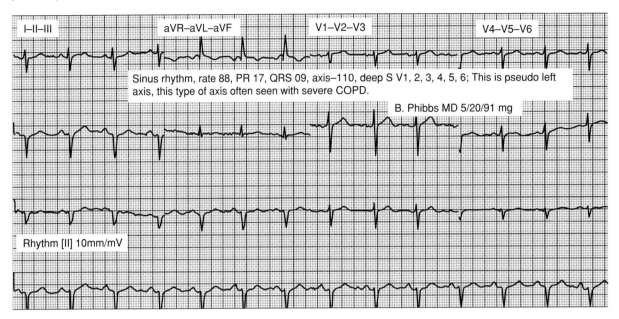

Sinus rhythm, rate 88, PR 17, QRS 09, axis–110, deep S V1, 2, 3, 4, 5, 6; This is pseudo left axis, this type of axis often seen with severe COPD.

B. Phibbs MD 5/20/91 mg

References

1. Romhilt DW, Estes EH. Point-score system for the ECG diagnosis of left ventricular hypertrophy. Am Heart J 1968;75:752.
2. Sokolow M, Lyons TP. Ventricular complex in left ventricular hypertrophy as obtained by unipolar precordial and limb leads. Am Heart J 1949;37:161.
3. Cumming G, Proudfit W. High-voltage QRS complexes in the absence of left ventricular hypertrophy. Circulation 1959;29:406–409.
4. Reicheck R, Devereux M. Left ventricular hypertrophy: Relationship to anatomic, echocardiographic and electrocardiographic findings. Circulation 1981;63:1391.
5. Chou T, Helm R. Clinical Vectorcardiography. New York: Grune & Stratton, 1967:77–99.

Twenty-two

"Nonspecific" Myocardial Pathology

It's time to consider limitations. It's safe to say that about 75% of all electrocardiogram (ECG) abnormalities do not fall into any of the specific disease categories described in the last three chapters. The honest electrocardiographer will recognize the limitations of the ECG and will use the term *nonspecific* many times a day. Properly interpreted, this means that the ECG is recording the presence of some kind of myocardial pathology. The term means further that it's not possible to say what kind of pathology is present or how severe it is. Don't try. Restraint and modesty are the hallmarks of the competent electrocardiographer; a special kind of medicolegal and diagnostic Hell awaits those who "over-read."

A great many diseases and toxins can attack the myocardium, all with the same unfortunate outcome: myocardial cells die and are replaced by scar tissue. These changes may be reflected in the ECG, and when they are, they'll appear as nonspecific abnormalities.

Coronary artery disease can cause diffuse myocardial scarring even though there has never been an actual infarct. A postmortem on any patient with prolonged angina pectoris will always reveal many small areas of scarring scattered throughout the heart muscle. This is the basis of *ischemic cardiomyopathy*. Sometimes there will even be localized masses of scar tissue—the phenomenon Dr. J. Willis Hurst referred to as *hunk disease* because there's a "hunk" of scar tissue that formed quietly, without infarction.

Viral infections, including acquired immunodeficiency syndrome (AIDS), lupus erythematosus, polyarteritis nodosa, sarcoidosis, and scleroderma; drugs like cocaine; and toxins like beryllium can all leave scarred, nonfunctioning myocardium. In addition, there's a substantial group of patients who turn up with evidence of cardiomyopathy for no discernible reason—the idiopathic cardiomyopathies.

There are no specific ECG patterns in this group of diseases. You'll see changes in the ECG that permit you to make the diagnosis of myocardial pathology, and at that point you put down the dictating machine and stop.

Electrocardiogram Diagnosis

Most of the time, these changes will be in the T waves. You've already learned about the "specific" patterns of S-T-T deformity in myocardial infarction, pericarditis, and hypertrophy. It's time to learn the rules about "nonspecific" T wave deformity.

The T waves should be upright in *most* leads. A flat, diphasic, or inverted T wave is abnormal in *most* leads. Note that I said "most," not "all." There are some leads where it's normal to see inverted T waves. Normal individuals will always have inverted T waves in aVR. They may have inverted T waves in lead III and in V1 or V2 (Fig. 22–1). When you see diphasic or inverted T waves without QRS or T wave change in any other leads, the reading is "nonspecific T wave deformity consistent with myocardial pathology." Stop right there. That's all you can say.

Figure 22–1.
Leads in which an inverted
T wave is a normal finding.

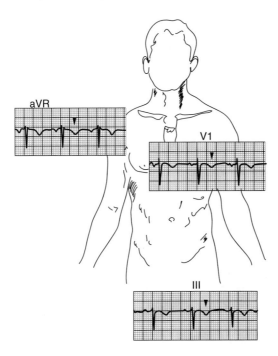

This is a very sound set of rules based on observation of millions of ECGs by every qual-
ified observer in the field. For an intelligent physician, that's not enough. It's necessary to
know why it's normal to have deformed T waves in some leads and not in others.

Look at Figure 22–2. This explains the inverted T waves in aVR and sometimes in V1
and V2. Think of the inside, or "cavity," of the heart as negatively charged. When you float
an electrode into the superior vena cava, for instance, all deflections will be negative because
you'll be recording from the negatively charged "cavity" of the heart. To put it another way,
all the activating waves are moving away from the recording electrode because of its position
above the heart. The aVR lead always "looks down" into the cavity of the heart—hence the

Figure 22–2.
Anatomic basis for the
cavity potential. The aVR
and V1 leads look down
from above into the
negatively charged interior
of the heart. They record a
negative or "cavity"
potential. That's why it's
normal for T waves to be
inverted in these leads.
Sometimes V2 records a
cavity potential as well,
with a normal inverted T
wave.

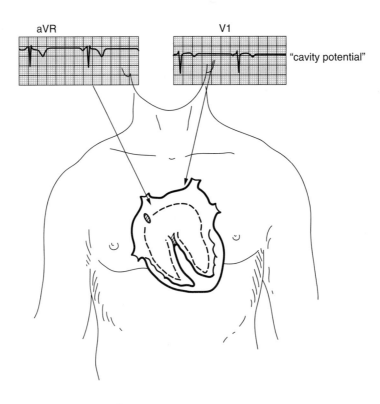

negative deflections. V1 and V2 can record the same kind of cavity potential, depending on the position of the heart in the chest.

How about lead III? This trips up many cardiologists, so it should be explained at some length. In about 15% of normal individuals, you'll see a significant Q wave in lead III. You'll see inverted T waves in about the same percentage of normal individuals, and often you'll see the Q and the inverted T together—a combination that has created many an imaginary infarct.

The simplest way to find whether a Q or an inverted T in III means anything is to look at aVF. If you don't see these deflections in aVF, forget them. They're a normal variant that appears only in lead III. Why only in lead III? Think about how leads I, II, and III are set up. They're bipolar leads, which means that they measure the difference in potential between two points. They're like the simple galvanometer you set up in high school physics with a positive pole and a negative pole. Lead III is set up to measure the difference in potential between the left leg (aVF) and the left arm (aVL). The left leg is the "positive" electrode. This means that when the left leg is positive *compared with the left arm,* there will be an upward deflection in lead III. When the left leg is negative *compared with the left arm,* there will be a downward deflection in lead III. Remember that in a bipolar system "negative" can simply mean "less positive." Thus, if aVF is registering a force of 1 mm while aVL is registering a force of 4 mm, there will be a downward deflection in III—not because there's any real negativity anywhere but simply because the left leg is recording a smaller positive potential than the left arm. In other words, lead III equals aVF − aVL or +1 − (+4) = −3. You're looking at "signed numbers" just as you did in the fifth grade. *Whenever the T in aVL is larger than the T in aVF, there will be an inverted T III even though T aVF and T aVL are both positive.* Figures 22–3 and 22–4 illustrate this simple point.

You won't see this effect in leads I or II because the indifferent electrode is the right arm, or aVR, where everything is negative. There's no positive potential to subtract as there is in aVL. That's why you see this curious effect only in lead III.

For the same reason, a Q in III doesn't mean anything unless you also see it in aVF. In Figure 22–5, you'll note that the initial part of the QRS is a tiny "septal" q, followed by a small, slurred, slowly rising r. In aVL, on the other hand, there's a sharply rising R. In other words, aVL is positive compared with aVF all through the first half of the QRS. Lead III obediently records a downward deflection all this time—hence the deep Q that doesn't mean anything. All it's telling you is that there's a stronger positive potential at the left arm

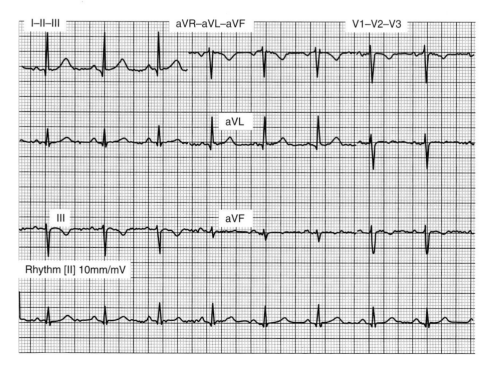

Figure 22–3.
A "physiologic" inverted T III. T aVF is flat, whereas T aVL is large and upright. Lead III equals the electric difference between aVF and aVL. In other words, you derive T III by subtracting T aVL from T aVF. T aVF is flat, whereas T aVL encloses an area of about 4.5 mm². When you subtract 4.5 from 0 you get −4.5, that is, a negative T in III. All the negative T III means is that the T in aVL is larger than the T in aVF.

Figure 22–4.
Same phenomenon. T aVF is small—about 1.5 mm² in area. T aVL is much larger, about 4 mm². Subtracting aVL from aVF leaves you with a negative T III even though the actual T potentials at both the left leg and left arm are positive.

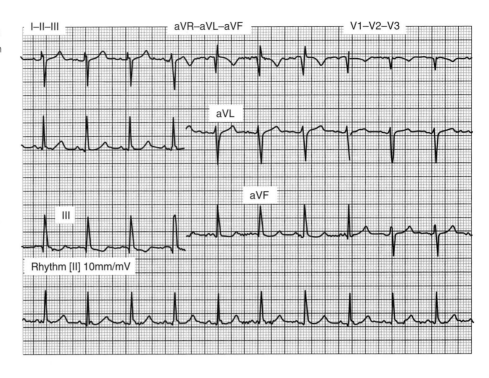

Figure 22–5.
The "physiologic Q" of lead III. Lead aVF records a small initial R, whereas aVL records a tall one. Lead III records a negative deflection or Q wave until the potential in aVL falls below the potential in aVF in the last part of the QRS. *Moral:* When you see a Q III, always look at aVF to see what caused it.

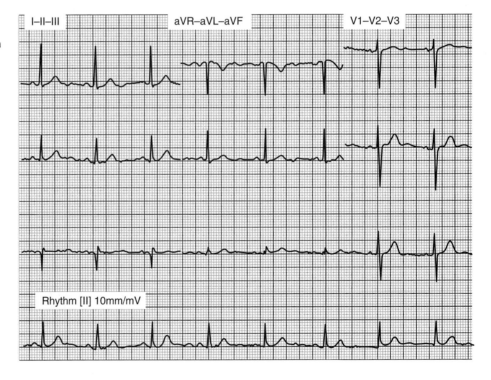

than at the left leg all through the first part of depolarization. This is of course a normal variant, and that's why you'll see wide Q waves in 15% of normal individuals.

You may ask, "Why bother to record the bipolar limb leads at all? Why not just record aVR, aVL, and aVF because those are the actual isolated potentials at the right shoulder, left shoulder, and left leg?" Good question. The augmented unipolar limb leads contain all the information you need, and we go on recording I, II, and III out of habit.

Figures 22–6 through 22–11 are examples of nonspecific T wave deformity. Obviously, the various types of cardiac pathology can affect the ventricular conducting network, and any kind of intraventricular delay may appear. There are some statistical associations—for example, in Chagas' cardiomyopathy, right bundle-branch block is common—but, overall, delay in intraventricular conduction must be classed as a nonspecific finding that may be a result of anything from ischemic cardiomyopathy to leishmaniasis. Look outside the ECG for specific causes!

Figure 22–6.

Diffuse T wave deformity in lateral, inferior, and anterior leads. Note the change in S-T-T morphology with the premature atrial beats in V1 to V3. You're seeing a kind of one-beat stress test with more deformity at a more rapid rate. The symmetrical inversion of the T waves suggests a "coronary" configuration, but it's only suggestive, not diagnostic.

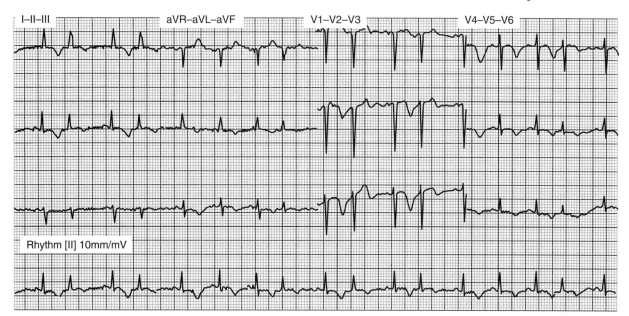

Figure 22–7.

Proper diagnosis: "anterior and lateral S-T-T deformity consistent with myocardial pathology." Period. End of diagnosis.

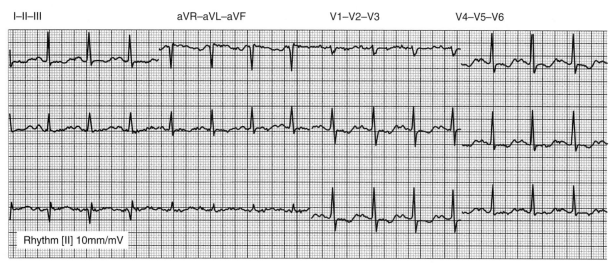

Figure 22–8.

Some of the criteria of left ventricular hypertrophy are here: increased voltage, left axis, hockey-stick S-T-T. Diagnosis: "some criteria for left ventricular hypertrophy. S-T-T deformity may be the result of hypertrophy, ischemia, or both."

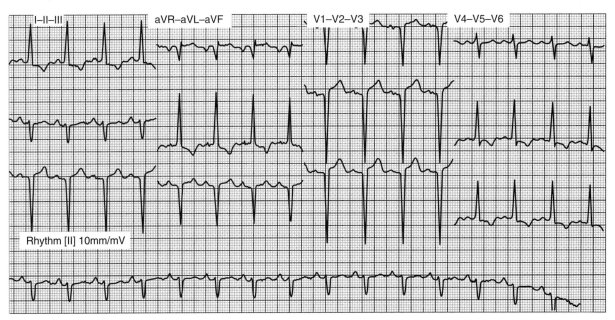

Figure 22–9.

Diffuse T wave flattening in lateral, inferior, and anterolateral leads. A flat T wave in one lead may not be significant, but diffuse T wave flattening in two or more lead systems is always significant and may be the result of myocardial pathology. It may also be the result of extracardiac metabolic or toxic factors.

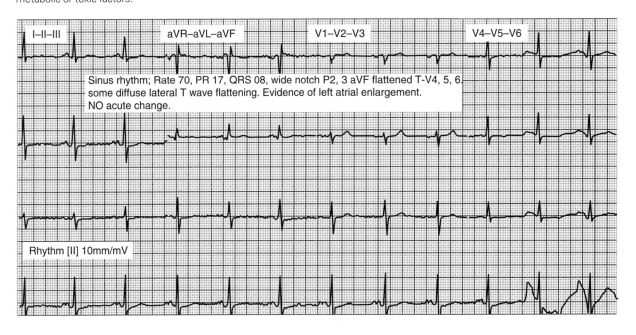

Figure 22–10.
Diagnosis: "abnormal tracing. Right axis deviation. Inferolateral S-T-T deformity consistent with myocardial pathology."

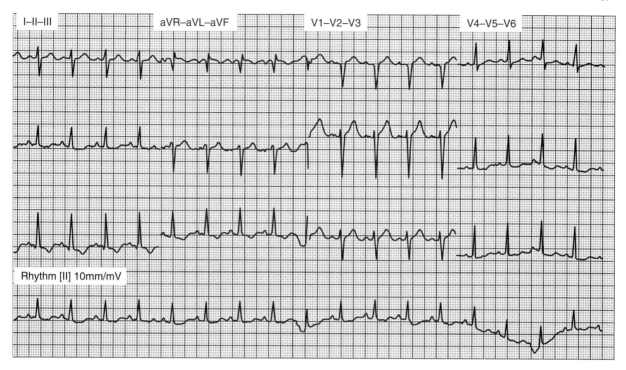

Figure 22–11.
Diagnosis: "diffuse S-T-T deformity with S-T depression in inferior and lateral leads, T wave inversion V3 to V4. Findings consistent with myocardial pathology."

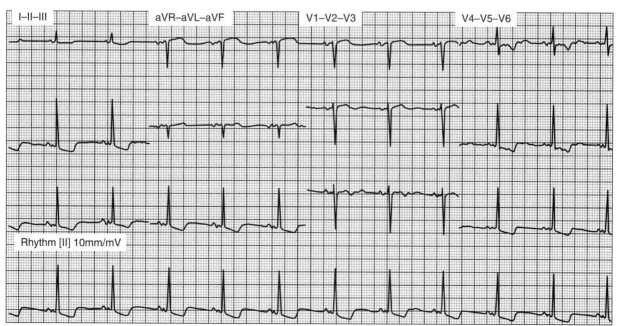

Twenty-three

Electrolytes and Drugs

Electrolytes

Changes in the levels of serum calcium and potassium can affect the electrocardiogram (ECG). Think of calcium as the "energizer" of the heart. After all, it is the movement of calcium into the myocardial cells that begins the chemistry of contraction. With an elevated serum calcium, the Q-T interval is shortened. In other words, with a high level of calcium, the heart is activated more quickly than normal (Fig. 23–1).

Hypocalcemia has exactly the opposite effect: the Q-T interval is prolonged (Fig. 23–2). Note that the prolongation is in the S-T segment, not in the T wave. This is an important point when differentiating quinidine effect from hypocalcemia.

Potassium has been described as the "soothing syrup" of the heart. Too much of it puts all the pacemaking and conducting tissues to sleep. Hyperkalemia depresses atrioventricular (AV) and intraventricular conduction and, in higher levels, can completely suppress the sinus node. There are progressive levels of change, depending on the level of serum potassium. Moderate elevation of K produces tall, peaked T waves (Figs. 23–3 and 23–4). Severe elevation of K causes depression of conduction in the bundle-branch system. Various types of QRS prolongation appear as serum K reaches levels of 8 to 9 mEq/L (Figs. 23–5, 23–6, and 23–7). With very severe elevation of K, there may be depression of sinus node function. The P waves become sparse or actually disappear. Life is maintained by idiojunctional or idioventricular rhythms (Fig. 23–8). Lethal elevation of K at levels around 12 mEq/L are likely to produce ventricular fibrillation or standstill.

Hypokalemia produces depression of the S-T segment similar to digitalis effect. There are also prominent U waves. The giant U waves often merge with the T waves to give an illusion of a prolonged Q-T, but this is an artifact; in fact, the Q-T interval doesn't change (Fig. 23–9).

Drugs

The digitalis-toxic arrhythmias have been described in Chapter 16. They're so common, so dangerous, and so specific in terms of treatment that they deserve a chapter of their own. Digitalis compounds commonly cause depression of the S-T segments with the "wet noodle" bowing as illustrated in Figures 23–10, 23–11, and 23–12. This kind of S-T depression is *not* a sign of digitalis toxicity; it should be described only as "digitalis effect." Minimal prolongation of the P-R is common with digitalis therapy. Like S-T depression, it should be described only as digitalis effect, not as digitalis toxicity. If you see a fixed P-R of 0.22 to 0.24 second, it doesn't mean you have to discontinue digitalis.

Figure 23–1.
Hypercalcemia. Q-T
interval, 0.21 second.

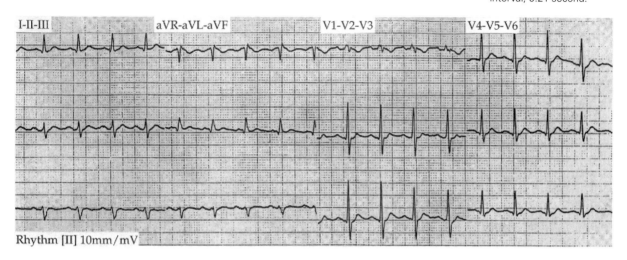

Figure 23–2.
Hypocalcemia. Q-T
interval, 0.56 second.

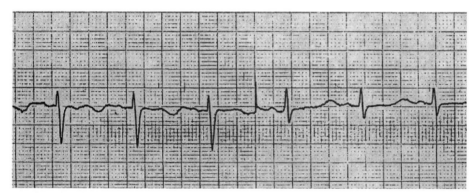

Figure 23–3.
Hyperpotassemia,
moderate. Note tall,
peaked T waves in V2, V3,
and V4. (*Rule of thumb:* A
tall, peaked T becomes
significant when it's more
than half the amplitude of
the R in a lead that
consists entirely of an R.)

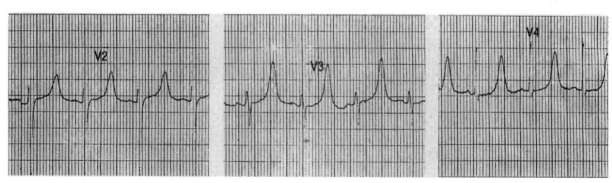

Figure 23–4.
More severe elevation of K. Prolonged P-R interval and giant, peaked T waves.

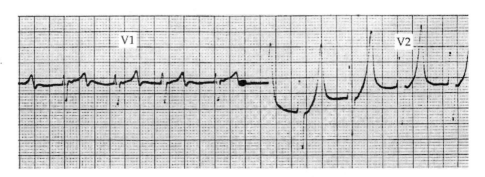

Figure 23–5.
Serum K of 8.8 mEq/L. Prolonged P-R, widened QRS, peaked T waves.

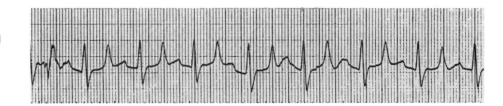

Figure 23–6.
Dangerous elevation of K at 10 mEq/L; extremely slow intraventricular conduction with QRS of 0.25 second.

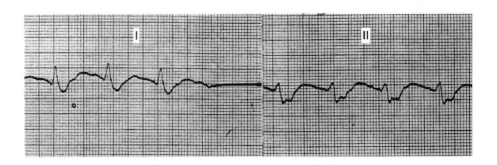

Figure 23–7.
Dangerous elevation of K, more than 10 mEq/L; P-R 0.26, QRS 0.26. Obvious extreme delay in intraventricular conduction.

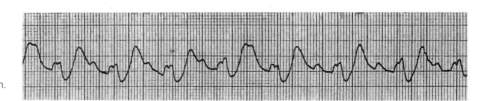

Figure 23–8.
K in excess of 10 mEq/L; complete suppression of sinus node activity. The junctional rhythm is life-saving.

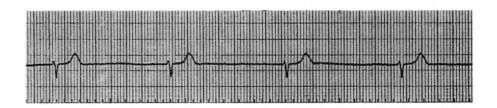

Figure 23–9.
Severe hypokalemia, 2.1 mEq/L. There is striking S-T depression, resembling digitalis effect. Prominent U waves give a false impression of prolongation of Q-T.

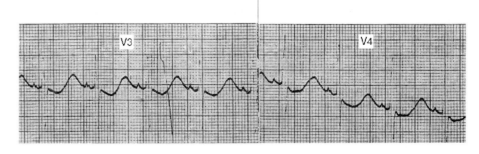

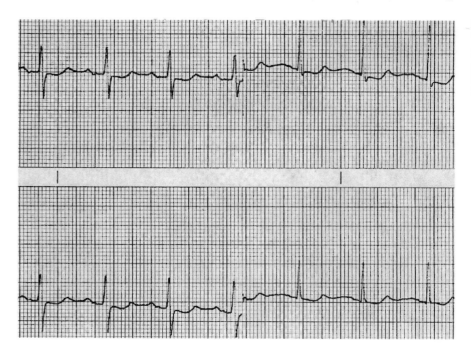

Figure 23–10.
Typical sagging of S-T segments seen in practically all patients taking digitalis for any length of time.

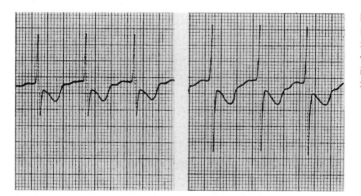

Figure 23–11.
Digitalis effect striking S-T-T deformity, with T waves "swallowed up" in the depressed S-T segments.

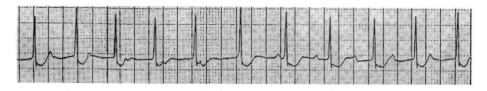

Figure 23–12.
A combination of digitalis *effect* (the sagging S-T segments) with digitalis *toxicity* (the accelerated junctional rhythm with complete AV dissociation).

Quinidine

Quinidine has a straightforward effect: it's a depressant. It depresses impulse formation and conduction everywhere in the heart. In the AV node, there's a diphasic effect. In small doses, quinidine opposes the vagus and accelerates AV nodal conduction; in the presence of atrial fibrillation or flutter, there may be an increase in ventricular rate with quinidine. Quinidine sometimes leads to 1:1 conduction in the presence of flutter with dangerous results, but the vagolytic effect is minor in this setting. The real problem with quinidine in flutter is that it slows the flutter rate in the atria so that every atrial impulse is conducted to the ventricles. Look at the flutter rate next time you give a patient quinidine, and you'll see for yourself: the atrial rate may slow from 300 to 215 or thereabouts. In higher concentrations, quinidine depresses AV nodal conduction and can produce any kind of AV nodal block.

The most common ECG manifestation of quinidine effect is prolongation of the Q-T interval. There is almost always some prolongation of Q-T with therapeutic levels of quinidine, and this is not per se an indication to stop the drug (Fig. 23–13). Extreme prolongation of Q-T, however, increases the danger of torsade; in fact, it's likely that this is the sole significant basis for the cardiac toxicity of quinidine (Fig. 23–14). The word *extreme* cannot be

Figure 23–13.
Minimal quinidine effect on Q-T interval. The interval is approximately 0.4 second, which is prolonged for a rate of 93. This degree of prolongation is very common and is not a reason to discontinue the drug. Quinidine can produce sagging of the S-T segment that looks exactly like digitalis effect.

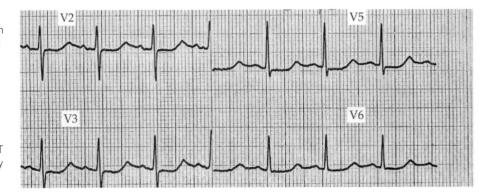

Figure 23–14.
Pronounced quinidine effect with Q-T interval of 0.54 second, at a rate of 86. Note the depressed S-T segments. Part of the large wave that runs all the way to the next P may be a U wave incorporated in the T.

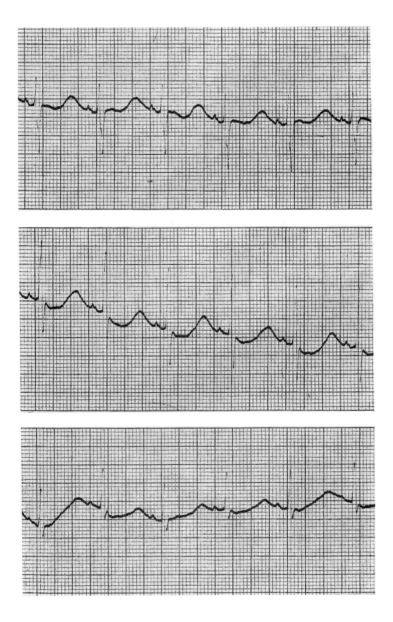

defined precisely at this time, but a reasonable rough guess would be that any Q-T prolongation more than 25% above the calculated maximum for age and sex presents a real hazard; the drug should probably be discontinued. Quinidine depresses the cells in the bundle-branch system and delays intraventricular conduction. If quinidine causes widening of the QRS to more than 15% above baseline, the drug should be stopped.

It's customary to warn about giving the drug to patients with bundle-branch block for fear that conduction in the other bundle branch might fail. This is a warning that probably has no basis in fact. In 50 years of administering quinidine, I have never seen serious depression of intraventricular conduction. I suppose it happens, but it's very, very rare. I can't remember the last time I saw significant QRS widening caused by quinidine, and all current studies bear this out. This particular hazard has been grossly exaggerated; the presence of bundle-branch block or other intraventricular conduction defect is not a contraindication to the use of quinidine. The real hazard with quinidine, to reiterate, is Q-T prolongation leading to torsade. Other 1A drugs, such as procainamide and disopyramide, can prolong the Q-T interval, with the attendant danger of torsade.

Tricyclic Antidepressants

Any drug in this category can depress conduction within the ventricles. Nonspecific widening of the QRS, frank bundle-branch block, or AV block caused by failure of both bundle branches can result. Like quinidine, these drugs can also affect AV nodal conduction, producing any variety of AV nodal block, although this is less common than delay in the bundle-branch system.

Phenothiazines

The phenothiazines as a group have effects much like quinidine: prolongation of Q-T interval and depression of conduction within the ventricles. AV block has occasionally occurred with overdoses of these drugs. Sudden death in apparently healthy individuals taking these drugs is doubtless the result of torsade following Q-T prolongation.

Twenty-four

Two Special Cases: Pulmonary Emboli and Hypothermia

Pulmonary Emboli

The most important thing to remember about pulmonary emboli is that most of them have no effect on the electrocardiogram (ECG) at all. Never rule out a pulmonary embolus just because the ECG remains normal! The reason for this is obvious: the lungs have such an abundant blood supply that an embolus must compromise a really major segment of the lung before it has any effect on pressure in the pulmonary artery. An embolus that compromises a large segment of a lung can create high pressures in the pulmonary artery and in the right heart. The ECG will reflect that sudden rise in pressure in the lesser circulation. The changes are quite predictable:

1. There will be a sudden swing of the axis to the right, often with a deep S in I. A small septal q will usually be present in III, which gave rise to the old "SI-Q-III" combination you still read about in textbooks. That phrase is a hangover from the primitive days in electrocardiography when we had only leads I, II, and III and didn't really know what a septal q was. The simple fact is that the sudden rise in pulmonary artery and right ventricular pressures swings the axis rightward, just as you'd expect; whether there's a small q in III is irrelevant.

2. There may be an incomplete right bundle-branch block pattern. This is usually seen in more extreme cases with significant elevation of pulmonary artery and right ventricular pressures. This will be accompanied by a right axis of the initial forces (Fig. 24–1).

3. There may be a peculiar type of S-T depression in the limb leads. There is a horizontal depression of the S-T with an abrupt, almost vertical rise into the T. The shape of the S-T-T complex gave rise to the German term *Treppe* or "steps," and in fact the S-T-T complex does resemble a staircase. This peculiar configuration is rarely seen in any other setting. In other words, it's not at all sensitive, but it's very specific. In Figure 24–2, there is a typical example of the Treppe type of S-T-T deformity combined with a right axis that had appeared abruptly at the time of symptoms. This was a major pulmonary embolus with a fatal outcome.

Pulmonary emboli can also produce S–T–T deformities of the "nonspecific" variety described in Chapter 22.

Figure 24–1.
Incomplete right bundle-branch block with rightward axis of initial forces in the limb leads. This is a typical configuration seen with a massive pulmonary embolus.

Hypothermia

There is one specific deformity associated with hypothermia: a deflection of the late forces of the QRS called an *Osborne wave*. A wide, slurred deflection appears at the end of the downstroke of the R (Fig. 24–3). This is a relatively mild example; sometimes an Osborne wave can be enormous, constituting most of the ventricular complex.

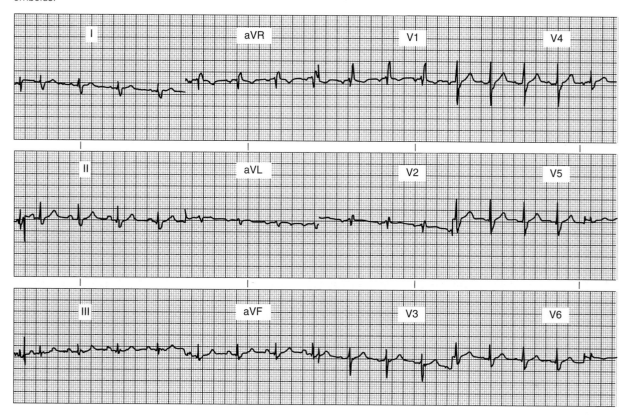

Figure 24–2.
Classic findings with
a pulmonary embolus.
A deep S has appeared
in lead I, and there's a
small septal q in III. The
sharp angle where the
depressed S-T joins the
T in leads I and aVL is
the typical Treppe or
"staircase" deformity.

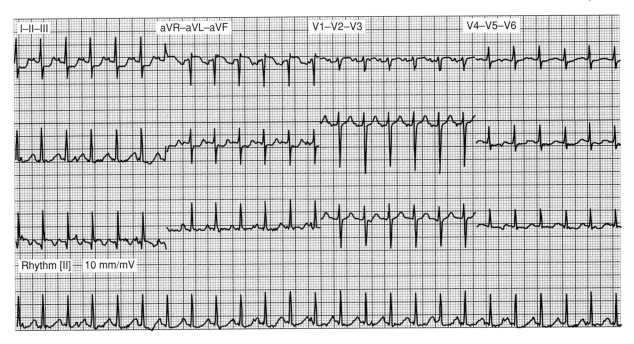

Figure 24–3.
The Osborne wave of
hypothermia. These are
leads V2 to V5. The wide,
slurred terminal portion of
the R is the characteristic
deformity of hypothermia.

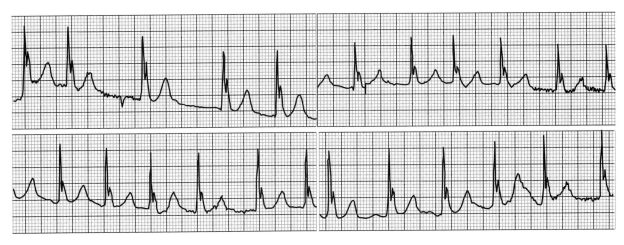

Self-Assessment III

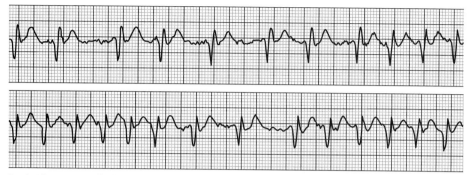

Figure SAIII–1.

1. A physician calls for help. She's been treating this patient's chronic atrial fibrillation with digoxin, but she notes that the pulse has become more rapid and that the patient is in distress. Giving more digoxin only seems to make it worse. Cause? Treatment?

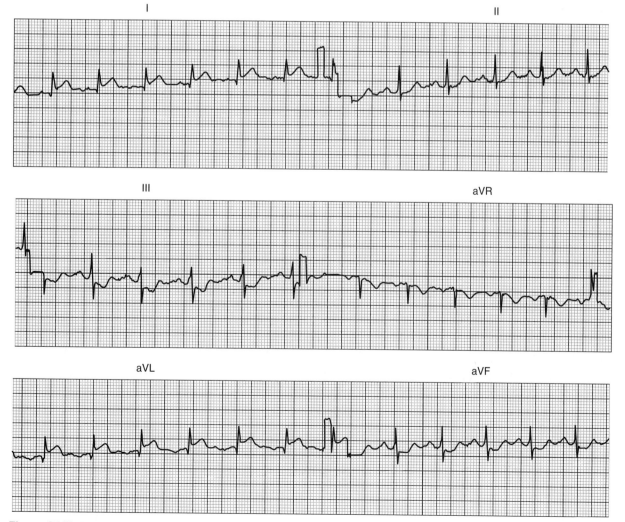

Figure SAIII–2. 2. Diagnosis? Number of criteria to support the diagnosis?

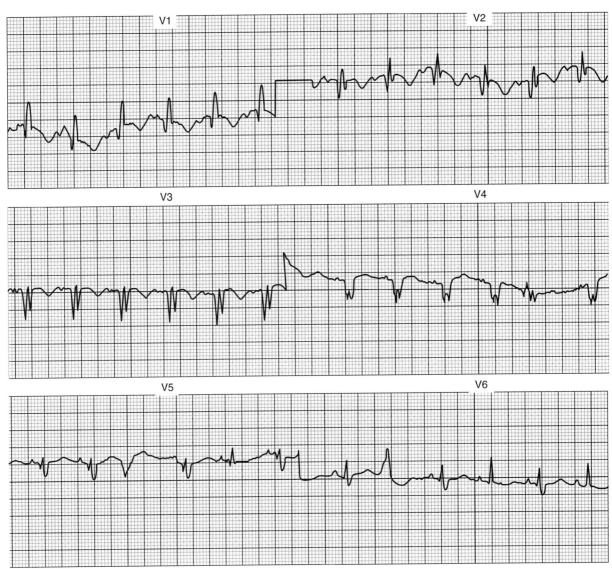

Figure SAIII–3. 3. Two diagnoses, please. Tracing recorded during chest pain in a patient who had a normal ECG a month ago. Prognosis? What's happening in V6?

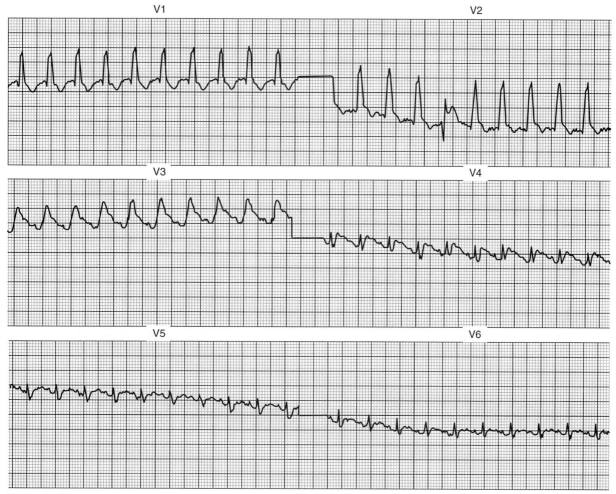

Figure SAIII–4. 4. Tracing handed to you from the emergency room. Two diagnoses and proof?

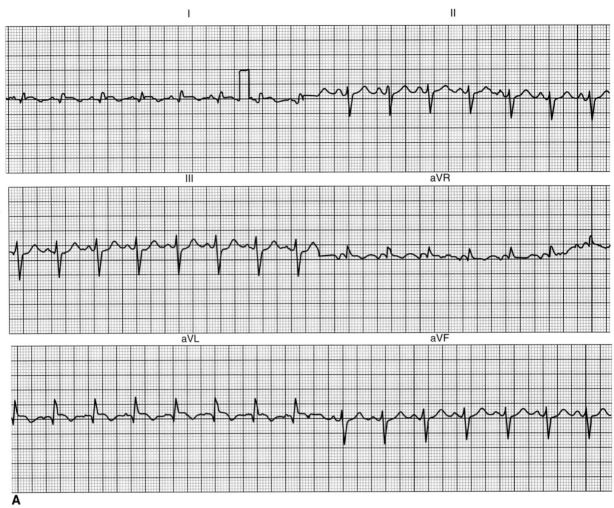

Figure SAIII–5A.   5. The patient had a normal ECG with normal axis 2 weeks ago. Diagnosis? How supported?
Additional feature?

(Continued)

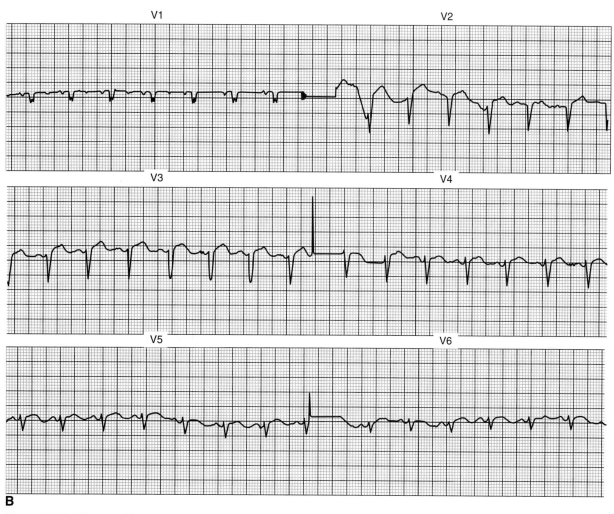

B

Figure SAIII–5B   cont'd.

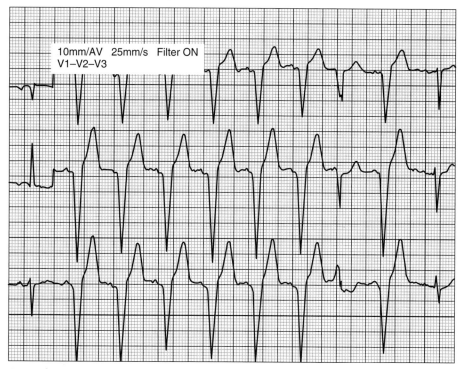

Figure SAIII–6.

6. Leads, V1, V2, and V3. Wide beats followed by narrow beats. Diagnosis?

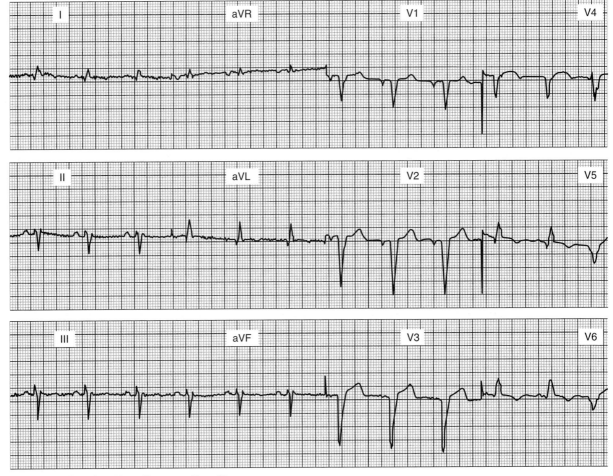

Figure SAIII–7.   7.   Two diagnoses. Proof?

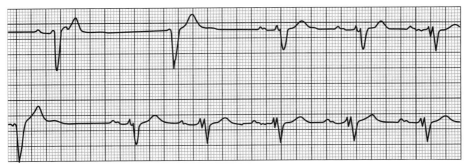

Figure SAIII–8.

8. Just from this rhythm strip, what symptoms would you anticipate? What clinical diagnosis? What cause would you rule out as a first step in treatment?

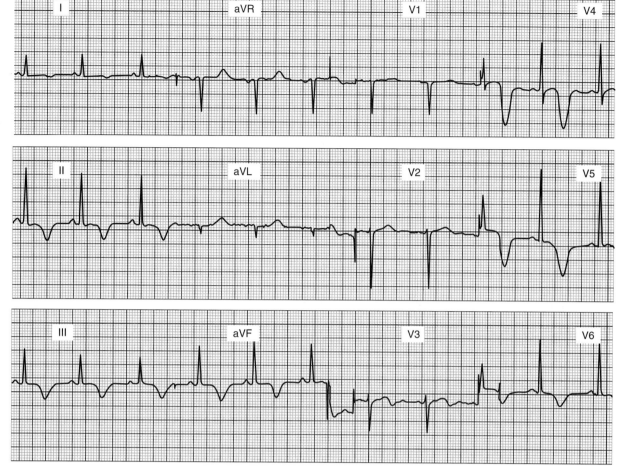

Figure SAIII–9. 9. What statement can you make about this ECG? What statement(s) can you not make?

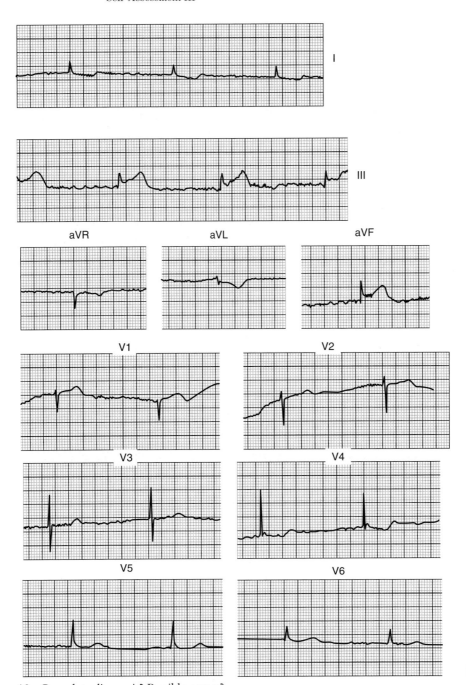

I

III

aVR   aVL   aVF

V1   V2

V3   V4

V5   V6

Figure SAIII–10.

10. Complete diagnosis? Possible causes?

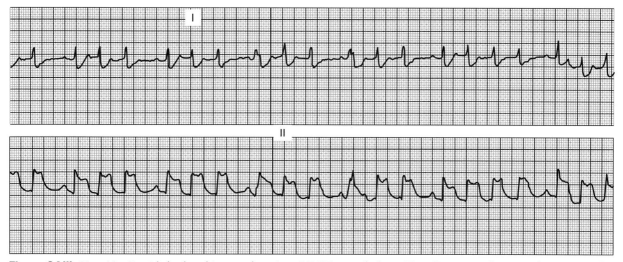

Figure SAIII–11.   11. Rapid rhythm; bizarre, changing QRST morphology. Two diagnoses, please (each a matter of life or death here).

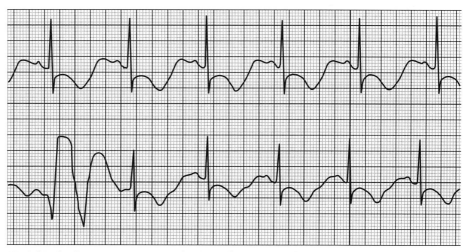

Figure SAIII–12.

12. This rhythm strip pops up in the critical care unit. What danger confronts this patient? Probable cause? Treatment?

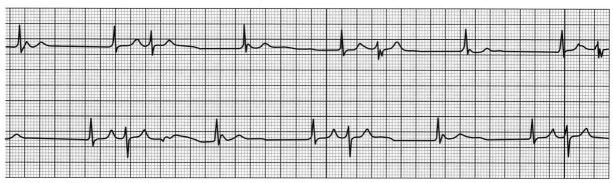

Figure SAIII–13.   13. This calls for tough reasoning. There's an obvious diagnosis here, but you have to use deductive logic to find it. Cause of the arrhythmia? Source of the P waves? State of AV conduction? Clinical entity?

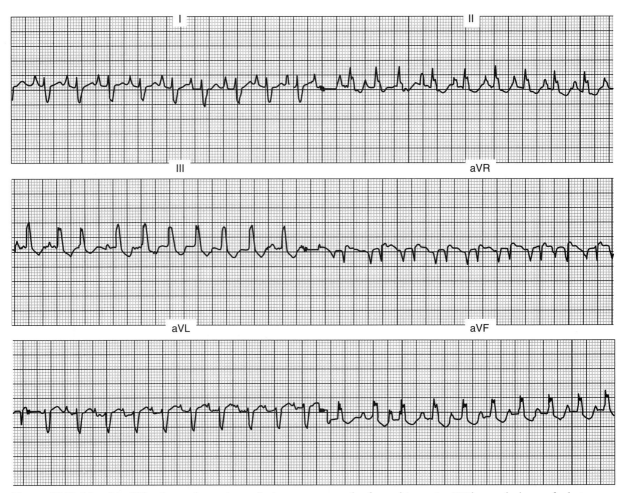

Figure SAIII–14.   14. What hemodynamic prediction can you make from this tracing? What pathology of what chambers?

(*Continued*)

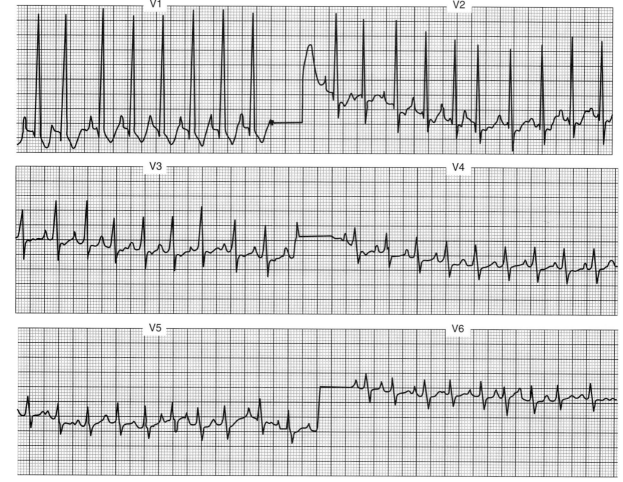

Figure SAIII–14   cont'd.

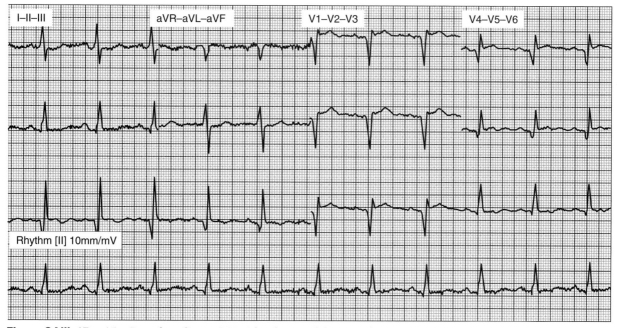

Figure SAIII–15.   15. Complete diagnosis? With what confidence? Why?

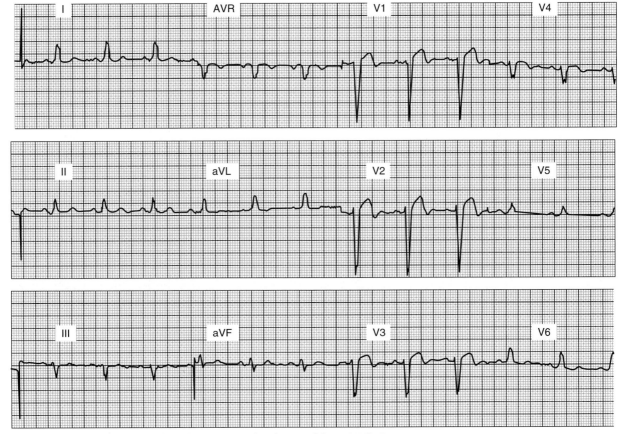

Figure SAIII–16.   16. Complete diagnosis? With what confidence? Why?

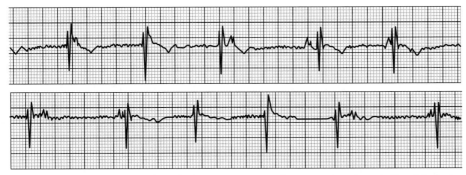

Figure SAIII–17.

17. This tracing came over the telephone transmitter from a remote hospital's critical care
     unit. Mechanism? Cause of pauses? State of AV conduction?

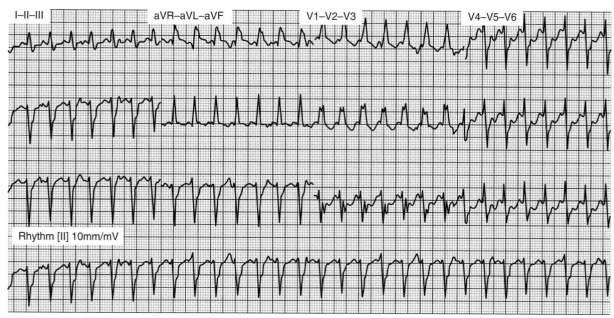

I–II–III   aVR–aVL–aVF   V1–V2–V3   V4–V5–V6

Rhythm [II] 10mm/mV

Figure SAIII–18.   18. Wide-beat tachycardia. Precise diagnosis? Significance?

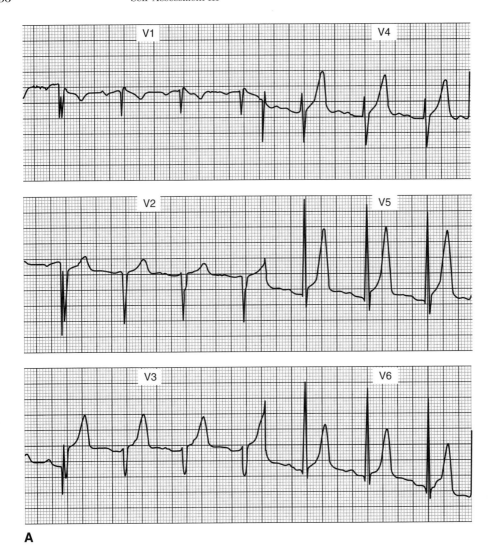

A

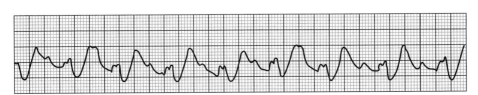

B

19. Tracings **A** and **B** illustrate different stages of the same abnormality.
    What is it and how is it treated ?

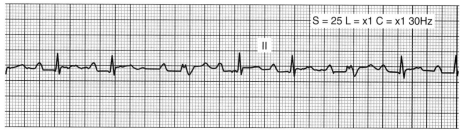

Figure SAIII–20.

20. Just to keep you honest: narrow beats and wide beats. Cause of the two wide beats?

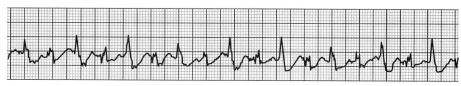

Figure SAIII–21.

21. Here's a test of your powers of observation. This specific arrhythmia isn't described in the text. What do you see? (Rare and dangerous.)

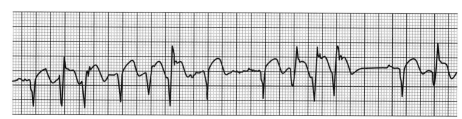

Figure SAIII–22.

22. This arrhythmia appeared on the monitor in the critical care unit. The patient had been admitted with a diagnosis of "probable anterior MI." Rhythm? Morphologic change? Significance?

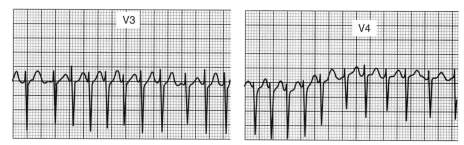

Figure SAIII–23.

23. Rhythm strip in the emergency room. Diagnosis? Possibility or probability of special pathophysiology? Steps to clarify? Treatment?

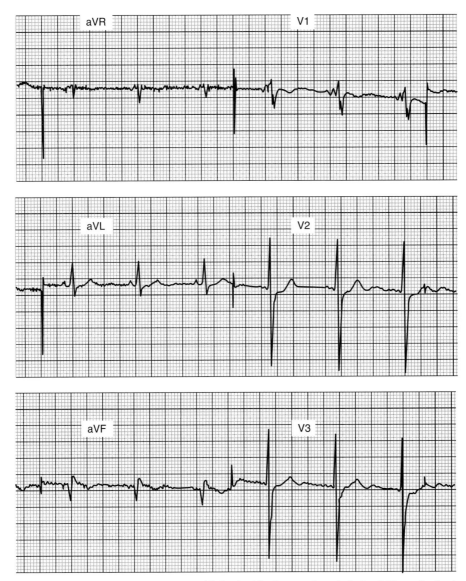

Figure SAIII–24.

24. The asymptomatic patient was told she had had a previous inferior MI on the basis of this tracing. Comment?

Answers

1. The periods of regular rhythm, rate 152, obviously represent runs of junctional tachycardia interrupting atrial fibrillation. This is one of the most common manifestations of digitalis toxicity.

2. Lateral wall MI, acute. There's a pathologic Q in aVL and obvious reciprocal S-T deviation in electrically opposed limb leads. The diagnosis is established beyond question.

3. Right bundle-branch block and anterior MI. The pathologic Q waves establish the diagnosis: pathologic Q waves are never produced by RBBB per se. There are occasional VPCs arising in the right ventricle. The fifth beat in lead V5 represents normalizing fusion. The narrow beats in V6 may represent normalizing fusion or intermittent bundle-branch block. Prognosis grave! New-onset bundle-branch block with MI implies 50% mortality.

4. Right bundle-branch block and acute anterior MI. The S-T elevation in V2 to V4 could not possibly be produced by the RBBB; it's characteristic of acute anterior ischemia.

5. Anterior and lateral MI, acute. In the frontal plane leads, there is obvious reciprocal S-T deviation and a lateral Q in aVL, all consistent with a lateral MI. There's left anterior hemiblock that appeared acutely with the MI. The precordial leads are a good example of a "Q-equivalent" deflection with no R wave progression at all from V2 to V6. The term "poor R-wave progression" is overused and much abused, but as you see it here, it's really significant. With left anterior hemiblock, it is common to see diminished R wave progression across the precordial leads, but here there are hardly any R waves at all, even in V5 to V6.

6. Intermittent WPW (Wolff-Parkinson White), type B. Look at the P-R intervals of the wide beats!

7. Left bundle-branch block with anterior MI. The pathologic Q waves in the midprecordium and the typical "tombstone" curve of S-T-T in V4 to V6 are diagnostic. Neither deformity will ever be produced by LBBB.

8. Subnormal sinus node function. Symptoms probably would be vertigo, presyncope, or frank syncope. The wide beats on the left-hand side of the strip are an idioventricular rhythm. There are no visible P waves during this period. The sinus beats on the right-hand side of the strip are conducted with first-degree AV block. If this isn't caused by drugs and if the patient is symptomatic, sick sinus syndrome is present.

9. You can say that this is an abnormal tracing with evidence of myocardial pathology. Period. That's all you can say. You can't say whether the pathology is ischemic or myopathic or degenerative. The symmetrical shape of the inverted T waves makes coronary disease with ischemic pathology more likely than other possibilities, but these are in fact nonspecific T wave deformities, and that's all you can call them.

10. Atrial fibrillation with complete AV block and inferior MI. The possible causes include the AV nodal block commonly seen with inferior MIs or—as in this case—overdose of digoxin.

11. Here and there you see obvious P waves. They appear every three or four beats. If you look at the S-T-T contour of the subsequent beats, you will see that there's a dramatic change in the shape of the T waves. The Q-T interval seems to shorten. Remember that the leopard doesn't change its spots, and the T wave doesn't change its shape. Neither does the Q-T interval shorten from beat to beat as it seems to be doing here. When you see either phenomenon, there's a P wave hidden in the T, and that's what's producing the changing morphology. If you measure those odd bumps in the T waves, you'll see that they "march out" precisely, yielding an atrial rate of about 152. In other words, PAT is present. Note that each P wave moves closer to the preceding R; this means that the P-R is getting longer, of course. Wenckebach block is present. Put the two diagnoses together, and you have PAT with block! Note the dramatic reciprocal S-T deviation; the diagnosis of an acute inferior MI is also obvious.

12. Prolonged Q-T interval. The immediate danger is torsade, and the most common cause is a 1A drug like quinidine. Treatment: discontinue the drug. Treatment of torsade: magnesium sulfate in large intravenous doses; also speeding of atrial rate by atrial pacing or atropine.

13. Tough reasoning. There are many narrow QRS complexes that are clearly junctional. There are also P waves. Are these sinus P waves, or do they represent retrograde conduction from the junction? Is there any sinus node activity at all? The first beat is clearly junctional: it's followed by a P wave that produces a response. Beat 3 is also junctional, with a P wave half-buried in it. Beat 4 repeats the pattern of beat 1, and so on throughout the strip. In other words, a P wave comes just after one junctional beat and then comes longer after the next junctional beat. After this long R-P, there's always an early QRS. Could these P waves be dissociated sinus beats? Of course not—they're always associated with junctional beats! If these were dissociated sinus beats, they'd occur all through the heart cycle, independent of the sinus impulses. This is retrograde Wenckebach from the junction. The first R-P is very short—the P is almost hidden in the QRS. The second R-P is longer, so the AV node has time to recover and conduct back down—reciprocal beating. Full diagnosis: junctional rhythm with retrograde Wenckebach and reciprocal beating. AV nodal conduction is normal—both retrograde and antegrade. There is no sinus node activity. Sick sinus!

14. The most pronounced form of RVH (type A). There is also evidence of right atrial enlargement. This type of RVH indicates right-sided pressures close to or equal to arterial pressures. Pulmonic stenosis or severe pulmonary hypertension secondary to Eisenmenger's pathophysiology will produce this pattern.

15. LBBB with anterior and inferior infarction. LBBB or not, those Q waves are still pathologic and specific!

16. LBBB with unmistakable Pardee (tombstone) configuration of S-T-T in V1 to V4. LBBB per se will never produce that configuration! Anterior ischemic process, presumably infarction.

17. There's a junctional rhythm with dissociated P waves and three long pauses. The pauses occur when the P wave comes a long time after the QRS. Concealed conduction! When the P wave comes long enough after the junctional beat, it finds the upper nodal tissues out of their refractory period; the sinus impulse penetrates to the site of the junctional pacemaker and resets it. That produces the pause. The lower node is still refractory, so the impulse never reaches the ventricles. Hence, the pause. Is complete AV block present? Of course not. The sinus impulse can penetrate to the junctional site to reset it, and the junctional site can reach the ventricles, so there's obviously a track from atria to ventricles. It's just a matter of timing.

18. Wide-beat tachycardia with RBBB configuration and extreme left axis. Fascicular ventricular tachycardia—a distinct entity in terms of mechanism, prognosis, and treatment. These tachycardias are often called "idiopathic ventricular tachycardias," but I think *fascicular* is a better term because it describes the origin and propagation of the impulse.

19. Strip **A** shows tall, peaked T waves, V3 to V6. Good working rule: When a T wave is more than half the height of an R in a lead that consists primarily of an R, it's significant. Hyperkalemia. Strip **B** shows sinus rhythm with very wide QRS complexes (about 0.24 second). This kind of extreme widening of QRS is strongly suggestive of hyperkalemia, which was in fact present.

20. The wide beats appear after sinus pauses, when the rate slows for one beat. Bradycardia-dependent aberrancy.

21. Wide-beat tachycardia without P waves. Note the alternans in shape and size. This is paroxysmal ventricular tachycardia with electrical alternans, a rare and dangerous arrhythmia usually produced by near-terminal digitalis toxicity.

22. Sinus rhythm with short runs of junctional tachycardia. Note the dramatic increase in S-T elevation with the rapid beating. You're seeing a kind of instant stress test—the more rapid rate is obviously producing increasing ischemia. Slowing the rate will probably be life-saving; obviously, there's a critical lesion in the LAD (left anterior descending coronary artery), and this patient is going to need very close attention if not intervention.

23. Atrial fibrillation with very rapid ventricular response. Some of the R-R intervals are equivalent to a rate of 250 or higher. This always arouses suspicion of preexcitation. Simple test: give adenosine. If the rate slows, there's no preexcitation; if it speeds, there is. If preexcitation is present, of course, avoid anything that depresses conduction through the AV node.

Warning! When you administer adenosine for possible preexcitation, have a defibrillator ready on standby. During the 6 seconds of AV nodal blockade, the bypass tract can drive the ventricles into ventricular fibrillation. Two such cases have been reported already (see Chapter 11).

24. *False alarm!* Look at V1, and there's obvious preexcitation. You can also see an obvious delta-R in aVL. The Q in aVF is simply the "delta force" of preexcitation, exactly opposite in polarity to the way it appears in aVL and V1.

Twenty-five

Graduation Exercise

This is a mini-atlas of complex arrhythmias. To analyze them, you don't need to learn anything new; you can reach a diagnosis in every case by using the elements you've learned in the text. The trick now is to apply these elements in a logical manner. Each step in the reasoning process is simple, but at the end, you'll find you have arrived at the diagnosis, prognosis, and treatment for a set of arrhythmias guaranteed to give most of your colleagues a throbbing sense of insecurity.

Figure 25–1.

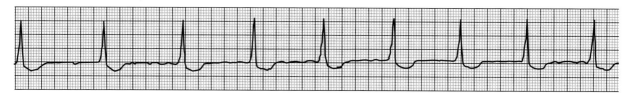

The rhythm in Figure 25–1 appeared in the setting of chronic atrial fibrillation. The patient was taking a variety of "heart medicines" but wasn't sure what they were. He presented in the emergency room complaining of "feeling faint" as if he were "going to pass out." Are impulses from the fibrillating atria reaching the ventricles? If not, what's the rhythm? Is it regular, and if not, is there any pattern? Is atrioventricular (AV) block present, and if so, where and what kind? How many levels of block do you see?

Answers: First, this is not the helter-skelter ventricular rhythm you expect if the ventricles are responding to fibrillating atria. The rate is slow and the rhythm is almost, but not quite, regular. Impulses from the fibrillating atria are obviously not reaching the ventricles.

Conclusion 1: This is some kind of idiorhythm, presumably arising in the AV junction. It is completely dissociated from the fibrillating atria.

Problem: Junctional rhythms are characteristically completely regular, but this one isn't. If you measure closely, you see that the ventricular complexes come progressively closer together, reading from left to right. In fact, the R-R intervals make a nice mathematical progression, measured in seconds: 1.28, 1.20, 1.15, 1.10, 1.05, 1.02, 1.0, 1.0, 0.09. When you see a progressive shortening of R-R intervals, what do you think of? Simple answer: You think of the "typical" form of Wenckebach block! (See Chapter 7 and note item 8 on page 75.)

Conclusion 2: There is a completely dissociated junctional rhythm, and the junctional beats are encountering Wenckebach block in the lower AV node.

Conclusion 3: The R-R intervals at the beginning of the strip equal a rate of 47. You therefore have the criteria for *complete heart block:* complete AV dissociation, a slow ventricular rate, and no capture by an ample number of atrial impulses (about 425 a minute if this is an average atrial fibrillation).

Conclusion 4: There are two levels of AV block:

> 1. **There is complete block between the fibrillating atria and the site of the junctional pacemaker.**
>
> 2. **There is Wenckebach block in the lower node, below the site of the junctional pacemaker.**

Final conclusion: The "heart medicine" almost certainly included digitalis, and the treatment simply consisted of withholding the drug. (Note that the digoxin level was 2.2, but the block disappeared completely after the drug was stopped, illustrating once more that you cannot depend on serum levels to diagnose digitalis toxicity. You have to look at the electrocardiogram [ECG] and the patient!)

Figure 25–2.

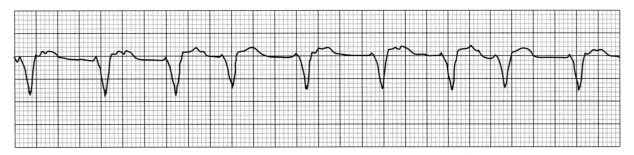

The ECG in Figure 25–2 reveals wide QRS complexes *not* preceded by P waves; the rate is normal, and the rhythm is slightly irregular. This pattern appeared 12 hours out in the course of a myocardial infarction; all previous QRS complexes had been narrow.

Differential diagnosis: There are two possibilities:

> 1. **Idioventricular rhythm (benign)**
>
> 2. **Junctional rhythm with new bundle-branch block (bad news: 50% mortality)**

The differentiation is critical. You can make it from this strip.

Observation 1: There are obvious atrial complexes. These are diphasic deflections appearing at different intervals after the QRS. Again there are two possibilities: these might be dissociated sinus P waves or retrograde P waves from the ectopic focus.

Answer: If these were dissociated sinus P waves, they would "wander through" the strip with no fixed relation to the QRS. In fact, they're always associated with a QRS: If you look closely, you see that they come at progressively longer intervals after the QRS. In other words, there's a progressive prolongation of the R–P—a *reverse Wenckebach* phenomenon, or as one of my bright students put it, a "Backenwenck." The retrograde P appears as a notch on the first part of the T in beat I, it's farther out into the T in beat II, and it comes at the end of the T in beat III. This pattern repeats itself in the strip, so it can't be accidental. These have to be retrograde P waves.

Observation 2: This is really the key. *Beat IV comes early.* The same pattern is repeated in the next four beats; after the longest R–P, there's an early QRS. This is reciprocal beating. The retrograde impulse takes so long traveling back up to the atria that the AV tissues have time to recover, and the impulse is conducted back down to the ventricles, producing the early beat. The sequence is ventricles–atria–ventricles. The reciprocal beat shows you the pattern of *normal antegrade conduction* just as if it were a normal sinus beat. The QRS of the reciprocal beat is wide, with exactly the same configuration as all the other beats.

Conclusion: The wide beats are the result of bundle-branch block. The pressing clinical problem is solved. This is in fact a junctional rhythm with newly acquired bundle-branch block. The reciprocal beat is the key to the whole diagnosis.

One more refinement: The QRS complexes appear in four-beat cycles. The last beat of each cycle is the reciprocal beat, and of course it's early. Measure the other R–R intervals carefully, and you'll find that beats II and III are always closer together than I and II. Again you see that diminishing R–R interval just as in the previous tracing: Wenckebach block! There is antegrade Wenckebach block in the lower node, below the site of the junctional pacemaker.

Final diagnosis: Junctional rhythm with newly acquired bundle-branch block with antegrade and retrograde Wenckebach block and reciprocal beating.

Figure 25–3.

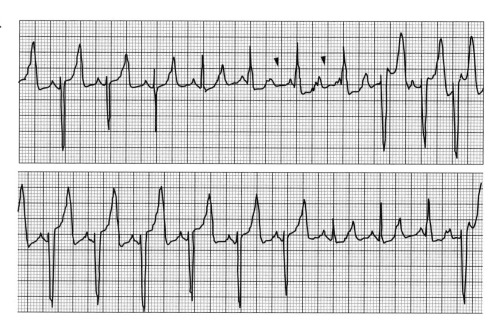

The patient in Figure 25–3 was sweating, hypotensive, and obviously very sick. He was an elderly member of the Tohono O'Tham tribe (formerly Papagos) and didn't speak much English. He had been taking some kind of medicine he obtained at a free clinic, but nobody knew what it was. The pulse was regular with a rate of 100. The two strips start with a series of beats with a normal P–R (three in the top strip, six on the bottom). Note that the shape of the QRS in these strips changes as you scan from left to right: The QRS becomes progressively narrower and then changes from negative to upright. The beats that consist of an R wave appear at exactly the same rate as the others—they're regular. Now look at the P waves in the series of beats that consist of an R wave. The P–R interval is changing—it seems to be shortening, whereas the ventricular rhythm is regular. A changing P–R interval with a regular ventricular rhythm means dissociation. AV dissociation can take place only when there's an ectopic rhythm. Therefore, there must be an idioventricular or idiojunctional rhythm here.

Between the ectopic beats, at the points indicated by arrowheads, you now see something different—the key to the whole arrhythmia. You see two P waves between each set of ventricular complexes. You now have a chance to measure the atrial rate; it's 250. March your calipers back through the tracing, and you can find this same rapid atrial rate all the way. In the beats that consist of a predominant S wave in the first part of each strip, the alternate P waves appear as a notch on the upslope of the T.

Now answer two questions:

> 1. **What are the atria doing? They are firing rapidly and regularly at a rate of 215.** *Diagnosis:* **paroxysmal atrial tachycardia.**
>
> 2. **Are all the atrial impulses reaching the ventricles? Obviously not. There's 2:1 block in the first part of the tracing and complete dissociation for a period of more than 2 seconds.** *Diagnosis:* **AV block.**

Put them together: paroxysmal atrial tachycardia (PAT) with block!

The peculiar change in QRS morphology is the result of progressive fusion between the sinus impulses and the ectopic rhythm. Because there's fusion, you now know that the ectopic rhythm is an idioventricular rhythm. The normalizing fusion with the narrowing of the QRS tells you that there's really bundle-branch block, even though part of the QRS is hidden in the baseline. (At the right-hand end of each strip, AV conduction resumes with Wenckebach periods.) Stop the digoxin; start the potassium!

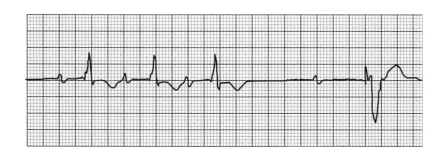

Figure 25–4.

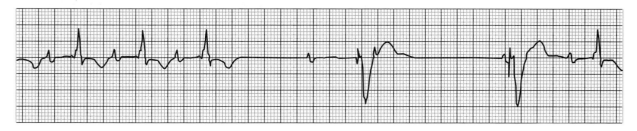

A pacemaker was implanted two years ago for unknown reasons in the patient in Figure 25–4. (They often are!) Now the patient presents with "presyncope"—a slovenly term meaning that sometimes the patient felt some blurring of consciousness "as if he was going to pass out." The ECG tells the whole story. There's a first-degree AV block with bundle-branch block. After three beats, there's an abrupt sinus pause. The pause is almost exactly equal to two sinus intervals, so it's true sinoatrial exit block (see Chapter 15). After the sinus pause, there's a blocked P wave followed by a paced beat. The same thing happens in the bottom strip—the P wave that comes after a long pause is blocked, and the pacemaker discharges.

Here's an odd phenomenon: The atrial complexes that come *late* are blocked; the ones that come earlier are normally conducted. You're looking at bradycardia-dependent refractoriness (see Chapter 6). More commonly, this phenomenon produces bradycardia-dependent aberrancy, but it can produce bradycardia-dependent block. Because one bundle branch is blocked, there's only one functioning strand connecting atria and ventricles—a strand consisting of the AV node and the normal bundle branch. The prolonged P-R interval may be the result of delay in the one functioning bundle branch or even in the one functioning fascicle if bifascicular block is present. If bradycardia-dependent refractoriness arises in that one functioning strand, AV conduction will fail when the rate slows, and that's what you're seeing here.

Because this is really intermittent bilateral bundle-branch block, it is in fact a variation of Mobitz-II block, and it has the same dangerous connotations. The patient really needs that pacemaker, but it's not functioning normally. It's firing too slowly (rate about 32) and too late (escape interval about 1.8 seconds). The pacemaker is in urgent need of readjustment or replacement.

Figure 25–5.

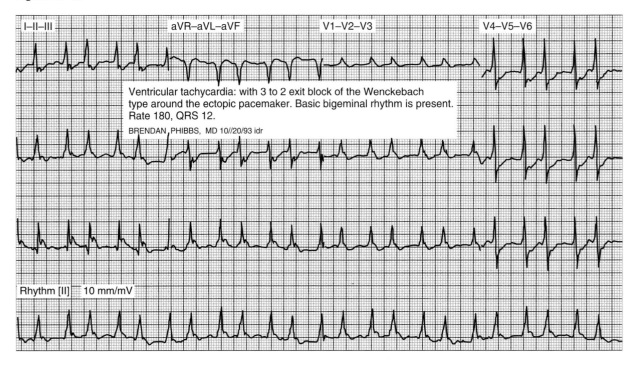

The old bugbear: A wide-beat tachycardia without P waves. The patient in Figure 25–5 had normal narrow QRS complexes on the tracing recorded a few hours previously; this arrhythmia arose in the course of hospitalization for crescendo angina. The ECG presents a simple pattern: it consists entirely of wide QRS complexes appearing in pairs. There are no atrial complexes anywhere. The beats appear at an interval equal to a rate of 166 (9 squares), then there's a pause that's *less* than double that interval (11 squares).

Answer: Ventricular tachycardia with Wenckebach exit block around the ectopic focus. Why Wenckebach? Remember that with 3:2 Wenckebach block, you see two QRS complexes followed by a pause. In any Wenckebach block, there's always recovery after the pause; in AV nodal Wenckebach, the P–R interval after the pause *shortens*—it "pulls in" the QRS—so that the pause is less than the sum of the two preceding beats. Same thing with Wenckebach exit block: the pause will always be less than a double interval of the basic rate.

Speculation: When you see exit block during a paroxysmal tachycardia, it's likely that the mechanism is parasystole, rather than reentry. It's easier to conceive of Wenckebach periods around a single ectopic focus than in a reentry loop.

That was a reasonably straightforward wide-beat tachycardia problem. Now try something challenging. The patient in Figure 25–6 again was severely distressed, with hypotension, sweating, and apprehension. There was a long-standing history of hypertensive heart disease, coronary artery disease, and congestive heart failure, all treated with many drugs by a number of physicians. When the patient presented to the emergency room, he wasn't quite sure which of his numerous medications he'd been taking, but he thought they included digoxin.

In this tracing, you see narrow and wide QRS complexes, appearing rapidly. The narrow complexes are clearly the result of some kind of supraventricular tachycardia; they appear at a rate of 150. The wide complexes appear at a rate of 125. Those two numbers are the key to

Figure 25–6.

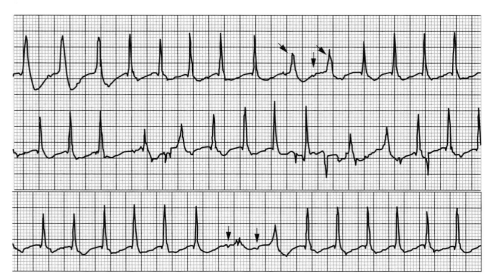

the whole arrhythmia. When you see wide QRS complexes, there are two possibilities: ventricular ectopic firing or aberrant conduction. The common type of sustained aberrancy is *rate-dependent aberrancy*. Here, the wide QRS complexes appear at a *slower rate* than the narrow ones. You can't invoke aberrancy to explain the wide QRS complexes—they have to be ventricular.

Diagnosis 1: supraventricular tachycardia interrupted by short runs of ventricular tachycardia. Digitalis toxicity is the presumptive diagnosis. What kind of supraventricular tachycardia? Look at the arrows, and you'll see some tiny but well-defined P waves that give you the answer. They appear at exactly the same rate as the narrow complexes. If you look closely, you'll see the same tiny P waves in other parts of the strip. The two QRS complexes following the marked P waves are intermediate in shape and size between the wide complexes and the narrow ones. They're *fusion beats,* and that absolutely identifies the wide-beat tachycardia as ventricular.

Now look at the P-R interval of those two beats. It's getting longer. Wenckebach! Look at the T waves of the next five narrow beats, and you see small but clearcut changes as the P moves closer to the preceding T until one is blocked. The P-R is getting longer, and the R-P of course is getting shorter. Wenckebach again!

You have now diagnosed the frightening combination of PAT with block and intermittent ventricular tachycardia. This is a potentially lethal combination of digitalis-toxic rhythms.

Treatment: Potassium for the PAT with block and diphenylhydantoin for the ventricular tachycardia (it's specific in this setting).

Atrial flutter with a bigeminal rhythm: Remember that in about one third of all cases of atrial flutter, the ventricular rhythm is irregular: The ratio of conduction to the ventricles changes from second to second, producing an "irregular irregularity" of the pulse that can't be distinguished from atrial fibrillation at the bedside. Here you have atrial flutter with a "bigeminal," or coupled, rhythm. This coupled rhythm isn't caused by extra systoles because there is a recurring precise pattern of relationship of flutter waves to QRS throughout. There's a flutter wave about 0.23 second ahead of the first QRS of each pair and a flutter wave 0.08 second ahead of the second QRS. This precise repetition cannot be accidental. What's going on?

Start with what you know about ordinary 2:1 flutter. Every other flutter wave dies at the AV junction because the AV tissues are refractory—fortunately for the patient. If every flutter wave came through, the heart would race itself to death. The nonconducted flutter waves don't penetrate the AV node at all. Often the flutter impulses that do travel down the AV node will encounter some kind of block. To diagnose the block, you must concentrate on the flutter waves that penetrate the AV node; in other words, the alternate flutter waves. You ignore the waves that die at the AV junction.

Figure 25–7.

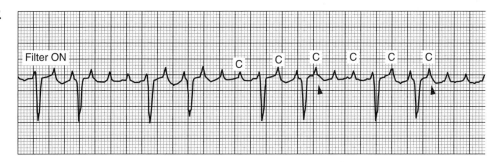

In Figure 25–7, the flutter waves that are conducted down the AV node are marked C. Look at the relation of those waves to the QRS, and ignore the other flutter waves because they never really leave the atria. The first C is conducted with a P-R of 0.23 second. The second is conducted with a P-R of 0.25 second. The third is blocked (arrowhead). The pattern is repeated precisely in the next three C beats. You're looking at Wenckebach block of the alternate flutter waves that travel down the AV node. In other words, it's an "every-other-beat Wenckebach."

Again you see two levels of block: one between the atria and the AV node, and the other down in the AV node itself.

Figure 25–8.

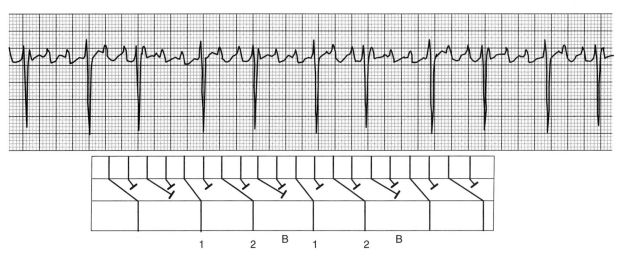

Figure 25–8 is a schematic diagram of the same phenomenon. The beats labeled 1 are the first beat of a Wenckebach cycle, the beats labeled 2 are the second, and the blocked beat, of course, is labeled B. Note that you ignore the alternate flutter waves that don't penetrate the AV node. When you're analyzing AV nodal block in the presence of atrial flutter, this is an important concept to keep in mind.

Figure 25–9.

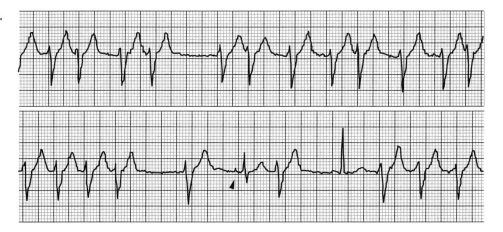

Figure 25–9 is a really rare bird. It's the only one of its kind I've ever seen, but it illustrates a couple of very basic principles in the diagnosis of wide-beat tachycardia. This woman presented to our clinic describing "dizziness and palpitations."

Most of this tracing is taken up with a totally irregular wide-beat tachycardia without P waves. At first blush, you'd think of atrial fibrillation with bundle-branch block. Look again. About two thirds of the way across the bottom strip, you see a normal sinus beat with a narrow QRS.

Next logical question: Why not paroxysmal atrial fibrillation with rate-dependent bundle-branch block? Look at the pause between the fourth and fifth beats in the top strip, and you see a long R–R interval—much longer than the one preceding the narrow sinus beat. If rate-dependent bundle-branch block was causing the wide beats, it should have disappeared after that pause. There's another long pause in the bottom strip, but the wide QRS persists. You have therefore ruled out rate-dependent aberrancy as a cause of the wide QRS complexes. Always be prepared to make this observation when you're analyzing intermittent wide-beat rhythms.

The only other possible cause of a wide QRS is ventricular ectopy. Irregular ventricular tachycardia? It seems unlikely, but look at the beat indicated by the arrowhead. It's narrow, but the shape of the QRS is definitely different from the two normal beats. The P-R interval is shorter than the P-R of the two normal beats.

Answer: Fusion! You have detected the 100% marker for ventricular ectopy. You have made the very rare but precise diagnosis of "unstable or erratic or variable-rate ventricular tachycardia." This is probably caused by a parasystolic focus with varying degrees of exit block. The principles you used in this rare tracing are the same basic principles you use in analysis of any complex wide-beat tachycardia.

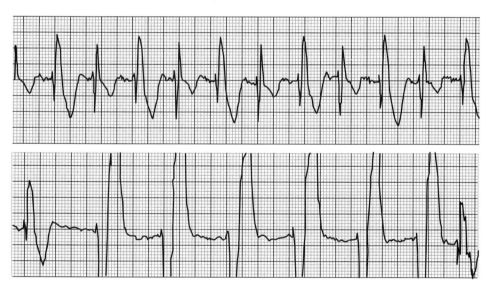

Figure 25–10.

An intern or a colleague brings you the rhythm strip of Figure 25–10, muttering about wide beats and some funny kind of ventricular tachycardia. You discover that it was recorded on an elderly patient with severe hypertensive heart disease and an exacerbation of congestive heart failure. The patient had been on many cardiac medications, including antihypertensives, digoxin, and diuretics, in varying combinations at other centers. No previous ECGs are available. Through most of the tracing, wide beats and narrower beats alternate. In the second strip, there is a pause punctuated by very wide QRS complexes with a different configuration and a slower rate. Diagnosis? Probable cause? Treatment?

1. **There are no P waves anywhere in the tracing, even in the long pause where there should be plenty of time to see them. Presumptive diagnosis: atrial fibrillation.**

2. **Put your calipers on the *beginning* of the alternating wide and narrow beats and you'll see that the rhythm is absolutely regular.**

Conclusion: The wide beats and the narrow beats are coming from the same focus. The narrow beats are too narrow to be ventricular, so they must be junctional.

This is an accelerated junctional rhythm with 2:1 right bundle-branch block (RBBB). The pattern varies from an "incomplete" to a "complete" RBBB on alternate beats. Accelerated junctional rhythm is the most common sustained digitalis-toxic tachyarrhythmia.

In the pause in the second strip, you see a slow rate with very wide QRS complexes. It looks like typical atrial fibrillation, but if you look closely, you'll see that the QRS complexes are quite regular except for the last one, which comes a little early. Clearly, this is not the pattern of random conduction from fibrillating atria; this is an idioventricular rhythm. There must be a high degree of AV block because the rate is 68—plenty of time to allow fibrillary impulses to reach the ventricles if the AV tissues were conducting normally. In fact, there's no evidence of conduction from the fibrillating atria to the ventricles anywhere in the tracing. The rhythm is set by two ectopic pacemakers—one junctional and one ventricular. *One more time:* Digitalis toxicity!

Figure 25–11.

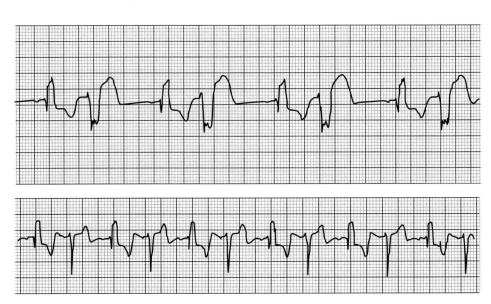

The top strip of Figure 25–11 is lead V1, showing RBBB. Ventricular ectopic beats form a bigeminal rhythm. Or are they junctional ectopic beats with Ashman aberrancy?

Next day: The bottom strip is still V1, still showing RBBB, but the premature beats are narrow!

Analysis: The sinus rate in the top strip is slow. If you count the visible P waves—the little inverted notches ahead of the RBBB beats—it's 40. There might be a P wave hidden in the ventricular premature contractions (VPCs), which would give you a sinus rate of 80. In the bottom strip, the sinus rate is much faster—about 106. The right bundle branch is blocked. The VPCs have a left bunch-branch block configuration, which means they arise in the right ventricle.

What's happening: In the second strip, the rate is much faster. The atrial impulses "get ahead" of the VPCs, so that the normal impulse is coming down the right bundle at the same instant that the VPC is activating the left ventricle. Both chambers are discharged at almost the same instant, eradicating the effect of the bundle-branch block for that beat.

It must be normalizing fusion (see Chapter 5)! As with any fusion, the P-R of the fused beat is a little shorter than the P-R of the sinus beats. Those premature beats are infallibly identified as ventricular.

Graduation!

Twenty-six

How to Take a Board
Examination

If you are an intern preparing for boards or a cardiologist preparing for subspecialty boards, or if you want electrocardiogram (ECG) reading privileges at any hospital of any size, you're going to have to take a qualifying examination in electrocardiography. Get used to the idea and prepare for it.

I was the one who launched the idea of the American College of Cardiology (ACC) qualifying examination back in the 1970s when I served on the continuing education committee of the ACC, and I helped to nurture the project in its early stages as a member of the ECG interpretation committee of the ACC. Under the subsequent able leadership of Drs. Nancy Flowers and Jay Mason, the examination has become an institution. The plan now is to offer it to hospital staffs to qualify physicians for ECG reading privileges, which was what I wanted to do with it in the first place. Dr. H. J. C. Marriott has been offering a similar service to hospitals nationwide for some time, and the enthusiastic reception of his efforts attests a strongly felt need.

Here are some hints on how to approach this kind of examination.

Describe *everything* on the tracing. There will almost always be a number of specific diagnostic deformities, and you'll be graded by the number you recognize.

Diagnosis: Figure 26–1.

1. **Complete atrioventricular (AV) block, nodal**

2. **Inferior myocardial infarction (MI), acute**

That one was easy.

Here you'll get in trouble unless you look at the rhythm strip on the bottom of Figure 26–2. The first beat is a normal sinus beat. It's followed by three ventricular beats at a rate of 150. All across the rhythm strip, there are occasional sinus beats followed by runs of ventricular ectopic beats and many fusion beats. Now look at the QRST configuration. The whole diagnosis is as follows:

1. **Sinus rhythm**

2. **Ventricular tachycardia, transient, recurrent**

3. **Frequent fusion beats**

4. **Anterior MI, hyperacute**

The term *hyperacute,* of course, refers to the extreme S–T elevation; it's interesting and significant that this elevation is apparent even in the ventricular ectopic impulses. You'll never see S–T elevation like this as part of a ventricular premature contraction (VPC) per se.

Figure 26–1.

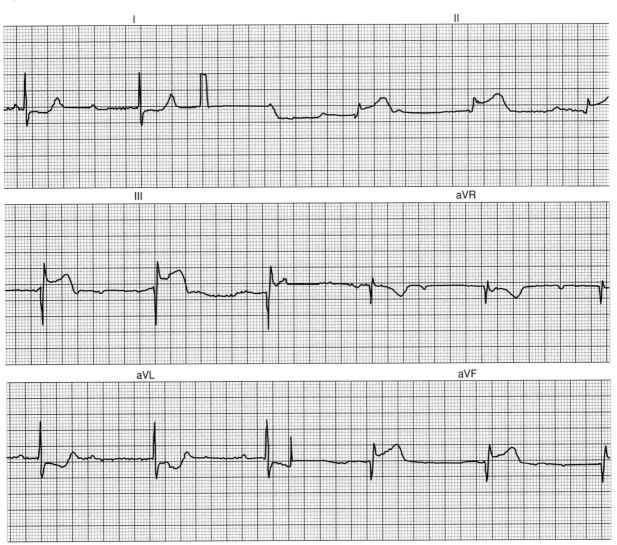

Figure 26–2.

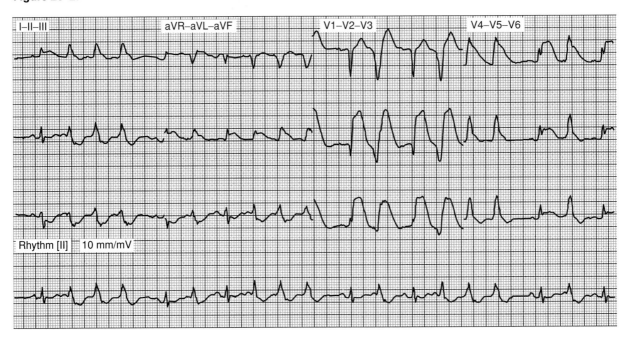

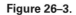

Figure 26–3.

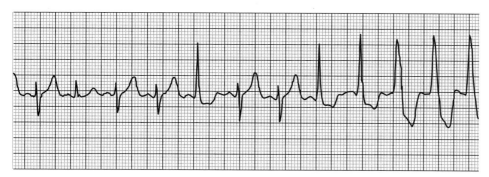

Figure 26–3 is a tracing that will probably bring a question about treatment. This tracing is recorded in an asymptomatic patient. Diagnosis? Pathophysiologic mechanism? Treatment?

1. **Sinus rhythm**

2. **Ventricular ectopic discharge with:**
   a. **A five-beat run of accelerated idioventricular rhythm with shortening R-R caused by type 1 exit block.**
   b. **Many fusion beats**

3. **Mechanism parasystole. Note varying coupling intervals and interectopic intervals.**

4. **Treatment: none. (You'll probably be presented with a tempting menu, including isoproterenol and pacing. Don't be fooled.)**

Figure 26–4.

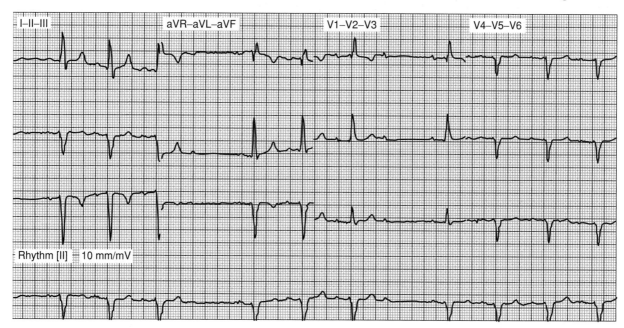

Figure 26–4 was recorded on a patient complaining of paroxysms of vertigo.

1. **Right bundle-branch block (RBBB)**

2. **Left anterior fascicular block**

3. **Mobitz-II block. (Look at the rhythm strip.)**

Figure 26–5.

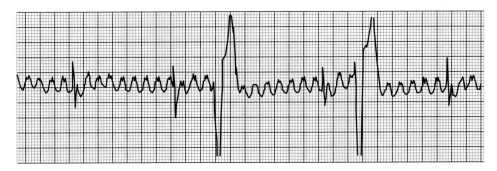

In Figure 26–5, the Mobitz–II block is a manifestation of *intermittent trifascicular block*. The patient has only one fascicle left, and that's failing now and then.

> 1. **Atrial flutter**
> 2. **High-degree or complete AV nodal block**
> 3. **Ventricular ectopic beats**

Warning: Whenever you're considering atrial flutter or fibrillation, always assess the degree of AV block—it's a favorite trap.

Figure 26–6.

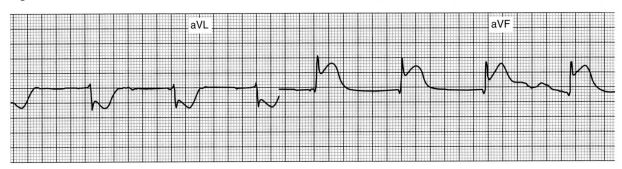

In Figure 26–6, the point is to recognize the acute sinus node suppression, the real cause of the junctional rhythm—a common complication of inferior MI.

> 1. **Junctional rhythm**
> 2. **Inferior MI, acute**
> 3. **Complete sinus arrest**

Figure 26–7

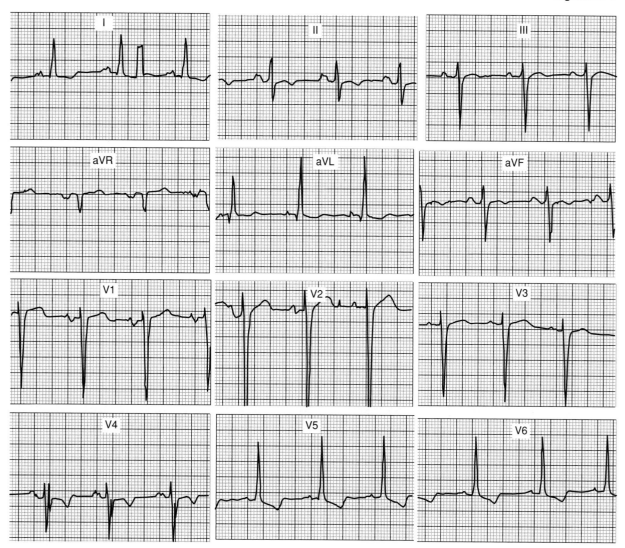

Figure 26–7 shows left ventricular hypertrophy based on:

1. **Increased voltage**
2. **"Strain" pattern in S-T-T**
3. **Left axis, 30 degrees**
4. **Left atrial enlargement**

Don't forget the left atrial enlargement as part of the final diagnosis or you'll lose points.

Figure 26–8.

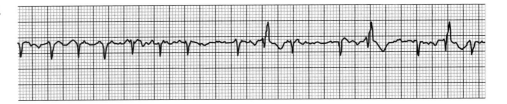

Look at Figure 26–8:

> 1. **Atrial fibrillation**
>
> 2. **Paroxysms of junctional tachycardia (note the absolutely regular tachycardia in the first part of the strip with a rate of 155)**
>
> 3. **Aberrantly conducted junctional ectopic beats (Ashman phenomenon). Note the constant linkage of the wide beats to the preceding narrow beat—this indicates that these are reentrant junctional beats, not random beats from the fibrillating atria.**
>
> 4. **Presumptive diagnosis: digitalis toxicity**

Figure 26–9.

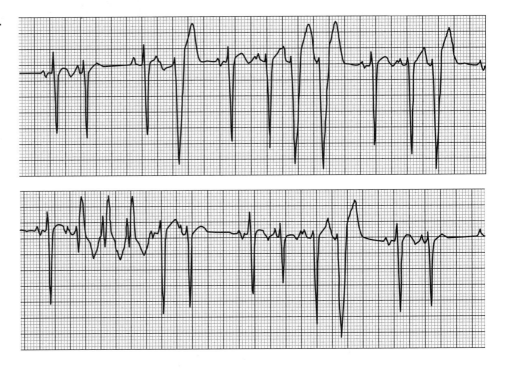

Figure 26–9 shows runs of paroxysmal atrial tachycardia with RBBB and left bundle-branch block (LBBB) aberrancy. Note the obvious P waves at the beginning of each episode and the numerous visible P waves during the runs of LBBB tachycardia. The RBBB tachycardia follows an Ashman pattern with normalization of QRS at the same rate after the three-beat run in the left bottom strip, whereas the LBBB aberrancy, as usual, is simply rate dependent. If the examination asks about the type of aberrancy, point out both.

Figure 26–10.

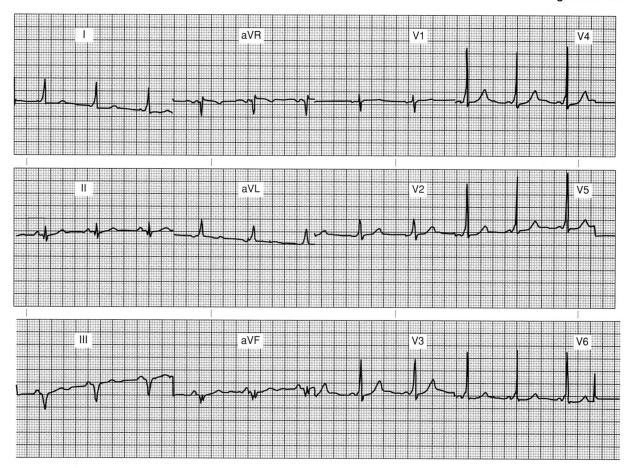

Favorite booby-trap: Don't call the strip in Figure 26–10 inferior MI. It's WPW preexcitation, and the apparent pathologic Q in III and aVF is simply the delta force of preexcitation.

Figure 26–11.

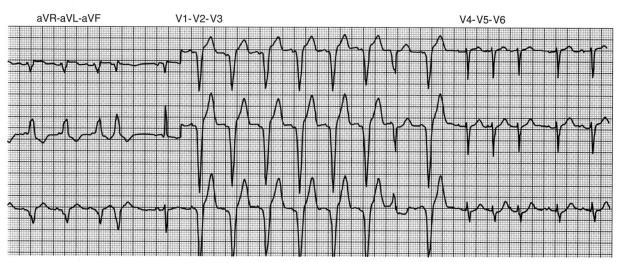

Examiners love intermittent preexcitation. Don't be misled into calling the tracing in Figure 26–11 a ventricular rhythm—the short P-R and wide QRS are obvious once you're alerted.

Figure 26–12.

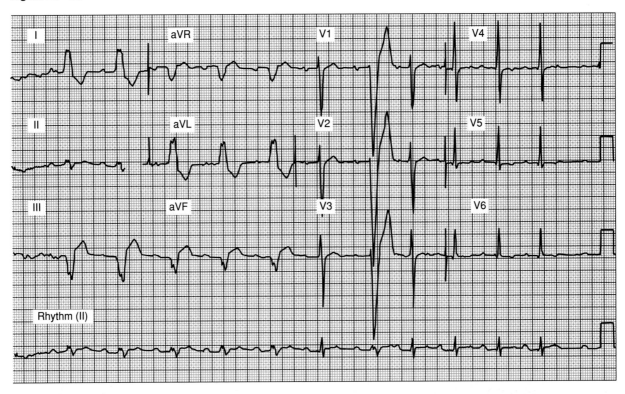

More about aberrancy: You'll probably see a 12-lead ECG like the one in Figure 26–12. The wide complexes appear at a rate of 68. When the rate speeds to 88, the QRS is normal. This is bradycardia–dependent aberrancy, *not* fixed LBBB.

Figure 26–13.

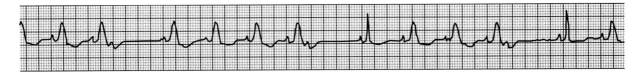

Still on the topic of aberrancy: Figure 26–13.

1. **Nonconducted premature atrial beats**
2. **Rate-dependent aberrancy**

Figure 26–14.

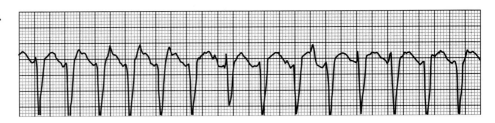

Ventricular tachycardia: Figure 26–14. In any wide-beat tachycardia, be sure to look for evidence of AV dissociation and capture beats with fusion, the two markers for ventricular tachycardia as opposed to aberrancy. The dissociated P waves are obvious, and there's an equally obvious capture beat with fusion right in the middle of the strip.

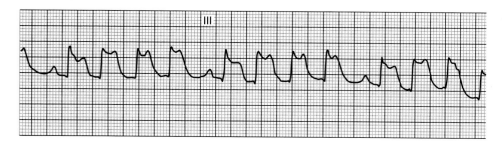

Figure 26–15.

They might get tricky on the cardiology boards and hand you something like this strip in Figure 26–15. First, note the obvious P waves in the pauses. Second, note the way the apparent Q-T interval shortens. This means that there's a P wave in the T wave moving progressively closer to the preceding QRS as the P-R prolongs. Note also how the R-R interval shortens in each run. Wenckebach!

1. **Sinus tachycardia**

2. **Type I (Wenckebach) AV block**

3. **Inferior MI with hyperacute changes**

Figure 26–16.

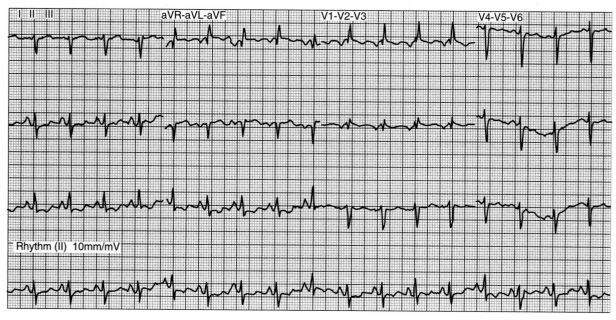

Have a look at Figure 26–16:

1. **Right ventricular hypertrophy**

2. **Right atrial hypertrophy**

Type A RVH; findings consistent with severe pulmonary hypertension.

Figure 26–17.

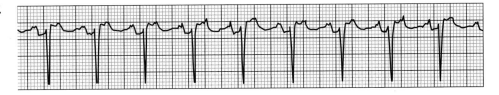

You're bound to get one of these strips like in Figure 26–17. Look for these two elements:

1. **A rapid regular atrial rate in the 150 to 250 range**

2. ***Any* degree of AV block: in this case, it's 2:1.**

PAT with block!

One more: Figure 26–18.

Figure 26–18.

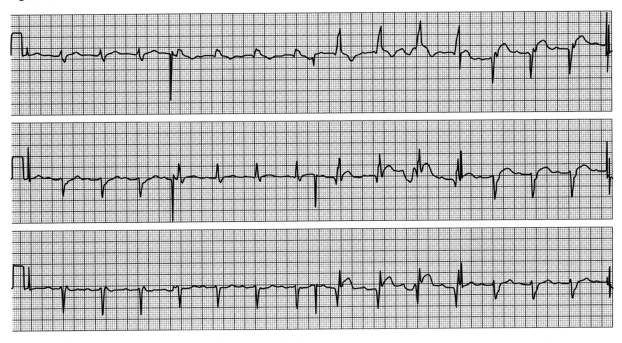

1. **RBBB**

2. **Left anterior fascicular block—left anterior hemiblock.**

3. **First-degree AV block—trifascicular block**

4. **Anterior MI**

Don't neglect any of these four items in your diagnosis!

Be sure to review all the infarct patterns and the major arrhythmias in their uncomplicated manifestations. Any examination will consist chiefly of combinations of these elements. Good luck!

Appendix I

Indications for Pacing in the Bradyarrhythmias

The incredibly sophisticated pacemakers available today are a triumph of technology. These instruments can sense the patient's atrial or ventricular complexes and can discharge on demand when the normal rhythm fails for a given period. They can track the patient's own sinus rhythm and can activate the ventricles with a preset P-R interval. They can be programmed to change modes when various rapid rhythms appear, thus protecting the ventricular rate. For those of us who remember the time when there were no such instruments, they are miraculous.

As always, there's another face to the coin. Any time you implant a foreign body in the heart, you have to accept a certain percentage of complications. A permanent pacemaker involves a power pack implanted under the skin and one or, more often, two wires in the heart. Occasional bacteremia and a tendency for blood to clot around foreign bodies must be accepted as a part of the human condition that modern science has not been able to alter. Thus, infection of the pacing apparatus and thrombosis must be anticipated as possible complications.

Most ventricular pacing wires will become permanently attached to the ventricular wall. Like infection around any foreign body, infection of an entrapped pacemaker lead is often resistant to antibiotic therapy and can be controlled only by removing the lead wire. Happily, newer methods of electrode removal by special catheters have reduced the risk inherent in this situation.

In a review that Dr. H. J. C. Marriott and I wrote in the *New England Journal of Medicine* (1985;312:1428–1432), we noted that the risk for late infection after implantation ranged from 1% to 7% in various reports. A later review by Dr. Seymour Furman, an acknowledged leader in the field of pacemaker technology, documented an 8% risk for infection of lead wires entrapped in the right ventricle in more than 130 patients.

Thrombosis can produce superior vena cava obstruction, massive brachial obstruction, or pulmonary embolization with an overall risk of about 4%.

Socioeconomic implications are serious. Patients wearing permanent pacemakers cannot obtain life insurance or individual health insurance. Many employers are reluctant to hire patients with pacemakers. Many high-frequency energy sources must be avoided (including microwaves).

In other words, the decision to implant a pacemaker must never be made lightly. It's a decision that can alter a patient's whole life.

In the early 1980s, I had the privilege of serving as chairman of a committee of distinguished cardiologists who completed a study published under the title "Indications for Pacing in the Treatment of Bradyarrhythmias" (published in the *Journal of the American Medical Association,* 1984;252:1307–1311). The guidelines that follow are derived largely from that report.

In reaching the decision to implant a permanent pacemaker:

1. Rule out drug effect. Repeat that to yourself about a hundred times. Many drugs in common use can depress sinus node function as well as atrioventricular (AV) and intraventricular conduction. I've tried to emphasize the effects of these drugs in the chapters on heart block and the sick sinus syndrome.

2. Make sure the condition is permanent. Many temporary conditions can affect impulse formation and conduction. Infarcts involving the right coronary artery commonly produce AV nodal block; they can also depress the sinus node. These effects are *always* transient; the patient will *never* need a permanent pacemaker.

3. Rule out extracardiac causes. Electrolyte abnormalities and extreme depression of thyroid function are two obvious examples.

In brief, make sure the condition is stable, permanent, and intrinsic to the heart, then proceed with your decision.

There are only two conditions that warrant pacing in the absence of symptoms:

1. Mobitz-II block localized in the bundle-branch system
2. Complete heart-block localized in the bundle-branch system

Either of these conditions represents a real and present danger to life: the first symptom may be the last. As one example, the rate of catastrophic events with true Mobitz-II block is about 30% per annum. Permanent pacing is indicated whether there are symptoms or not. (That's why we spent so much time in the chapter on heart block talking about these two diagnoses.)

In the conditions listed below, pacing is justified only if the disorder produces symptoms or compromises hemodynamics. "Symptoms" will almost always mean vertigo or syncope; sometimes a sustained slow heart rate will produce chronic fatigue. "Compromised hemodynamics" refers to depressed left ventricular function, usually with some evidence of congestive heart failure.

Complete AV Nodal Block

This is less ominous than complete block localized in the bundle-branch system—that is, it is less likely to lead to syncope or sudden death. Even so, complete AV nodal block will usually require pacing because the criteria for "complete heart block" include a ventricular rate of 45 or less. Nobody can tolerate a rate that slow forever, and you can be sure there will be symptoms sooner or later. As long as you're quite sure the block is permanent and not caused by extracardiac factors like drugs, pacing is reasonable.

Second-Degree AV Nodal Block

As the student knows, this can take the form of Wenckebach periods or fixed-ratio block with 2:1 or other conduction. Pacing in this setting is justified only if the block is clearly producing symptoms.

First-Degree AV Nodal Block

First-degree block never justifies pacing.

Atrial Fibrillation with Slow Ventricular Rate

Review the diagnosis of AV block in the setting of atrial fibrillation. If the ventricular rate is slow enough to cause symptoms and if the condition is clearly permanent, pacing is indicated.

Special Categories

Bifascicular Block with Syncope

When bifascicular block is present, conduction from atria to ventricles is reduced to one strand—the one functioning fascicle of the left bundle. If such a patient turns up with recurrent syncope, you might wonder about intermittent failure of that one strand. Careful studies have shown, however, that the risk for this kind of conduction failure is very small. Syncope in the presence of bifascicular block is very rarely the result of a failure of AV conduction. This combination is not per se an indication for pacing.

Trifascicular Block with Syncope

If a patient has right bundle-branch block with hemiblock and if P-R prolongation then appears, it's possible that the delay in AV conduction is in the last remaining fascicle; the term *trifascicular block* is used. Again, careful studies have shown that the risk for progression to Mobitz-II or complete block is small. Pacing is indicated only if actual failure of AV conduction can be demonstrated.

Sick Sinus Syndrome

The sick sinus syndrome, properly defined, is always an indication for pacing. There is no other adequate treatment. When you're considering the diagnosis of brady-tachy syndrome, be sure you demonstrate a significant "brady" stage between the episodes of tachyarrhythmia. If you see a normal healthy sinus rhythm in the periods between paroxysms of atrial tachycardia, fibrillation, or flutter, the patient certainly does not need a pacemaker!

Carotid Sinus Syncope

This is a very rare condition. Accidental stimulation of the carotid sinus by movements of the head or neck or by accidental pressure, such as during shaving, will produce abrupt standstill with syncope. In another variation of the syndrome, carotid sinus stimulation causes a drop in blood pressure with syncope. If the bradycardia type of carotid sinus syncope is in fact present, pacing is indicated.

Warning: Massaging the carotid sinus will often produce long pauses in the sinus rate. This doesn't mean that carotid sinus syncope is present. It's common to see pauses of 3 seconds or more after carotid massage in perfectly normal people who have never fainted in their lives. In one large series, only 5% of people with pauses of 3 seconds or longer after massage of the carotid sinus actually had clinical carotid sinus syndrome. Drugs that accentuate vagal effect, like digitalis or beta blockers, will produce exaggerated pauses after carotid sinus stimulation.

You can diagnose carotid sinus syncope only when accidental stimulation of the carotid sinus by normal activity causes a pause in heart rhythm or a fall in blood pressure.

Nonindications, Waste Motion, and Booby Traps

In the 1970s and 1980s, there was a wave of enthusiasm for invasive electrophysiologic studies to assess syncope. This led to some spurious indications for pacing, now known to be worthless.

Prolonged H-V Interval

It's possible to measure the interval from the beginning of activation of the His bundle to the beginning of ventricular activation. This interval, also called the H-V interval, is about the last third of the P-R. It is now established beyond question that prolongation of the H-V interval per se doesn't mean a thing. Even in the presence of bifascicular block, prolongation of H-V does not indicate increased risk and is not an indication for pacing.

Invasive EP Study of AV Nodal Function

Wenckebach Periods Induced by Atrial Pacing. If you place a pacing wire in the right atrium and pace the heart, you'll produce type I block in almost everybody. In some, the block will appear at rates as low as 75 to 80, whereas in others, it won't appear until the rate is more than 150. Wenckebach block induced by artificial pacing is a meaningless finding. It has no correlation with intrinsic block in the AV node. The rate at which Wenckebach periods appear—the so-called Wenckebach number—has no significance in terms of AV nodal function in real life.

Invasive Electrophysiologic Measurement of Functional and Effective AV Nodal Refractory Periods. If the P-R interval on the surface electrocardiogram (ECG) is normal and remains normal throughout any and every variation of rate, there's nothing wrong with the AV node. That's all you need to know about the AV node. Invasive measurements of AV nodal refractory periods serve no useful purpose and have no predictive or prognostic value.

"Chronotropic Incompetence." This is a mysterious entity that was used to justify many pacemaker implantations a few years back. The idea was that the sinus node couldn't speed up on demand the way it was supposed to, so that a patient might feel weak or dizzy with exertion because the heart rate was too slow to meet the increased demand. There never was any evidence for the existence of such a syndrome, and the notion has been discarded, but you may still encounter patients wearing pacemakers for treatment of this mythical disorder.

Invasive Electrophysiologic Measurement of Sinus Node Function. Several methods were devised to measure sinus node function in questionable cases of sick sinus syndrome. These included measurement of the pause after rapid pacing and estimation of conduction time from sinus node to atria. Neither of these measurements was very reliable, and the invention of event recorders has made them obsolete. To diagnose sick sinus syndrome, you record sinus node slowing during symptoms by means of Holter recording or with the event recorder—that's the gold standard. Invasive measurements are useless and may be misleading.

Appendix II

How to Determine Axis

You've probably learned some of the "shorthand" ways of determining frontal plane axis. Thus, the axis will be at right angles to the lead that's isoelectric—in other words, the lead that has a total amplitude sum of zero. That's correct, but limited. Sometimes there's no lead like that. You may have learned to derive axis from leads I and aVF, but when you combine a standard lead with an augmented limb lead, it's like combining centimeters and inches: the leads represent different electric magnitudes, and you'll be off by exactly 10 degrees. Sometimes that can be a significant error.

Here's the right way to go about it. Start with the triaxial system, with all leads reduced to a common center (Fig. A–1). Look at the electrocardiogram (ECG) illustrated in the upper left corner of Figure A–2 and go through the drill outlined there. You simply determine the algebraic sum of deflections in any two leads and mark off that amount on the appropriate lead. Remember that the left arm is plus in lead I and the left leg is plus in leads II and III. Now drop perpendiculars from the points you've measured to the point of intersection, and

Figure A–1.

The triaxial system with all leads reduced to a common center.

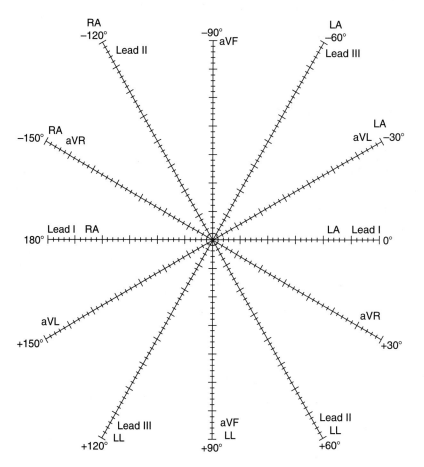

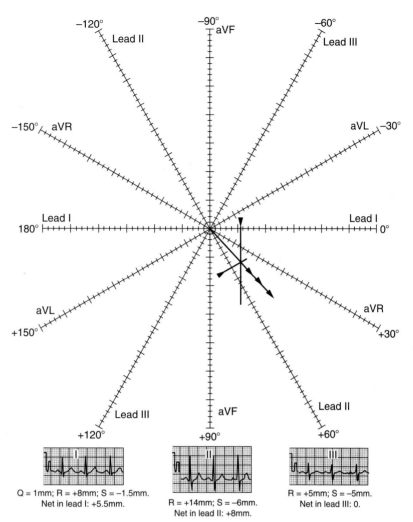

Figure A–2.
This is "normal" axis. Many texts state that a "normal" axis lies between 0 and +90 degrees. This is dangerously misleading. You have to correct for age and body habitus before you decide whether an axis is normal.

Q = 1mm; R = +8mm; S = –1.5mm.
Net in lead I: +5.5mm.

R = +14mm; S = –6mm.
Net in lead II: +8mm.

R = +5mm; S = –5mm.
Net in lead III: 0.

draw an arrow from the center to that point. That's the mean axis. It's really the simple vector analysis you learned in high school to determine the mean vector of two forces.

Now consider left axis deviation as in Figure A–3. Leads I and III give exactly the same value, except that lead I is plus and lead III is minus. Plot the values, drop the perpendiculars, and you'll find you've bisected the angle between 0 and 60 degrees: 30 degrees. *Next important point:* The value of lead II is exactly zero. Draw a perpendicular from the zero point on lead II, and you're pointing right out at minus 30 degrees. This time the isoelectric lead trick worked.

Extreme left axis is illustrated in Figure A–4. *Rule:* When the negative value of lead III is greater than the plus value of lead I, the axis will lie leftward of minus 30 degrees. Lead II will always be negative in this setting. Try various values on the triaxial sheet, and you'll see how it works.

Right axis deviation (Fig. A–5). Some simple rules:

1. If lead I is exactly zero, the axis must point straight up or straight down—plus or minus 90 degrees.
2. If II and III are plus, the axis must point down, at plus 90 degrees.
3. If lead I is negative and leads II and III are plus, the axis must lie to the right of 90 degrees—about plus 12 degrees in the example here.
4. If lead II is exactly zero, lead I is negative, and lead III is plus, the axis will be at right angles to lead II, or plus 150 degrees.

And so on. Play around with some values on a sheet with the triaxial lead system, and you'll be able to derive axis by simple inspection very accurately.

Figure A–3.

Left axis deviation. The plus value in lead I is the same as the minus value in lead III. You're bisecting the angle between lead I (0) and lead III (–60), just the way you did in high school geometry. Lead II is exactly zero. The perpendicular from lead II points out along the –30 line. This is the other way you can diagnose an axis of –30. Remember, the axis will always be at right angles to the lead that equals zero, just the way it is here. If lead II is zero, the axis will be ±30 degrees. If lead I is zero, the axis will be ±90 degrees. The other leads will tell you at once whether the value is plus or minus either way.

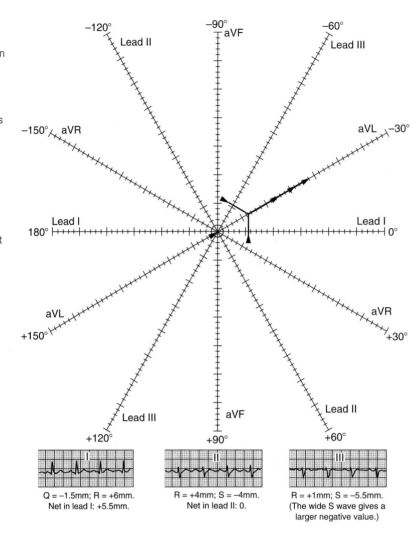

Q = –1.5mm; R = +6mm.
Net in lead I: +5.5mm.

R = +4mm; S = –4mm.
Net in lead II: 0.

R = +1mm; S = –5.5mm.
(The wide S wave gives a larger negative value.)

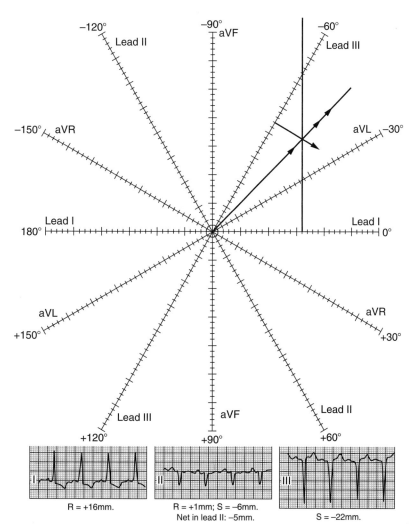

R = +16mm.

R = +1mm; S = −6mm.
Net in lead II: −5mm.

S = −22mm.

Figure A–4.
Extreme left axis deviation. The minus (negative) value in III is greater than the plus (positive) value in I. Lead II is negative. By looking at the graph, you'll see at once that both these findings put the axis leftward of −30 degrees— up in the range of −45 degrees or higher. (Remember, "higher" means "more leftward.")

Figure A–5.

Right axis deviation. Whenever lead I is minus and leads II and III are plus, the way they are here, the axis has to be somewhere to the right of +90 degrees. Try moving the lead I value farther to the minus side, and you'll see values of +110, +120, and so on. Simple concept.

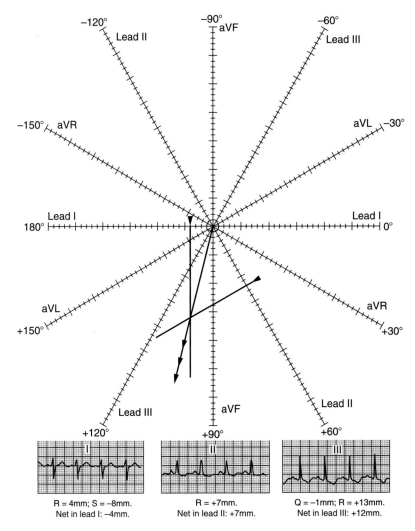

R = 4mm; S = –8mm.
Net in lead I: –4mm.

R = +7mm.
Net in lead II: +7mm.

Q = –1mm; R = +13mm.
Net in lead III: +12mm.

Index

Page numbers followed by f refer to figures. Page numbers followed by t refer to tables. Page numbers followed by sa refer to self assesment chapters.